MAKING PHONOLOGY FUNCTIONAL

**Butterworth–Heinemann
Series in Communication Disorders**

Charlena M. Seymour, Ph.D., Series Editor

Battle, D.E. *Communication Disorders in Multicultural Populations, Second Edition* (1998)

Billeaud, F.P. *Communication Disorders in Infants and Toddlers: Assessment and Intervention, Second Edition* (1998)

Huntley, R.A. and Helfer, K.S. *Communication in Later Life* (1995)

Kricos, P.B. and Lesner, S.A. *Hearing Care for the Older Adult: Audiologic Rehabilitation* (1995)

Maxon, A.B. and Brackett, D. *The Hearing-Impaired Child: Infancy Through High School Years* (1992)

Wall, L.G. *Hearing for the Speech-Language Pathologist and Health Care Professional* (1995)

Wallace, G.L. *Adult Aphasia Rehabilitation* (1996)

Velleman, S.L. *Making Phonology Functional: What Do I Do First?* (1998)

MAKING PHONOLOGY FUNCTIONAL

What Do I Do First?

Shelley L. Velleman, Ph.D., CCC-SLP

Assistant Professor of Communication Sciences
and Disorders, Elms College, Chicopee;
Pediatric Speech-Language Pathologist,
Baystate Medical Center,
Springfield, Massachusetts

Foreword by
Carol Stoel-Gammon, Ph.D.
Professor, Department of Speech and Hearing
Sciences, University of Washington, Seattle

Butterworth–Heinemann

Boston   Oxford   Johannesburg   Melbourne   New Delhi   Singapore

Library of Congress Cataloging-in-Publication Data

Velleman, Shelley Lynne.
    Making phonology functional : what do I do first? / Shelley L.
Velleman.
       p.   cm. -- (Butterworth-Heinemann series in communication
disorders)
    Includes bibliographical references and index.
    ISBN 0-7506-9525-0
    1. Articulation disorders in children. I. Title. II. Series:
Butterworth-Heinemann series in communications disorders.
    [DNLM: 1. Articulation Disorders--in infancy & childhood.
2. Speech-Language Pathology. WL 340.2 V439m 1998]
RJ496.S7V45 1998
618.92'855--dc21
DNLM/DLC
for Library of Congress
                                          97-52015
                                           CIP

British Library Cataloguing-in-Publication Data
A catalogue record for this book is available from the British Library.

The publisher offers special discounts on bulk orders of this book.
For information, please contact:
Manager of Special Sales
Butterworth–Heinemann
225 Wildwood Avenue
Woburn, MA 01801-2041
Tel: 781-904-2500
Fax: 781-904-2620

For information on all Butterworth–Heinemann publications available,
contact our World Wide Web home page at: http://www.bh.com

10 9 8 7 6 5 4 3 2 1

Printed in the United States of America

For Dan

Contents

Foreword

Learning to talk is one of the most amazing feats that occurs during childhood. Before the appearance of words, babies communicate through gestures and vocalizations that attract the attention of adults in their world. With words, however, the sophistication of the communication increases enormously. The production of *mommy, daddy,* or *bye-bye* is a much heralded event in the baby's life. Within months of their first words, toddlers begin to produce short phrases and then longer sentences. The size and complexity of their vocabulary develop, and their ability to make themselves understood is enhanced. One of the most intriguing aspects of language development is the rapidity and apparent ease with which children acquire their mother tongue. Unlike adults studying a second language, children do not memorize lists of new vocabulary words or receive structured explanations of the pronunciation patterns and syntactic rules of their language; yet by the age of 5 years, American children are quite proficient speakers of English; Nigerian children can converse fluently in Yoruba; and Brazilian children have learned to speak Portuguese.

In some instances, however, language acquisition does not follow the normal developmental sequence: Some babies fail to produce recognizable words before their second birthday; some produce words but are not able to string them together to form coherent sentences; and some others produce sentences that do not conform to the syntactic and semantic patterns of the ambient language. The first step in trying to help such children is to determine the cause of the problem. Do they suffer from a hearing loss that prevents them from perceiving the speech of their parents, siblings, and peers? Do they have a cognitive deficit that interferes with the normal timetable of acquisition? Do they have a structural abnormality, such as tongue tie or cleft palate, that prevents them from being able to produce speech sounds correctly? Identifying the cause of the problem is an important step in developing an appropriate treatment plan.

In a majority of cases, children with speech and language disorders have normal hearing and cognitive abilities and no apparent structural or functional problems, making it difficult to pinpoint the underlying cause. In the area of phonology, such children for whom the cause cannot be identified are said to have a "functional phonological disorder." Although all children with this label exhibit problems with phonology, their production patterns vary substantially from one child to another: For some, the primary difficulty seems to be with individual consonants and vowels of their language; for others, the problem lies with an inability to produce particular sequences of sounds or to produce a sound in a particular position in a word; still others may have difficulty producing multisyllabic words or with correct placement of stress. Determining the nature and severity of the problem of a child with a functional phonological disorder represents a major challenge for practicing speech-language pathologists, a challenge that must be addressed through careful examination of the child's phonological system.

In this book, Shelley Velleman addresses this challenge using a comprehensive approach to the understanding of nonfunctional phonological systems and a multilevel approach to data analysis. Combining a strong background in theoretical linguistics with her extensive experience as a practicing speech-language pathologist, she is able to incorporate theory and practice in a unique way. Velleman believes it is important for clinicians to understand the normal processes underlying spoken language in children and adults; thus, she includes many examples from children with normal development. She also believes it is important to recognize the universal nature of phonological patterns and thus includes examples from other languages, some of which show that developmental patterns that may be viewed as deviant for children acquiring English occur regularly in the phonological systems of other languages.

Perhaps the most unique aspect of this book is that multiple perspectives are used in describing phonological data. Velleman includes discussions of independent and relational analyses, phonetic inventories and phonemic contrasts, and stress patterns and phonological processes. For each of these, she provides readers with analysis forms that can be used to document various aspects of a child's phonological system. These forms should be very useful for practicing speech-language pathologists. The book goes well beyond the usual assessment and treatment text, however, with the application of recent developments in phonological theory, including nonlinear phonology and optimality theory. An awareness of these approaches, even at an introductory level, allows the reader to see the promise of contributions from theoretical linguistics and furthers the understanding of nonfunctional phonologies from both theoretical and practical perspectives.

Carol Stoel-Gammon

Preface

This book was conceived in a supermarket. In the produce section, Charlena Seymour and I discussed the possibility of my writing the phonological disorders book for this series, of which she is the editor. As I considered whether I had a book in me, the first thought that came to mind was of my clinical colleagues, by whom I had often been approached with phonology test results and the question, "What do I do first?" I have found that my background in theoretical phonology has made it much easier for me to determine what is going on in a child's phonology and, if a disorder is indicated, what to do about it. Understanding how the phonologies of the languages of the world are pieced together and how all of those pieces function together as a unit helps me to view each child's phonology as a system, which may or may not be functional. For this reason, I consider my background in linguistics to be my most valuable clinical asset. I have always wondered why some concepts make the transition from linguistics into speech-language pathology and some do not. I realized as I stood there beside the green beans that I wanted to share this perspective of a phonology as a functional (or nonfunctional) system with my present and future clinical colleagues.

As a speech-language pathologist cum linguist, I walk the tightrope between the elegance of theory and the pressure of real clinical work. Over the years, I have coped with this by developing child phonology worksheets. I can use these do-it-yourself forms quickly when my stack of reports is high or carefully when I have a little bit of breathing space. Either way, they assist me in considering multiple aspects of each child's phonology and how these aspects complement or interfere with each other. These worksheets form the backbone of this book.

Chapter 1 is an overview of the concepts presented in later chapters. Each of Chapters 2–5 begins with a description of one component of phonology, including a discussion of how that component manifests itself in the languages of the world and in the phonologies of normally developing children. The discussion then turns to what can go wrong with that particular aspect of the phonological system and how one can tell something has gone wrong. The relevant worksheets are provided, with examples of real children drawn from the literature and from my own clinical experience. Appropriate goals are suggested. Each chapter ends with a brief overview of current phonological theory as it relates to that aspect of phonology. These final sections are optional; it is not assumed in later chapters that the reader has read the earlier theoretical portions. Chapter 6 delves into the phonology of one real child at two points in time, presenting a complete analysis of her dysfunctional phonological system at each age. Continuities over time within the functional and the dysfunctional aspects of her phonology are highlighted. Specific goals that were addressed in therapy are presented, with rationales and outcomes.

There are at least two potential audiences for this book: practicing speech-language pathologists who would like to understand their clients' phonologies better so that they may provide more efficient intervention, and students who have taken at least one course that includes an introduction to phonetics and phonology, including natural processes. Those who are relatively new to phonology or uncomfortable with this subject matter are likely to skip the theoretical sections at the ends of Chapters 2–5 on first reading, but it is my hope that they will eventually go back to them, and turn to further works, to deepen their understanding of phonologies as functioning systems.

I am grateful to the many parents and children with whom I have been privileged to work, who have provided so much fascinating phonological data over the years, and to many clinical colleagues who have brought other interesting cases to my attention.

Several people have been intimately involved in the conception and birth of this work. First, of course, is Charlena Seymour, without whose confidence in me I never would have considered whether or not I had a book to write. I am more grateful than I can say to Ruth Huntley Bahr and her students, who worked through earlier drafts of these chapters in a phonology seminar at the University of South Florida, tried out some of the worksheets and approaches with their own clients, and provided extremely thoughtful, constructive feedback. I owe deepest thanks to Denise Segal, too, who read and commented in detail on earlier drafts of several chapters and encouraged me throughout. Additionally, Margaret Kehoe's knowledgeable and insightful comments were quite helpful. Their input led to many improvements both in style and in content. Kristine Strand also tried out some of the worksheets and provided useful comments about them, as well as participating in innumerable stimulating dialogues about the phonologies of children with developmental verbal dyspraxia. My father; sixth-grade language arts teacher Ellen Stonehill; and professors Andrea Levitt, John McCarthy, and Carla Dunn originally inspired my interest in language, linguistics, and (child) phonology. My colleagues and good friends Marilyn Vihman, Carol Stoel-Gammon, and Barbara Davis have provided continuing moral support and encouragement, as well as engaging in many absorbing discussions about normal and disordered phonological development. Adrienne Terrizzi, Larry Shriberg, and Barbara Murphy have been incredibly patient and supportive throughout the lengthy, intense, final stages of the writing process.

Finally, although my husband, Dan Velleman, was not actually present at the moment of its conception, he has played a major role in the development of this work. He has been extremely generous with his expertise, critical eye, time, patience, and encouragement for far longer than either of us had imagined writing this book would take.

Many thanks to you all.

The author is grateful for the partial support of NIH grant # HUD 1 R01 HD26892-01 during the initial portion of the writing process.

SLV

CHAPTER ONE

Concepts and
Definitions

> Nothing is as practical as a good theory to enable you to make
> choices confidently and consistently, and to explain or defend
> why you are making the choices you make.

Larson & McKinley (1995)

Johnny has a functional phonological disorder. What does this mean? All speech-language pathologists use the term **functional phonological disorder** to refer to phonological disorders of no known physiological or neurological basis. The term describes a situation in which some components of a child's phonological system either are not functioning properly or are not interacting properly with one another, yielding a phonological system that is not adequate for the child's communicative needs. Unfortunately, the true meaning of the term has had little effect on approaches to remediation. One can easily be caught up in developmental norms and decisions regarding which phoneme to target first, or in advertised packages and the determination of whether to use a process approach or a feature analysis, forgetting that the true goal is actually very simple: function. The many analysis techniques and packages available to us for identifying phonological malfunctions are of secondary importance. They are merely convenient tools. The heart of the matter is that the child's phonology is functionally disordered—that is, his or her phonology is not properly performing its job of transmitting messages via sound. Our job as speech-language pathologists is to identify the nonfunctional aspects of the individual's current system and to determine the types of change that can be employed to make the system more functional.

All human beings have certain physiological, neurological, and cognitive limitations that have profound effects on their phonologies. As speakers, we cannot communicate by extrasensory perception, so, typically, we use our mouths and ears. There are limits to our fine motor coordination, and therefore the articulation of the various sounds we attempt must not be too similar or difficult. For example, because it cannot be incorporated quickly enough into a word, a raspberry (labiolingual trill) is not a speech sound in any language. Finally, we must breathe, so the number of words we produce without a pause is limited.

As listeners, we have neither unlimited memory nor unlimited attention, so the speaker must pause occasionally to let us reflect on what we are hearing. We cannot pay attention to more than a certain number of acoustic details, so the speaker must produce speech sounds as predictably and clearly as possible under the circumstances.

Such limitations, in conjunction with the characteristics of the language being learned by the child, the specific patterns of the speakers to whom the child is exposed (e.g., dialects, favorite expressions, characteristic tones of voice), and the child's own preferences and learning style, will combine to determine a particular learner's phonological patterns. The number of phonological patterns available to any human being is limited by the combination of these factors. Therefore, the phonological systems of all languages and all people must share the same components, and these components interact within the same systems in certain, usually predictable ways.

The similarities among the phonologies of individual children—and of individual languages—are far more numerous than are the differences. This book focuses on children with functional disorders. In these cases, there is no identifiable physiological basis for the disorder. Such children have what will be referred to here as **nonfunctional phonologies (NFPs)**. However, the issues to be discussed are appropriate for children with any type of disorder that interferes with the transmission of ideas via language. For example, young children with cleft palate have some specific physiological limitations to overcome, but the phonologies they develop must include the same components—and these must interact with one another in basically the same ways—as would the phonologies of the same children were they physically intact.

Because the deaf typically cannot use oral-aural communication as efficiently as can hearing individuals, they often use sign languages, which have their own manual phonological systems based on hand shapes and hand movements rather than oral articulatory positions and movements of the oral articulators. In fact, sign language phonologies parallel oral phonologies quite closely, their components being basically the same. Most of the differences are superficial ones induced by the change in perceptual modalities (vision versus hearing) and in articulators (hands and, to some extent, faces rather than oral structures). It is this author's assumption that the phonologies of children who are learning a manual language can be nonfunctional in ways that parallel the nonfunctional oral phonologies that are the focus of this book, although such cases have not been documented extensively. It is the functionality of these phonologies in the face of human limitations that interests us and that is far more relevant in this context than are the nonphonological causes of such limitations.

To truly understand what a functional phonology is, it is necessary to explore many phonological systems and to discuss how they work, including both functional and nonfunctional phonologies of adults and children. To understand the many different ways in which a phonology can function properly, one must consider the phonologies of other languages. Knowledge of phonological tendencies among the languages of the world can be extremely helpful to the speech-language pathologist for the following reasons:

- Those sounds and sound patterns that are most universal are easier to perceive or to articulate (or both) than those that are rare. They can therefore be assumed to be good targets for early remediation.
- Children who have been exposed to a particular language only may use word shapes, sounds, or phonological patterns that are not typically found in that language but that do occur in other languages. In some of these cases, the pattern chosen by the child may actually be more common within universal phonology than the pattern that happens to be used in the target language. Children who use patterns that are used in at least some languages are believed to have a better prognosis for improvement than those who use deviant patterns (i.e., patterns not found in any languages).

- By understanding the critical components of a phonological system and the ways in which those components interact, one can gain a better understanding of what has gone wrong in a particular child's phonological system. Because all components of a child's system are developing at the same time, these interactions sometimes are more difficult to discern in children's systems than they are in adult phonologies. By exploring the components of adult phonologies, it is easier to identify the types of interactions that may be present.

In 1982, Schwartz and Leonard demonstrated that individual children are more likely to attempt new words if the words fit within their existing phonological systems. The children tried to say these "in" words in imitation and learned to use them spontaneously in fewer sessions than it took for them to learn "out" words that did not fit their current systems. Understanding which words are in and out of a child's phonology requires that one have a thorough intuitive grasp of what a phonology is. Although many different types of phonological patterns are discussed here, an effort will also be made to take a broad scope whenever possible, so that the reader will not feel overwhelmed by the many details.

The goals of this book are as follows:

1. To divide phonology into its various components and to develop an understanding of each component and the ways that each interacts with the others, in order to analyze what a functioning phonological system is
2. To present methods for assessing the functioning of those parts both separately and together
3. To illustrate the piecing together of the components into a whole system, so that those missing pieces having the greatest impact on the functioning of the entire system can be easily identified and targeted in therapy

Once the functioning (and malfunctioning) aspects of a child's phonological system have been identified, it is far easier to determine which of these aspects must be targeted in remediation to improve that child's communicative effectiveness. One can easily be drawn into the procedural details of a particular system of phonological analysis and so overlook the phonological system as a whole. A more general assessment will yield a deeper understanding of the nature of the communication disorder. Once a broad pattern of malfunction has been identified, phonological analysis becomes a tool rather than an additional source of confusion; the clinician can see more clearly ways in which to approach the problem and can prioritize these methods of remediation.

IMPORTANT CONCEPTS FROM LINGUISTICS

Many linguistic concepts are important in child phonology. Although some of these concepts are very familiar to most speech-language pathologists, others have not been carried successfully from linguistics to the study of communication disorders. Some of these terms have different uses and even different definitions within various theories. Because the reader's understanding of each author's intent in his or her use of such terms is important, the most central terms are defined here. Readers who are unfamiliar with many of these concepts should not concern themselves with understanding every detail in this chapter. These definitions are elaborated and exemplified further later in this book. Other terms that are peripheral to this topic or for which there are generally known and agreed-upon definitions are defined as needed.

Phonology

Phonology is the term most critically in need of definition. Crystal (1991, p. 261) defines phonology as:

a branch of linguistics which studies the sound systems of languages. ... Putting this another way, phonology is concerned with the range and function of sounds in specific languages ... and with the rules which can be written to show the types of phonetic relationships that relate and contrast words and other linguistic units.

As Crystal points out, this term often is used in different ways by different phonologists. In many models, some of the components that are described here—especially the phonetic repertoire and the optional fast-speech rules—are omitted from the phonology proper.[1] In this book, however, *phonology* is used to encompass all actions, patterns, elements, and linguistic structures relating to the use of sound in speech production. This term will also be used to include the compensatory strategies employed by children with physiological, cognitive, neurological, perceptual, or articulatory limitations. Thus, in this context, it is irrelevant to ask whether one is dealing with phonology or articulation. Rather, the critical question that must be answered in regard to a child's phonology is, "What aspects of this system are interfering most with its effective functioning?"

Another vital point is that phonology has both input and output components as well as central organization. A child may not perceive as important some aspects of adult phonology. Therefore, he or she might either screen out those aspects when storing words or ignore them when planning for word production. This can occur even if the child is perfectly capable of hearing every phonological distinction and possibly is even capable of producing them under certain circumstances. It is important to realize that the child may not be attempting to produce a word as adult speakers of the language expect it to be produced. (This is discussed further in Chapter 4.) The word **target** will be used to refer to the adult production of a word, but this should *not* be construed as implying that the adult production of the word actually is the child's current target. Rather, it is *the therapist's* eventual intervention target on behalf of the child.

---

[1]For an argument against this practice, see Kingston and Diehl (1994).

Phonological Elements

Some elements that are relevant to phonology include words, phones, phonemes, allophones, features, and syllables.

Words

To define other phonological elements, it often is necessary to refer to the **word**. Crystal (1991, p. 380) explains that words are "the most stable of all linguistic units." That is, the subcomponents of each particular word have a fixed order. For example, the parts of the word *rearrangement* cannot be rearranged into *mentarrangere* and still have meaning. Words typically are not interrupted by pauses within the flow of speech unless the speaker stutters or revises the utterance. To be considered a word—a unit of meaning that may contain several smaller units of meaning—the unit must be able to express that meaning on its own. Thus, *is* is a word, but *-ist* is not because it has meaning only when added to another unit of meaning (such as *commun-*).

Words come in many shapes and sizes, depending on the number of meaning units that they contain, the number of syllables that they contain, and the consonants and vowels that make up these smaller elements. A one-syllable word is **monosyllabic**, a two-syllable word is **disyllabic**, and a word with three or more syllables is **multisyllabic**.

Phones

Phones are those sounds that are used by a child (or by any speaker), regardless of whether they are used contrastively and regardless of whether the target language uses them. Phones are enclosed in square brackets: [d], [b], [u],[2] and so on. The adjective used to refer to phones or analyses of phones is **phonetic**. **Phonetic repertoires** (i.e., the sets of sounds that are available within a particular speaker's phonological system) are discussed in Chapter 3.

Phonemes

Phonemes are those sounds that are used contrastively by a language or a speaker. For example, the fact that the English language includes the words *bat, hat, cat, fat, mat, gnat, sat, rat,* and *vat* and that each of these words has a different meaning tells us that each of the consonant sounds *b, h, k, f, m, n, s, r,* and *v* is a separate phoneme in this language. Phonemes are enclosed in slashes: /b/, /h/, /k/, /f/, /m/, /n/, /s/, /r/, /v/. Phonemic repertoires, and phonological contrast in general, are discussed in more depth in Chapter 4.

Allophones

Allophones are variants of phonemes that do not change meaning. For example, the way that Americans pronounce the /t/ in *pot* can vary. In casual speech, it may be produced very slightly, or as a glottal stop ([ʔ]; the sound in the middle of *uh-oh* and *button*). In more formal speech, it is pronounced completely, usually with a burst of air

known as **aspiration** ([tʰ]). The different pronunciations do not change the meaning of the word in any way. Thus, these pronunciations are all allophones of the phoneme /t/. Allophones are enclosed in square brackets, as they are a special kind of phone—for example, [t], [ʔ], [tʰ].

Features

Features are articulatory or perceptual differences between phones, such as voicing (e.g., [p] versus [b]), aspiration (e.g., [tʰ] in *top* versus [t] in *stop*), and rounding (e.g., [o] versus [e]). Those features that help distinguish phonemes in a language's or a child's system are often referred to as **distinctive features**. For example, voicing is a distinctive feature of English because it does differentiate phonemes, such as /d/ versus /t/ (*dot* versus *tot*), and /b/ versus /p/ (*cab* versus *cap*).

Phones or phonemes sometimes are labeled with features by the use of a plus (+) or a minus (−) sign to indicate whether that feature is present. For example, the phonemes /d/ and /t/ could be differentiated with distinctive features as follows:

$$/d/ \quad \begin{bmatrix} C \\ +\text{alveolar} \\ +\text{voice} \end{bmatrix}$$

$$/t/ \quad \begin{bmatrix} C \\ +\text{alveolar} \\ -\text{voice} \end{bmatrix}$$

The phoneme /d/ is produced with the tongue tip elevated to the alveolar ridge and with voicing; the phoneme /t/ is articulated similarly but is produced without voicing. Features are discussed in more detail in Chapter 3.

Syllables

The **syllable** is a very difficult entity to define, despite the fact that native speakers of any language usually are very good at counting the syllables in their own words. Crystal (1991, p. 338) tells us that a syllable is "a unit of pronunciation typically larger than a single sound and smaller than a word." Most syllables have a component that is very sonorous and is produced with a relatively open vocal tract (such as a vowel) and edges that are less sonorous and produced with a more closed vocal tract (such as a consonant). In more recent phonological theories, the first consonant (or set of consonants) is referred to as the **onset** and the final consonant (or set of consonants) as the **coda**; the sonorous portion is called the **nucleus**. The nucleus and coda together form the **rhyme** (Crystal, 1991).

The Components of Phonological Systems

In considering how any mechanical system is built, one tends to think first about its parts—switches, gears, cranks, wires, nuts, and bolts. However, at least as important to the proper functioning of the system are several other factors: the ways in which the parts are connected to one another to form functional subcomponents; the mechanical process (the way

---

[2]International Phonetic Alphabet (IPA) symbols that have pronunciations that differ from the pronunciations of English orthography are given and exemplified in Appendix C, as are the phonetic diacritics used in this book.

each part's function interacts with the functions of others and contributes to the functioning of the whole); and, finally, the rate and intensity of the work done by the system.

Like any other functional system, phonological systems include basic elements (features, which combine to form phones) with assigned roles (transforming them into phonemes), which are combined in specific ways into larger units (syllables and words). All of these elements interact in certain ways (referred to as **processes**, **rules**, or **constraints**, as defined in Chapter 5) at specified rates and intensity levels (the **prosody**) to achieve the final result, spoken language. Furthermore, all of these elements, levels, and interactions can be defined in terms of the questions they answer about the phonological system:

- The **phonotactic repertoire**: What syllable and word shapes are available for use?
- The **phonetic repertoire**: What sounds (and features) are available to form the content of those syllable and word shapes?
- The **phonemic repertoire**: What is each sound's role in the language, or, more specifically, how do the sounds contrast to yield distinctive words?
- **Phonological patterns** (**processes**, **rules**, or **constraints**): How do the syllable, word, and phrase shapes interact with the sounds and contrasts to yield the final pronunciation of the utterance? What influence does the morphology of the language have on the pronunciation of different types of words and endings? What types of phonetic or articulatory "slop" are allowed in the final pronunciations of words and utterances in fast or casual speech?
- **Suprasegmental patterns** or **prosody**: Where in the word or the sentence does the stress fall? Is stress marked by the loudness, the pitch, the duration of the segments, or some combination of these three? Are relatively unstressed syllables timed approximately equally or do they follow some other rhythmic pattern? What other purposes do loudness, pitch, or durations serve in the language? How does the morphology of the language influence the prosody?

As noted by Fee (1996), all levels of phonological organization are simplified in a child's phonology, but all are relevant. Unless all of the phonological subcomponents and the ways that they interact are considered, therapists will be agonizing needlessly over intervention priorities. Including all aspects of the phonological system in assessment and planning may appear to be extra work, but it will simplify goal setting and assessment of progress to a remarkable degree and can often be accomplished fairly simply and quickly.

Summary

Phonology is used here as a cover term to refer to a child's phones, phonemes, allophones, and syllable and word shapes, and the patterning of these in rules, processes, or constraints. Any strategy a child uses to convey meaning by sound, including strategies that are inspired by physiological limitations (such as cleft palate), will be considered to be part of that child's phonology. A phonology (child or adult) has several components, each of which can function in various ways both independently and interactively with other components. However, phonologies must also be considered in their entireties. We cannot look at any one component alone and draw adequate conclusions about phonological malfunction without considering every other aspect of the child's phonology as well. Assessment of the functions and interactions of all of these components will reveal the source of the phonological malfunction and facilitate identification and prioritization of remediation goals.

IMPORTANT CONCEPTS FROM CHILD PHONOLOGY

The functionality of a child's phonology needs to be considered in light of all of the subcomponents and elements that are used in adult phonologies. In addition, some special issues arise in the discussion of immature phonologies. Most of these issues have their source in the fact that, while no phonology remains unchanged for any long period of time, a child's phonology is in a state of rapid flux, as are the child's body and mind. Although an immature phonology may be functional for the child at one point in time, new cognitive, physical, or environmental factors may make additional communicative demands on the child at any moment. Similarly, new cognitive, physical, or environmental developments may increase the child's potential for phonological development. In this section, some of the consequences of these conditions are addressed. Again, the concepts presented here are described in further detail in later chapters.

Presystematic Versus Systematic Phonology

Children's very early phonologies differ in some important ways from their later phonologies. Many studies have shown that the first words are learned with very little phonological regularity. For example, the presumed target /f/ in initial position in one word may be stopped ([p]), whereas another target-initial /f/ may be produced quite accurately. It may not appear as though the child has any particular way to produce [f]; he or she is simply attempting to produce **words**. If one word is short and simple, the child may be able to get all the details right. If another is longer or more complex, the child may grasp the gist of it without worrying about the individual phones. Almost like parrots, children at this age are learning chunks of language in memorized words and phrases, without recognizing many relationships among the sounds in different words. If an analysis of a child's system is attempted at this stage, consistency or patterns may be unidentifiable (see, e.g., Velleman 1996a).

Typically, when children's vocabularies reach 25–100 words, often at the same time that they begin to combine words (approximately 18 months), systematization becomes apparent. Children identify those word shapes they are comfortable producing and focus on those. Thus, the typical signs of such systematization are the selective learning of words that fit preferred production patterns (i.e., that fit the system) and the avoidance of words that are understood but that cannot be adapted to the preferred word shape. For example, Vihman's (1976) daughter, "V," for months avoided saying the words for *mommy* and *daddy* in her native Estonian because she knew how to handle only words containing a low vowel followed by a high vowel (as in the English words *mommy* and *daddy*). The Estonian words ([ema] and [isa]) have the opposite pattern of a higher vowel followed by a lower one, which the child could not (or would not) produce. It is important to consider such selection and avoidance patterns when attempting to increase the expressive vocabularies of such children.

Another sign of systematization is that we can begin to identify clear phonological patterns in a child's speech. These patterns may be phonetic, phonemic, or phonotactic, but they are often pervasive. When they are spread to words with different adult forms, they are referred to as **word recipes**. For example, one child appeared to decide that she liked words that end with a nasal + vowel syllable (such as *funny*, *mommy*, *Grandma*) so much that she changed other words to fit this pattern—saying, for example, [ɪnni] for Nicky (Vihman & Velleman, 1989). Similarly, Vihman's daughter eventually changed the Estonian words for *mommy* and *daddy* so that she could pronounce them, saying [ami] for *ema* and [asi] for *isa*.

The establishment of such patterns, while it may lead to more adultlike productions of some words, may lead to apparently worse productions of other words. Words that previously were distinct may become homonyms; words that previously were clear may seem garbled. Parents may express concern because their child seems to be regressing phonologically.

This apparent regression is not regression at all. Just as children who begin to overgeneralize the regular past tense, plural, and the like at a certain age (saying *eated* for *ate*, *tooths* for *teeth*, etc.) do so because they are searching for regularities in the morphology; children who begin to demonstrate phonological systematicity are demonstrating that they are rule learners in this respect too. Such children have hit on a phonological pattern that (in most cases) is viable for a subgroup of the words of their language (just as *-ed* is for the past tense), and they are trying to make all words fit that pattern. Although this may be frustrating to us or to parents, it is a very good sign. These children have discovered the basic truth that language in general and phonology in particular are **rule governed**. Such children now have a phonological system.

Phonological Idioms

Children's early words that do not fit with other aspects of their phonological patterns are referred to as **phonological idioms**. Phonological idioms may be advanced in comparison to the rest of a child's system, or they may be simpler. One child said *pretty* very accurately very early in her word learning, even though this is expected to be a very difficult word (Leopold, 1947). Another may hang onto a very early gross simplification of some word even when he is phonologically capable of producing similar words more accurately. For example, one child named Mickey called herself [didi]. This was one of her very first words, so it was not a surprise that she simplified it. However, this was not a result of a perceptual confusion; she never responded if she was called "Deedee" by others. Yet, even when she was able to produce more difficult, similar words (such as *monkey*), Mickey persisted in saying her own name as [didi].

These characteristics of early phonology must be kept in mind when we are analyzing the phonologies of children with small vocabularies. At an early stage, lack of a system, or persistence in using words that are not consistent with a system, may be perfectly normal (Stoel-Gammon & Stone, 1991). However, this lack of system does not mean that it is impossible for the speech-language pathologist to carry out any type of phonological analysis. It is in just such cases that the ability to assess other aspects of the child's phonology, especially the phonotactic and phonetic repertoires, can play a vital role. Phonetic, phonotactic, and suprasegmental characteristics can be assessed, even in children who are still in the babbling or jargoning stages. A very young child just before the onset of word learning should still produce a variety of phones (typically four to six), usually in a few different word shapes (e.g., consonant-vowel [CV], VC, CVCV, CVC), with pitch patterns that are appropriate to the context (question, request, demand, etc.). As the child's vocabulary grows, there should be signs of emerging systematicity.

It has been suggested (Leonard, 1992; Leonard et al., 1989; Leonard & McGregor, 1991) that children with phonological disorders may be even more likely than children whose phonologies are developing normally to demonstrate idiosyncratic phonological patterns as their systems develop. Leonard (1992) suggests that this tendency may be due, in part, to the children's efforts to acquire larger lexicons using less sophisticated phonological systems.

Summary

At the beginnings of word learning, children's phonologies may be unsystematic, having no detectable regularities. As children begin to systematize, selection, avoidance, and preferred production patterns (or word recipes) may be identified. Phonological idioms may occur as either surprisingly sophisticated early productions or as simplified forms that do not improve even as the child's phonology changes to accommodate more phones and word shapes. Similar patterns may be seen and may be even more pervasive in the phonologies of children with phonological disorders.

ASSESSMENT

The **identification** of a moderate to severe phonological delay or disorder is relatively simple; often one can make this diagnosis on the basis of 2 minutes of observation.

The challenge is to find the time to analyze the phonological system of a child with such a disorder thoroughly enough that effective goals can be set. Whatever tool is used to identify a phonological disorder, more detail is likely to be needed for the establishment of intervention targets. This level of detail often is not available from any one standardized instrument but can be obtained from such instruments or from speech samples if one understands well what is being sought.

Relational Versus Independent Analysis

Relational Analysis

The tests that most speech-language pathologists use are relational (i.e., contrastive); they consider only how a child's phonology compares with the adult system. In other words, they identify a child's **errors**, from an adult point of view. For example, in a **relational analysis**, a child's accurate production of adult word and syllable shapes (e.g., clusters, multisyllabic words) is calculated. A relational analysis compares a child's output with the adult form to identify those elements that must be changed in order for the child's phonology to sound adultlike. Substitutions, omissions, and distortions—predictable patterns in which a certain presumed target phoneme or class of phonemes is produced in some other way or is omitted completely by the child—are documented or are classified as phonological rules or processes. However, the rules or processes are not necessarily taking place within the child's system. If a child thinks he is producing the form correctly, then as far as he is concerned, no rule or process is involved.

Relational rules and processes are merely descriptions of the differences between a child's productions and the adult, presumed target productions. In many cases, the adult pattern may actually *be* a particular child's internal phonological target and, under those circumstances, the pattern describes both a rule or process within the child's phonology and a description of the difference between the child's pronunciation and the adult's. Nonetheless, one cannot make this assumption without first conducting a careful analysis of the child's own system.

Independent Analysis

An **independent analysis** evaluates the child's system independently of the adult target system. Such an analysis considers the child's system as a phonological system in its own right, which may or may not be functioning well. In an independent analysis, the word and syllable shapes that the child actually *does* produce are determined. Any phonological system must be sufficiently rich (i.e., sufficiently complex) for the level of communication of its user. A child who attempts only 10 words might easily get away with one or two consonant phonemes and one or two vowel phonemes but, as she attempts to acquire more words, her system must become more complex.

A variety of options are available for expanding a phonological system. Complexity can be phonotactic (number of word and syllable shapes available), phonetic (number of sounds available), phonemic (number of con-

trasts available), pattern-based (interactions of phones and phonemes), or prosodic (number of suprasegmental patterns available). Children may choose to add complexity to their systems in ways that have not been chosen for the adult phonology that surrounds them. In an independent analysis, this finding is irrelevant; the primary questions are whether the phonological system is appropriately rich and which subsystems are contributing to this complexity. If one subsystem is grossly underdeveloped compared with others (e.g., the child has many phonemes but all of her words are monosyllabic), that subsystem will be the target of the speech-language pathologist's intervention.

Thus, an independent analysis gives us a clearer picture of a child's actual phonological capabilities and limitations. One additional major advantage of an independent analysis is that it can be carried out without respect to the presumed target words. Thus, if a child is unintelligible or produces only babble or jargon, it still is possible to assess the components of his or her speech production to determine whether those components are age-appropriate or severely limited. For instance, one prelinguistic child may produce reduplicated canonical syllables only (e.g., [bababa]), whereas another may produce widely varied syllables, even including some primitive stop + glide clusters ([e.g., djædiwɑtʃu]).

Complementary Aspects of Two Types of Analysis

Both independent and relational analyses of the child's phonology are vitally important for establishing intervention goals. Although the ultimate long-term goal is to make the child's phonology adultlike, identification of the nonfunctional aspects of the child's current system *as a system* is critical before remediation can be attempted. Children who have NFPs may exhibit extreme deficits in one particular subcomponent or in the interactions among subcomponents, and then this subcomponent or this type of phonological interaction must be an important focus of therapy. On the other hand, the purpose of having an intact phonology is to communicate. For this reason, children ideally should have not only functional phonologies but also phonologies that are as similar as possible to that of their environment, so that people will understand them. Contrastive analysis will help to determine which aspects of a child's phonology are most deviant in this sense and will be a second major influence in the goal selection process.

Most of the assessment tools available to speech-language pathologists are relational. They compare the child's productions to the adult forms of the target words and rate the child's errors using developmental norms. Both articulation tests and phonological process analyses are of this type. Using such tools alone blinds the clinician to the child's phonological system as a system, which may be more or less functional. The various components of the system are not analyzed to determine which may be contributing the most (or the least) to the child's current level of communicative effectiveness. Such an approach might be compared to a mechanic evaluating a malfunctioning car by watching it drive down the road beside an intact vehicle. The mechanic may get some hints as to the general location of the problem—muffler versus carburetor, and the like—and the sight of the well-functioning car will remind her of her eventual goal for the ill-functioning vehicle. She cannot, however, determine the actual source of the malfunction until she opens the hood and examines the muffler, carburetor, and so on. Of course, an experienced mechanic may be able to identify which component is malfunctioning just by watching the car drive by. An experienced child phonologist also can often differentiate malfunctioning phonological components simply by listening to the child speak. To become an experienced mechanic, however, one first must learn to identify the components of the car and how they work both individually and together. Furthermore, even expert mechanics verify their hunches before beginning repairs. Many more examples of both types of analysis and their implications for intervention are given throughout this book.

Summary

Independent analysis allows the speech-language pathologist to look at the child's system as an entity and to identify nonfunctional components or poor interactions among components. Relational analysis reveals how the child's output differs from adults' output and helps to identify which of these differences has the most important impact on intelligibility.

Popular Assessment Tools

It is not the purpose of this book to review popular assessment tools or to recommend any one over another. It is assumed, however, that all clinicians systematically collect phonological data of some sort before attempting to set therapeutic goals. The majority of speech-language pathologists use marketed tools, often in conjunction with other analyses, for this purpose. These assessment materials fall into three broad categories: **articulation tests**, **process tests**, and more comprehensive **phonological analysis procedures**. Some basic differences among these three types of tools are highlighted here. Specific commercially available phonological assessment tools are discussed in more depth in Appendix A. This appendix reviews some specific materials by category and identifies ways in which these materials typically are used to determine remediation priorities.

Articulation Tests

The limitations of assessing a child's speech sounds one by one without considering more general phonological patterns have been clear for a decade or more, but many sound-based articulation tests remain popular nonetheless. These tests typically include a set of pictures that are to be labeled by the child so that the clinician can score the child's production of each sound in initial, medial, or final position, as appropriate. Each observed sound substitution is assessed as either developmentally appropriate or not, depending on the predetermined age of acquisition for the target sound.

Although the use of such tests may be sufficient for identifying a phonological disorder, most phonologists now believe that the data these tests yield are far too superficial for determining remediation targets. However, articulation test data can facilitate phonological analysis in some ways. The data gathered from such tests may be more useful if each of the child's word productions is transcribed in its entirety, rather than transcription of only the child's productions of the target sounds for each stimulus item. Using such transcriptions, especially if they can be supplemented by samples of spontaneous speech, the speech-language pathologist can conduct further analyses to investigate particular classes of sounds that occur (or do not occur) in initial, medial, or final positions or within clusters. In addition, some useful information may be gleaned from the child's productions of multisyllabic words, which also are included (rather unsystematically) in most articulation tests, despite the fact that no syllable production data are explicitly collected during standardized test administration.

Some real advantages and important limitations accompany the use of transcriptions of articulation test items for broader analysis. One advantage is that the picture stimuli already are gathered, with the intent of representing a variety of English sounds. The pictures have been designed to be attractive and recognizable to young children. Furthermore, when a child labels a picture, the clinician usually knows what the child's target word is. This can be very important when undertaking relational analysis of unintelligible children. A few tests provide stimulus sentences for immediate or delayed imitation; thus, phrase-level phonological effects (discussed in Chapter 2), which may complicate identification of target words as well as analysis, are either well controlled or absent in tests with only single-word productions. Finally, comparisons among children are facilitated by the fact that all the children tested label the same stimuli.

The limitations of using articulation tests include the small sets of words assessed, which tend to be restricted to nouns. Most phonemes are sampled only once in each word position, and some vowel phonemes or uncommon phonemes (such as /ʒ/) may not be sampled at all. Furthermore, word complexity may not be appropriately controlled. As mentioned earlier, these tests were designed to identify segmental errors (omissions, substitutions, and distortions of single segments and consonant clusters) only. Identification of whole-syllable and whole-word patterns may be more difficult for the clinician. If a test that does not include phrase- or sentence-level productions is used, the production of only single words may be a disadvantage as well as an advantage: The lack of phrase- or sentence-level effects enhances intelligibility and transcribability, but if these effects are not observed, they cannot be analyzed and treated. Finally, an articulation test's speech production context is not natural; younger, lower-class, and nonwhite children may be particularly unfamiliar with picture-naming tasks and may not demonstrate their true phonological capabilities. (See Shriberg & Kwiatkowski, 1980, for further discussion of these ideas. A matrix illustrating the inclusion of some of these factors in various articulation tests is included in Appendix A, Table A-1.)

Process Tests

Other tests have as their aim the identification of error **patterns**, most commonly called **phonological processes** (described in depth in Chapter 5). These tests typically include specific stimulus words that a child is to produce. Most often the words are to be produced singly and spontaneously, although some tests elicit entire sentences containing target sounds and, in some cases, imitative productions are expected or at least are considered to be acceptable. Once they have been elicited, these word productions are analyzed with respect to the presence or absence of specific patterns.

Like articulation tests, process tests generate a useful set of word productions that can be analyzed in ways other than those recommended in the manual. Furthermore, they can point us in the direction of the types of further analyses that might be appropriate.

Comprehensive Phonological Analysis Procedures

Several manuals are available for carrying out a more detailed phonological analysis on the basis of a longer transcribed free-speech sample. Each describes the process of thoroughly sampling and assessing various aspects of a child's speech production patterns, based on theoretical principles that reflect the individual author's views of child phonology. These procedures typically provide a fairly comprehensive view of a child's phonology. However, a lengthy sample of (preferably) spontaneous speech must be elicited from the child being tested and must be carefully transcribed by the clinician. The time required for obtaining and transcribing such a sample, when added to the time required for carrying out such detailed analyses, is viewed as prohibitive by many practicing clinicians.

Do-It-Yourself Analysis

In the best of all possible worlds, there would always be enough time for all speech-language pathologists to carry out an in-depth, quantitative phonological analysis of every child evaluated or seen for treatment. Unfortunately, reality is far from that ideal. Most of us have minimal time available for phonological analysis. Nonetheless, addressing inappropriate, inefficient, or unachievable goals is a true waste of valuable therapeutic time (and, in many cases, money).

If quantitative data (percentages) or age norms are not needed, many aspects of a child's phonological system can be assessed fairly simply and quickly using a speech sample obtained from spontaneous speech, from the administration of a standard articulation or process test or, preferably, from both. The combination provides a set of elicited single-word utterances with known targets plus a set of spontaneous utterances from a more natural context, some of which may be partially or totally unintelligible. Interesting differences may emerge from the comparison of conversational and elicited speech samples.

Most clinicians record a language sample, obtained either in conversation with a child or through observation of even more natural interactions (e.g., in the classroom or at play with another child). With practice, one can fairly quickly simply transcribe the taped language sample into the International Phonetic Alphabet (IPA), thus "killing two birds with one stone." Over time, a clinician can become proficient at transcribing much of the sample online, during the clinical session, using the tape to verify and to add in utterances that have been missed. Then the clinician can scan the transcribed words from the articulation test plus the language sample and indicate the results on a worksheet (as described later) to identify the phonological system used by the child being evaluated. Any immature or deviant patterns that are identified can be more thoroughly quantified later to establish baselines in therapy.

Most child phonologists, over their years of conducting phonological analyses, have developed their own worksheets, but the typical speech-language pathologist lacks the time and experience required for developing such protocols. Worksheets for do-it-yourself analyses of children's word productions are provided in each chapter of this book. These worksheets provide the clinician with "shortcut" ways in which to analyze different aspects of a child's speech in some detail without having to carry out an entire phonological analysis. The worksheets can be used either with spontaneous speech samples or with elicited word productions such as those that would be obtained through the administration of a traditional articulation test. Ideally, as noted earlier, the clinician would administer such a test *and* transcribe the child's language sample (or at least a portion of it) in IPA, in order to take advantage of the benefits of each data-gathering procedure. In this way, comparisons could be made between elicited and spontaneous speech.

Although these worksheets are not standardized and, at best, provide an overview of the child's phonological system, they do offer a means of sketching each aspect of phonology within a feasible time frame. Furthermore, they are far more user friendly than are many of the in-depth analysis procedures on the market. Finally, the worksheets provided in this book can be used at three different levels of accuracy, allowing the clinician to select the depth of analysis that is appropriate to the client, to the time available, and to the clinician's own experience level.

The use of do-it-yourself worksheets cannot replace in-depth phonological analysis in cases that require careful quantitative documentation, nor can it provide age equivalencies or scores. However, such worksheets can serve as efficient, flexible assessment tools that will facilitate goal setting and, later, reassessment.

Summary

A child's phonology can be assessed in a variety of different ways: by the use of an articulation test to score correct or incorrect productions of one target phoneme per word, a process test to identify patterns of errors in elicited words, or an in-depth analysis of spontaneous speech. The do-it-yourself worksheets provided in this book are intended to allow the speech-language pathologist to screen quickly all components of a child's phonological system, mainly within an independent analysis approach, either as a supplement to other testing or as an overview of the functioning of the child's entire phonology *as a system* in its own right.

Each of these procedures has its advantages and disadvantages. The real advantage of articulation tests is their simple format and scoring system. Many young or very active children cannot be induced to name more than a small set of large, colorful pictures and would therefore not be appropriate candidates for longer elicitation procedures. However, the amount of information that can be gleaned from one production of each phoneme in each position may be very limited. More in-depth analyses require one to obtain spontaneous connected speech, which is certainly more natural but also is far more challenging and time-consuming to transcribe. Furthermore, data from unintelligible children may often be difficult to use because the target words are unknown. Each clinician must assess each child's linguistic and behavioral capabilities as well as the clinician's own limitations in time and ability in order to determine the most efficient method for assessing that child's phonology.

Perspectives on Goal Setting

Two important factors that shape the phonology of every language are **ease of perception** and **ease of production**. The term *ease of perception* refers to the idea that a language must choose sounds and sound patterns that are distinct enough that the listener can distinguish them, even in running speech. The term *ease of production* refers to articulatory simplicity: All else being equal, a language will incorporate sounds that are easy to produce rather than sounds that are more difficult.

These factors are important in child phonology as well, although children appear to be far more motivated by ease of production than by ease of perception. Their babble and early words typically include those sounds that are the least difficult to articulate (see Chapter 3 for further details). Sounds that are easy to perceive but more difficult to produce, which are common in adult phonologies, are rare in child phonologies.

When considering therapeutic goals for a disordered child, the clinician must consider both ease of production and ease of perception. Obviously, those sounds, sound classes, and sound patterns that will be easier for the child to produce generally will be addressed before those that are more difficult to articulate are targeted. A given child's physiological limitations (e.g., cleft palate, low tone) and current phonological system must be taken into account. However, the phrase *ease of perception* has two interpretations—namely, ease for the listener and ease for the speaker—both of which must be considered. First, there is the question of which changes in a child's current phonological system are most likely to increase intelligibility, thereby easing the *listener's* burden and improving the child's communicative effectiveness. Second, the child's perceptual system must not be ignored: An attempt must be made to determine those sounds and sound patterns that appear to be most perceptually salient to the child. It may be a waste of time to attempt to facilitate a child's learning of a contrast on which the client does not place communicative value. Targeting a pattern of which the child is linguistically aware but that is not yet produced in an adultlike manner will yield a higher success rate.

CONCLUSION

A phonology is a functioning system having many subcomponents, each of which depends on various combinations of elements. Children begin the language acquisition process without such a system; they learn their first words, parrotlike, as unrelated wholes. Children who are normally developing, however, quickly begin to systematize.

To assess a child's phonology efficiently, one must view it as a system that may or may not be functioning adequately for the child's communication needs at this time. For this reason, independent phonological analyses are critical to effective goal setting.

CHAPTER TWO

Phonotactics: Word- and Syllable-Level Patterns

I
it
sit
spit
spite
spiteful
unspiteful
unspitefulness
unspitefulnesses

INTRODUCTORY CONCEPTS

Words come in all different shapes and sizes. The major components of any word are its syllables (defined in Chapter 1), which may range in number from 1 to more than 20. Syllables can also be of different shapes and sizes. The shapes and sizes of syllables and words are determined by a set of restrictions that are specific to each language. Every language in the world has certain preferred word or syllable patterns as well as other patterns that are not preferred or even not allowed. These patterns can reflect a variety of different factors, including the following:

- The numbers of syllables that tend to occur in each word
- The numbers, types, and locations of consonants in clusters
- The presence or absence of final consonants
- The presence or absence of diphthongs or long vowels
- **Harmony patterns**, in which consonants or vowels become more similar to each other
- **Phrase-level effects**, which change the pronunciations of sounds in phrases and sentences

There is a trade-off among the patterns that are allowed by the language. If the language is more restrictive in some ways, it must be less restrictive in others. These restrictions on word and syllable shapes and sizes are called the **phonotactic constraints** of the language. They are very important in the analysis of delayed or disordered phonology, as many children have developmentally inappropriate or unusual phonotactic constraints. Furthermore, many adult and child phonological patterns (processes, rules, or constraints) appear to operate at the syllable or word level rather than to affect particular segments in isolation. A phonotactic repertoire can often be described using notation that is not sound specific, such as *CV* to represent an open consonant (C) and vowel (V) syllable, or *#CC* to represent a word–initial consonant cluster (where # represents a word boundary—either the beginning or the ending edge of a word). However, phonotactic patterns also include effects of one part of the word on the other, such as harmony, assimilation, and reduplication. In this chapter, the discussion focuses on phonotactic constraints and other patterns that operate at the syllable level and above.

The critical significance of syllable-level and word-level analysis for describing and explaining child (and adult) phonologies in all languages has been increasingly recognized over the past two decades, beginning with Ferguson and Farwell (1975), Ferguson (1978), Macken (1979), and

others. Ingram (1978) listed four main reasons for focusing on syllable and word structure in child phonologies:

1. Some phonological patterns, such as consonant cluster reduction and final consonant omission, function primarily to simplify syllables.
2. Other processes, such as unstressed syllable deletion and reduplication (repetition of the same syllable, as in *boo-boo*), operate only on entire words.
3. The development of many segments differs according to their placement within the syllable or word (e.g., velars[1] often develop first in final position).
4. Segmental complexity (the difficulty and variety of sounds within the word) interacts with syllabic complexity (the shape of the syllable) and triggers word-level processes (such as harmony patterns, described later). As segmental complexity increases, syllabic complexity may decrease, and vice versa. In other words, the child may be able to produce either difficult sounds or difficult word shapes, but not both within the same word.

Many child phonologists believe that very early phonology, at least, is exclusively word- or syllable-based and that children's early phonological systems do not refer to the segmental level at all. Furthermore, many speech-language pathologists have found that clients of any age generalize their learning much better when sounds are targeted at the syllable or word level rather than in isolation.

PHONOTACTIC PATTERNS

Different languages have different phonotactic patterns, but there must always be a certain amount of phonotactic freedom within any language. Without a certain amount of flexibility, the vocabulary of a language would be either very limited or composed of nothing but homonyms. A language that allowed only monosyllabic words, with only **open CV syllables**, might be restricted to 200 or so possible different words, far too few for functional communication. This is the dilemma of many children with nonfunctional phonologies (NFPs): They have too many phonotactic constraints for the number of meanings they would like to express. As a result, to communicate they must restrict their vocabularies, produce many homonyms, or supplement their oral words with gestures and nonspeech sounds.

Phonotactic patterns are far from random. They are based on human speech production constraints. To permit communication, each language must incorporate some components (such as complex clusters or lengthy multisyllabic words) that are difficult to articulate, but

---

[1]Familiarity with basic English phonetic features (place and manner of articulation) and with the International Phonetic Alphabet (IPA) is assumed in this chapter. Readers who are not familiar with these concepts should refer to the introduction section of Chapter 3, especially Tables 3-1 through 3-4, and also to Appendix C.

every language has a limited number of these more challenging production patterns. The overall difficulty level of every language still is manageable by its speakers. If it becomes too difficult to be spoken, a language must either change or die. Furthermore, the most frequently used words in a language will be the shorter, simpler ones. Longer or more complex words that come into frequent use will be simplified (as *television* has been reduced to *TV* in English).

Phonotactic patterns are critically important in speakers' judgments (usually subconscious) of which words are or are not acceptable in their language. Often, for example, English speakers are capable of saying a foreign word—it is made up of phones that approximate English phones—but that word will not sound right to us because of its shape. For example, while traveling, this author recently had lunch in a sandwich shop called *Jreck*. The name was composed of the two owners' initials; presumably other options, such as *Jerck*, were ruled out. The chosen name is pronounceable but seems very strange to native speakers of English.

In many cases, native English speakers will mispronounce seemingly impossible words, especially those that are borrowed from foreign languages, in ways that more closely fit the phonotactic patterns of the English language. For example, the name *Schwarzkopf* usually is pronounced by most Americans without the penultimate *p* sound: [ʃwɑɚtskɔf]. Most English-speaking Americans actually have no trouble pronouncing a final *-pf* cluster. We even use this sequence of consonants medially in some words (e.g., *capful*). However, it is a cluster that is not allowed in English in final position; therefore, English speakers are not comfortable saying it in that position and simplify it to make it fit better within the concept of "English-ness." Similarly, the common Vietnamese name *Nguyen* is alien to English speakers because of its initial [ŋg], although English speakers produce [ŋg] medially in words such as *anger* and *longer*. Those who speak English typically make this name and others like it more English sounding by reducing the cluster and changing the place of articulation (as singleton [ŋ] is not allowed in initial position either), with the resulting pronunciation [nujen].

The preceding examples are all feature specific. Such feature-specific restrictions are one type of **distribution requirement**. Distribution requirements, in general, are restrictions on which types of sounds or syllables can occur in which positions in the word. They are discussed in greater depth later in this chapter and in Chapter 3.

Languages (and children) also have constraints at more basic levels. The Japanese language, for instance, avoids consonant clusters in any position and compensates for this with more multisyllabic words. When Japanese speakers attempt to produce English words with clusters in them, they epenthesize (insert) extra vowels (such as [u]) to make the words conform to Japanese phonotactic restrictions. In some words, this may double or even triple the number of syllables in the word, such as [pɑburikku] for *public* or [pɑrusu] for *pulse* (Hyman, 1975). Similarly, Japanese who practice English songs by [ʃinatəro fəranku-san] (Frank Sinatra) in their [karaoke

bɑksu] (karaoke "boxes," or practice rooms) sing their own version of "Smoke Gets in Your Eyes" (Reid, 1992):

...and [sʌmədeɪ] you'll [fɑɪnədo]
All true love is [bɛlɑɪnədo]...

The phonotactic constraints of any language are so ingrained in its speakers that they almost never violate them, although most people are not consciously aware of the constraints. Even in slips of the tongue, these rules rarely are broken. Speakers might interchange phonemes (as in "You hissed all my mystery lectures") or even, occasionally, features (as in the stop-affricate switch in "This is a wild juice case"). However, Shattuck-Hufnagel and Klatt (1979) demonstrated that speakers rarely produce errors that result in illegal word or syllable shapes. When an English speaker moves a phoneme to another place within a word or phrase, for example, its landing site will always be one that is allowed by English phonotactic restrictions. For instance, *mowing thrud* for *throwing mud* is a typical error; [θroʊɪm ŋʌd] or *thowing mrud* would be highly unexpected slips of the tongue because *mr-* is not a possible consonant cluster and [ŋ] is not allowed in syllable-initial position in English. Similarly, a Japanese person would never produce a slip of the tongue that resulted in an initial or final consonant cluster.

Children—whether or not they have an NFP—often have more restrictive phonotactic constraints than does the language that they are learning. This becomes a problem only when their constraints are very persistent or extremely restrictive while their vocabularies continue to grow. A different set of problems arises when a child's phonotactic system is more permissive than the target language's phonotactic system. As a result, the child may sound as though he or she has an accent. Examples of both types of systems are given in the "Child Phonology" portions of the following sections.

In summary, all languages have rules about allowable word and syllable shapes, and these rules are called *phonotactic constraints*. The constraints determine the types of words that are possible in the language.

Let us look in more detail at specific types of phonotactic patterns that may be found in some languages and in some children's phonological systems. The majority of these are production-based patterns—that is, they increase ease of production. Some clearly operate at the word level; others operate at either the word or the syllable level. The following factors that influence the phonotactic patterns of all languages are considered here:

- The number of syllables in a word
- The inclusion of a vowel as syllable nucleus
- The inclusion of a consonant as syllable onset
- The occurrence of open versus closed syllables
- Cluster constraints
- The inclusion of sequences of vowels
- Harmony, assimilation, and reduplication patterns
- Distribution requirements
- Suprasegmentals
- Phrase-level interactions
- Perception-based patterns

As each pattern is discussed in detail, examples will be drawn first from the languages of the world to establish the various ways in which functional adult phonotactic systems may work. Then, examples from functional or nonfunctional child phonologies in English and, if possible, other languages will be given.

Constraints on the Number of Syllables in a Word

Languages of the World
The most obvious evidence for processing at the level of the word comes from phonotactic constraints on the number of syllables that can occur in a word. Although no language has a specific upper limit on the number of possible syllables in a word, some languages (e.g., Japanese and Hawaiian) tend to have far more multisyllabic words than others (possibly to compensate for other phonotactic restrictions, as is discussed in "Open Versus Closed Syllables"). Other languages, such as English, tend to have shorter words *on average*. The number of syllables in a word is inversely proportional to its frequency of occurrence. In other words, the most commonly used words in any language are the monosyllabic ones (Crystal, 1987).

Child Phonology
Similarly, children seem to prefer monosyllables or disyllables to longer words. English-speaking children are especially partial to monosyllabic words, probably because English words tend to be short compared with those of other languages. However, Stoel-Gammon (1987) found that 79% of 34 English-speaking children at the age of 24 months used CVCV words at least some of the time; 67% used two-syllable words ending in a final consonant (CVCVC). The most common response to a preference for short words among English-learning children is to omit unstressed syllables, yielding forms such as [nænə] for *banana*, [waʊn] for *around*, and [bʌʔ] for *button*. Word-stress patterns affect this tendency, as is discussed in the section on suprasegmentals.

Vowel as Syllable Nucleus

Languages of the World
Many languages require a vowel at the heart (nucleus) of each syllable. English is one of the exceptions to this; it does allow a consonant that is nasal or liquid to carry an entire syllable in words such as *button* or *bottle*. Consonants that serve in this role are called **syllabic consonants**. Berber (a Moroccan language) goes even further in this direction than does English, according to Archangeli (1997). In this language, the third-person feminine singular prefix *t-* plays a similar role to the *-s* on the end of verbs in English, as in *plays, kicks, eats*, and the like. In consonant cluster–initial words to which this Berber prefix is added, the result is three consonants in a row. For example, the stem *-ldi* (to pull) may have the *t-* prefix added to express *(she) pulls*. The resulting pronunciation is a two-syllable word (with the syllable division indicated by a dot)—[tl.di]—of which the first syllable consists of two consonants.

Bell (1978) noted that, of the 182 languages representing the major language families and areas of the world that he had studied, 85 had some sort of syllabic consonants. Resonant consonants (nasals and liquids) were the most popular type of syllabics, occurring in 71 of the languages. Twenty-four of these allowed obstruent (stop or fricative, or both) syllabic consonants also; only 10 (including languages as geographically distant from one another as Hsiang Chinese and Wichita) allowed obstruents but not resonants to act as the nucleus of a syllable.

Child Phonology
Most English-speaking children include a vocalic nucleus in every syllable, with the exception of certain English words that allow a liquid or nasal to serve as a syllable (see earlier). In addition, a few motherese sound effects may be treated as words by some children (e.g., *shh, mmm, rrr*). Some children with disorders, especially developmental verbal dyspraxia (DVD), may exhibit particular difficulty in building consonant + vowel syllables. These children may use an unusually high number of words that consist of a single consonant without a vowel nucleus (or a single vowel without a consonant onset). A detailed example is given in the section on the phonotactics of DVD, later in this chapter.

Inclusion of Consonant as Syllable Onset

Languages of the World
All languages allow a syllable to begin with a consonant (i.e., have an **onset**). Many languages do not allow syllables that lack an onset—that is, syllables may not begin with a vowel (Prince & Smolensky, in press). According to Blevins (1995), languages that allow vowel-initial syllables are more common than languages that do not. Adult languages that do not allow them use various strategies for avoiding onsetless syllables that occur as the result of morphological changes, in borrowed words, and so on. These strategies include epenthesis (the insertion of a sound; in this case, the addition of an initial consonant to the syllable). Epenthesis is used for the purpose of avoiding onsetless syllables in languages such as Madurese[2] (McCarthy & Prince, 1995) and Axininca Campa (an Arawakan language of Peru; McCarthy & Prince, 1993).

Child Phonology
Demuth (1996), Demuth and Fee (1995), Fee (1996), and Fikkert (1994) have proposed CV as the **core syllable** with which children of all languages begin phonological acquisition. As in some adult languages, some young children epenthesize consonants at the beginnings of vowel-initial words. Other children may use other strategies, such as **metathesis** (the interchange of elements within a word; in this case, the moving around of consonants within the word) to ensure the presence of an onset. For

---

[2]Madurese is an Austronesian language spoken in Java, according to Crystal (1987).

example, Gnanadesikan (1995) describes a child, Gita, who avoided vowel-initial syllables in medial positions of words by moving the final consonant into the middle of the word. Thus, *going* was pronounced as [gonə] and *lion* as [jɑni].

However, this tendency for children to prefer syllables with onsets is not an absolute universal. For example, Freitas (1996) reported that children who are learning Portuguese as their native language do produce some vowel-initial syllables, even in the early stages of word learning. This author's experience with English-speaking children indicates that most occasionally produce onset-less syllables as well.

Open Versus Closed Syllables

Languages of the World

Another very basic restriction that languages place on their phonologies is a prohibition against closed syllables, which are those with one or more final consonants.[3] Such a phonology would have no CVC syllables. All languages have CV syllables (Crystal, 1991); very few have no CVCs because of the severe limitations that such a restriction places on word shapes. Hawaiian, for instance, permits only V and CV syllables; no syllable may have more than one consonant, and some have none. As a result, this language has only 162 possible syllables. Thai, in contrast, has 23,638 possible syllables (Crystal, 1987). Hawaiian compensates for its limited syllable variety with extremely long words.

Child Phonology

Many children, regardless of the language they are learning, enter into word production with only open CV (and V) syllables. Closed syllables may not emerge until a child is producing 8–11 different consonants, at approximately 2½ years of age (Grunwell, 1982). According to Stoel-Gammon (1987), 100% of English-speaking 2-year-olds produce CV syllables, and 97% produce CVC syllables at least some of the time. Branigan (1976, p. 128) stated that, "monosyllables are the first structures to be closed and … this operation occurs simultaneous with the production of bisyllables." The near co-occurrence of the development of two-syllable words and of final consonants has also been proposed by Demuth and Fee (1995) and Fee (1996). It is not known whether the developmental progression is the same in children with NFPs, but it is well established that syllable closure constraints often persist beyond age expectations in such children.

Metathesis may be motivated by restrictions on final consonants. Attempts to restrict consonants to initial position may result in productions such as [pʌ] for *up*, [fɔ] for *off*, or [gʌ] for *egg*. When complicated by omissions within the word, these forms can be quite confusing, such as the use of [kʌ] for *stuck*.

Cluster Constraints

Languages of the World

Languages may differ in the number of consecutive consonants that are allowed in various word positions and in the ordering of consonant types within clusters. The latter type of feature-specific distribution requirements are considered in depth in Chapter 3. For the moment, the focus will be on constraints on the *number* of consecutive consonants that the language will permit.

Some languages, such as Japanese, are far more restrictive than English with respect to sequences of consonants. Japanese has almost no consonant clusters and allows only one specific type of consonant (/n/) in final position. The language compensates for these limits by having many very long multisyllabic words. The syllables themselves are much simpler than in some other languages (such as English), but there are many more of them per word. Many common words that are monosyllabic in English are bi- or trisyllabic in Japanese, such as [kokoro] for *heart* and [ʔotoko] for *man* (Hyman, 1975).

Languages such as Japanese and Yawelmani (a Native American language from the U.S. West Coast) have entire sets of rules (**conspiracies**) designed to prevent the occurrence of clusters. The rules used by such languages to cope with clusters that would otherwise be too long include deletion and epenthesis. Deletion in this case involves removing one element of the illegal cluster, and epenthesis involves inserting a vowel between the consonants to break up the cluster. As demonstrated earlier, Japanese speakers rely heavily on epenthesis of vowels to help them to pronounce foreign words. Hawaiians also resort to epenthesis to avoid consonant clusters in borrowed words. For example, they pronounce the English word *flour* as *palooa*, and *velvet* as *weleweka* (Archangeli, 1997).

In English, a wide variety of clusters are allowed. However, English speakers tend to use deletion to simplify clusters in casual or fast speech. *Facts* may be pronounced without the [t], *fifths* without the [θ], or *library* without the first [r] (Clark & Yallop, 1995).

Long clusters that are created by adjoining two words into a phrase may also be simplified. American English speakers rarely pronounce all the medial consonants in a phrase such as "mashed potatoes," "stopped speaking" (Crystal, 1987), or "next stop." Typically, this latter phrase is produced with only one of the -*st*- sequences:

$$
\begin{array}{cccccccccccc}
\# & n & \varepsilon & k & s & t & \# & s & t & ɑ & p & \# & \rightarrow \\
\# & n & \varepsilon & k & \varnothing & \varnothing & \# & s & t & ɑ & p & \#
\end{array}
$$

Coalescence also is used in American English at times, in more casual speech. For example, the historical [d] and [j] of the medial cluster in *soldier* ([soldjɚ]) are merged in some dialects, yielding [soldʒɚ]. The same is true in some dialects for the word *Indian* (Clark & Yallop, 1995). Sometimes even whole words can be coalesced within a phrase. The most often cited example is the coalesced version of "Did you eat yet?"—[dʒiʔ jɛʔ]—to which the reply is supposed to be the also-coalesced "Did you?"—[dʒu].

---

[3]Syllables that are vowel-initial (e.g., VC syllables) are not considered to be open.

TABLE 2-1.
"Martin"'s Coalescence of Clusters

string	[fɪn, fɪm]
strawberries	[fɔberi]
swimming	[fɪmɪn]
thread	[fɛv]
tree	[fi]
sleeping	[fiʔm]
drinking	[fɪnʔɪn]

Source: Adapted from P Grunwell. *Clinical Phonology*. Rockville, MD: Aspen, 1982.

Child Phonology

Many children from any linguistic environment have phonotactic constraints against all or most clusters in any position, especially early in their phonological development. Stoel-Gammon (1987) reported that 58% of English-speaking 24-month-olds use initial two-element consonant clusters, 48% use such clusters in final position, and 30% use them in medial position. Children with reduced intelligibility often lack consonant clusters in their speech (Grunwell 1981; Hodson & Paden 1981). The simplifications that they use may include omissions, coalescence, epenthesis, metathesis, and migration, as detailed below.

OMISSIONS. Omission occurs when one or more elements of the cluster are not produced (e.g., [pɑt] for *spot*). According to Ingram (1989), children typically go through an initial stage in which neither member of the cluster is preserved, then another in which they preserve only one member of the cluster. Lleó and Prinz (1996) confirmed the latter pattern for German- and Spanish-speaking children as well.

COALESCENCE. In coalescence, the elements of the cluster are merged phonetically, and one phone—a combination of features from the original phones—is produced. For instance, the child might say [fɑt] for *spot*. In this case, the [f] is a combination of the frication of the [s] plus the labiality of the [p]. Other children attempt to produce [s] + nasal clusters by combining the voicelessness of the [s] with the nasality of the nasal, yielding a voiceless nasal. Thus, a word such as *snake* is pronounced as [n̥eɪk].

Once children, especially those with an NFP, have devised a coalescence pattern for some clusters, they may apply it to other clusters, regardless of whether it actually represents a coalescence of those other clusters. The use of [f] to represent a variety of clusters is especially common. The example of a 6-year-old named "Martin," given in Table 2-1, is typical (Grunwell, 1982). Martin initially used [f] as a coalescence of [s] plus [w]. The labiality of the [w] combined with the frication of the [s] to yield [f].

Martin's production of /r/ as [w] may have influenced him to extend this pattern to clusters with [s] and [r], such as *str-* (treating /r/ in the same way as /w/). However, eventually the pattern was extended also to other clusters with [s], such as *sl-*. It was extended additionally to other clusters with [r], such as *thr-, dr-,* and *tr-.* As a result, [f] ended up substituting for the majority of clusters, a difficult situation for listeners.

EPENTHESIS. **Epenthesis** is the insertion of one phonological element (e.g., a sound) into another (e.g., a word). With respect to clusters, it typically involves the insertion of a vowel between the consonants in the cluster (e.g., [bəlu] for "blue," [səpɑt] for "spot"). This addition is more common in the speech of speakers of other languages learning English than it is in the speech of English-speaking children. However, overeager speech-language pathologists or parents who encourage children to pronounce each element of the cluster separately, then attempt to blend them together, might inadvertently encourage children with an NFP to use this pattern. Some children with severe NFPs or with DVD may come up with this unfortunate strategy on their own, especially if they are literate and therefore aware of both elements of the cluster. Other children speak so slowly that it sounds as though they are inserting vowels between consonants or even extra consonants within clusters (e.g., [bəlu]).

METATHESIS. Sometimes the order rather than the number of consonants is problematic for the child developing a system. In such a case, the child may resort to changing the order. A stereotypical example of this (which occurs also in some dialects of American English) is metathesis of *-sk-* to *-ks-*, as in [ækst] for *asked* and [bæksɪt] for *basket*.

MIGRATION. Some children resort to moving one element of a cluster completely away from the other element, sometimes even crossing over a vowel. For instance, a child might say [kus] for *school* (Leonard & McGregor, 1991). This demonstrates again the importance of syllable-level analyses. One cannot hope to describe such a pattern without reference to the syllable or word as a whole. Referring to this pattern as a substitution of [s] for /l/ hardly describes what actually is happening.

Inclusion of Sequences of Vowels

Languages of the World

Perhaps one-third of the world's languages include diphthongs. Numerous languages also include long versus short vowels (Ladefoged & Maddieson, 1996). Languages that do not permit two consecutive vowels typically use either deletion or epenthesis to eliminate or separate the vowels when morphological patterns or borrowed words otherwise would require the production of such a sequence. For instance, one dialect of Basque (a Romance language spoken in western Spain) contains a suffix with a meaning similar to our word *the*. This suffix is sometimes pronounced [e]. If this suffix is added at the end of a vowel-final word, a sequence of two vowels results. However, in this case, a glide

German too is permissive with respect to consonant clusters. Although it does not permit some clusters that are acceptable in English, it does include some clusters that are not allowed in English, such as *ʃw-, ʃm-, ʃp-,* and *ʃpr-* in initial position and *-pf* in initial and final position.

([j] or [w], depending on the vowel) is epenthesized in between the two vowels to keep them apart. For example, *erri*, which means *village*, becomes *erriye* (*the village*), and *buru*, which means *head*, becomes *buruwe* (*the head*; Kenstowicz, 1994).

Deletion of one vowel from a sequence often occurs in phrases. This pattern is the basis for several contractions in English, such as *I'm, you're, he's*, and the like, and also in French, including *j'ai* (I have), *l'air* (the air), and the like (Clark & Yallop, 1995). In casual speech, American English speakers often delete one vowel or merge the two vowels in such phrases as *go away* ([go weɪ]) and *try again* ([trɑɪ gɛn]; Crystal 1987). (See also the discussion of French liaison in the section on phrase-level interactions.)

Child Phonology

Few researchers have made studies of diphthong production in children from any language background. However, Pollock and Keiser (1990) reported on the vowel production of 15 English-speaking children with phonological disorders. Fourteen of these subjects made errors on diphthongs. Nineteen percent of the children's total vowel errors were diphthong reductions. These findings suggest that children who are phonologically disordered, at least, prefer simple vowels. However, in 9% of cases, the children diphthongized simple vowels, and some diphthongs were substituted with other diphthongs (e.g., [ɔɪ] replaced with [oʊ]), so the picture is not as simple as one might hope. Pollock and Hall (1991) and Velleman et al. (1991) also found that diphthongs were particularly difficult for children with an NFP, including dyspraxia.

Stemberger (1988) described a child who omitted an initial vowel after a word ending with another vowel. In this case, his daughter, Gwendolyn, produced *How about him?* ([hɑu əbaʊt hɪm]) as [hou bɑ tʰɪm]. Clearly, far more work needs to be done in this area; it has been neglected sorely. Research is ongoing in Pollock's group.

Harmony, Assimilation, and Reduplication Patterns

Harmony, assimilation, and reduplication are among the phonological patterns most difficult to describe without referring to an entire syllable or word. All require one consonant or vowel to peek ahead or back at another segment so as to resemble it more closely. Consider a child who pronounces *doggie* as [gɔgi] but *doughnut* with appropriate alveolar consonants ([donʌt]). It is simply incorrect to say that this child is using a backing process (pronouncing alveolars too far back [i.e., at the velar place of articulation]). The child's velar and alveolar production patterns clearly depend on the phonology of the entire word, not simply on substitution of one phone for another.

Technically, **assimilation** describes *adjacent* elements becoming more alike, such as when the negative prefix *in-* is added to the word *possible* to yield *impossible*. By definition, **harmony** describes *more distant* units becoming more alike. In the *doggie* example, for instance, the /d/ and /g/ are separated by a vowel, but the /d/ harmonizes with the /g/ over the /ɔ/. Despite their technical definitions, in

TABLE 2-2.
Nasal Assimilation in English

inept
immobile
impossible
intolerant
indelible
incredible
illegal
illegitimate
irreverent
irresponsible

practice the terms *assimilation* and *harmony* often are used interchangeably to refer to word segments that come to resemble each other more closely.

Reduplication is the process whereby one syllable of the word is repeated, as in many English "baby-talk" words (so-called motherese; *boo-boo, tum-tum, pee-pee*, etc.).

Languages of the World

Due to ease of production (see Chapter 1), American English speakers tend to assimilate some clusters in casual speech. This phenomenon is partly responsible for the pronunciation in some dialects of *sandwich* as [sæmwɪtʃ] (inspiring the name of the Sam Witch Deli in Austin, TX). In this case, the [d] is deleted to simplify the cluster; then the nasal /n/ is labialized in anticipation of the labiovelar [w]. The assimilation continues the process of rendering a somewhat difficult medial cluster more manageable. This change makes the word easier because [m] and [w] share a place of articulation, whereas *-nd-* and [w] do not. Similarly, in some dialects, speakers say [pɪtʃɚ] for [pɪkʃɚ] (*picture*). It is easier for a speaker of any language to pronounce an alveolar immediately before a palatal (as the two locations are very close) than a velar before a palatal.

Some English assimilation patterns are morphophonological—that is, English speakers routinely assimilate the voicing of certain morphological endings, such as plural, although the assimilation is not reflected in our spelling. Examples include the following:

- *-s* plural: [kæts] versus [kɪdz] (cats, kids)
- third-person singular: [kɪks] versus [dʒɔgz] (kicks, jogs)
- possessive endings: [pɑps] versus [babz] (Pop's, Bob's)
- past tense: [kɪst] versus [bʌzd] (kissed, buzzed)

Some English morphological assimilations have become so standard that they even are spelled in their assimilated forms. The nasal in the negative morpheme *in-*, for example, assimilates to match the place of articulation—and sometimes even the manner of articulation—of any following consonant, not only of [p]. The words are spelled as English speakers say them to the extent that our alphabet allows,[4] as shown in Table 2-2.

---

[4]The English alphabet has no orthographic symbol for [ŋ] (as in [ɪŋkredɪbəl]), so this is spelled with *n*.

TABLE 2-3.
Turkish Vowel Harmony

Gloss	Turkish Pronunciation
I came	[geldim]
I stood	[durdum]
I laughed	[güldüm]

Note: The umlaut indicates a front-rounded vowel.
Source: Adapted from WJ Poser. Phonological representation and action-at-a-distance. In van der Hulst H, Smith N (eds). *The Structure of Phonological Representations: Part II*. Dordrecht, Holland: Foris, 1982, 121–158.

TABLE 2-4.
Warlpiri Reduplication

Singular		Plural	
kurdu	*child*	kurdu**kurdu**	*children*
kamina	*girl*	kamina**kamina**	*girls*
mardukuja	*woman*	mardukuja**mardukuja**	*women*

Note: Reduplicated portions are boldface for easy identification.
Source: Adapted from A Marantz. Re: Reduplication. *Linguistic Inquiry* 1982;13:435–482.

The morpheme retains its default form, [ɪn], before alveolars, as [n] also is alveolar. Often, nasals that assimilate to the following (or preceding) consonant are referred to as **homorganic**, in reference to the fact that they are articulatorily (i.e., organically) similar to the neighboring segment.

Generally, such assimilation patterns are optional or morpheme specific in English, as this language has no broad rules of assimilation as do some languages. The types of assimilation/harmony that may be obligatory in other languages' phonologies include consonant harmony or assimilation, vowel harmony, reduplication, and consonant-vowel assimilation. Each of these is described as it applies to adult and child phonologies.

CONSONANT HARMONY OR ASSIMILATION.   In some languages, certain consonants in certain types of words or syllables must share certain features. The most extreme restriction would prohibit words containing two (or more) different consonants; only one type of consonant per word would be allowed. This very strict limitation probably does not exist in adult phonologies. Most adult consonant harmony or assimilation is more limited, requiring that consonants adjacent to or near each other must share certain features (i.e., place or manner of articulation or voicing).

The examples of the English prefix *in-* and of the casual pronunciation of *sandwich* and *picture* fall within the category of adjacent consonants sharing place (and, in some cases, manner) of articulation, a process referred to as **place assimilation**. According to Cruttenden (1978), harmony (affecting nonadjacent consonants) is rare in adult phonologies. When harmony does occur, it affects consonants in similar syllable positions (e.g., a syllable-initial consonant harmonizes with another syllable-initial consonant).

A few cases of nonadjacent harmony do exist, such as the sibilant ([s] versus [ʃ]) harmony in a language called *Chumash*. In this language, all sibilants in the word must have the same degree of palatality. In other words, [s] and [ʃ] cannot both occur in the same word. If they would occur for some morphological reason, one of them will change to the other when the word is pronounced. Thus, /k + sunon + us/, which means *I obey him*, remains as such: [ksunonus]. However, /k + sunon + ʃ/, which means *I am obedient*, must change to [kʃunotʃ]. (The /n/ changes to [t] for other reasons.) Similarly, *I pay* is [saxtun], whereas *to be paid* is [ʃaxtunitʃ] (Poser, 1982).

In contrast to adult phonology, nonadjacent consonant harmony is quite common in child phonology.

VOWEL HARMONY.   In some languages, certain vowels in certain types of words or syllables must share certain features. In extreme cases, words cannot contain two different vowels; all vowels within the word must be identical. Far more commonly, vowels that occur in the same word must agree by having the same height (e.g., [i] and [ɑ] cannot occur in the same word), the same backness (e.g., [i] and [u] cannot occur in the same word), or the same roundness (e.g., [o] and [ɑ] cannot occur in the same word). Often, the vowel harmony applies only in certain morphological circumstances. Poser (1982) provided an example from Turkish in which the vowel in the past tense suffix *-dVm* (where *V* stands for a variety of vowels, as described), which is roughly equivalent to *-ed* in English, must agree with a previous vowel in the verb stem. The vowel is always high. However, if the previous vowel is front, the past-tense vowel will be front; if back, back; if round, round. Thus, when [e] is the stem vowel, the suffix is *-dim*, when [u] is the stem vowel, the suffix is *-dum*, and when [ü] is the stem vowel, the suffix is *-düm*, as shown in Table 2-3.

REDUPLICATION.   In a sense, reduplication is a combination of vowel and consonant harmony. Multisyllabic words are formed by repeating one syllable of the base word so that all consonants and vowels are the same. This pattern is found in baby-talk register in some languages, including English (*dada, mama, baba, boo-boo, no-no, nigh'-nigh'*, etc.).[5] Although English speakers may think of it as a frivolous type of phonological rule to be used only very casually, some languages use reduplication grammatically in their everyday words. In Warlpiri (a language spoken in Australia), for instance, the plurals of some nouns referring to human beings are made by **total reduplication**—that is, the entire word is repeated to indicate plurality (Marantz, 1982), even for multisyllabic words, as shown in Table 2-4.

In other languages, **partial reduplication** (e.g., repeating one syllable only) is used to express grammatical meanings. Speakers of Agta (who live near Mt. Pinatubo in the Philippines), for instance, use partial reduplication to express a plural or a more comprehensive meaning (Marantz, 1982), as shown in Table 2-5.

---

[5]Baby-talk rules are considered to be a special subset of the phonological rules of a language that one learns as one learns the language. Even preschool children demonstrate knowledge of this register by using it with younger siblings.

TABLE 2-5.
Agta Reduplication

Singular		Plural, Comprehensive	
bari	*body*	**bar**-bari-k kid-in	*my whole body*
mag-saddu	*leak* (verb)	mag-**sad**saddu	*leak in many places*
na-wakay	*lost*	na-**wak**wakay	*many things lost*

Note: Reduplicated portions are boldface.
Source: Adapted from A Marantz. Re: Reduplication. *Linguistic Inquiry* 1982;13:435–482.

TABLE 2-6.
Consonant-Vowel Assimilation

[ʃi]
[ʃe]
[su]
[so]
[sa]

Source: Adapted from LH Hyman. *Phonology: Theory and Analysis.* New York: Holt, Rinehart and Winston, 1975.

TABLE 2-7.
English Palatal Assimilation

nature	[netʃɚ] (not [netjɚ])
train	[tʃreɪn] (not [treɪn])
groceries	[groʃriz] (not [grosriz]; some dialects)
"**Did you** eat yet?"	[dʒɪʔjɛʔ] (not [dɪd ju ...])
"**Put your** shoes on."	[pʊtʃɚ ʃuz ɑn] (not [pʊt jɚ ...])

Note: Assimilated segments are boldface.

TABLE 2-8.
Feʔfeʔ-Bamileke Consonant-Vowel Assimilation

to whip	[vɑp]
to seek	[tʃɑk]
to eat	[fat]

Source: Adapted from LH Hyman. *Phonology: Theory and Analysis.* New York: Holt, Rinehart and Winston, 1975.

TABLE 2-9.
Child Consonant Harmony

doggie	[dʌdi]
diaper	[bɑpi]
thank you	[gɛgo], [dɛ:do:]
tractor	[gogi]

Note: The colon represents increased segment duration.
Source: Adapted from L Menn. *Pattern, Control, and Contrast in Beginning Speech: A Case Study in the Development of Word Form and Word Function.* Bloomington, IN: Indiana University Linguistics Club, 1978a.

TABLE 2-10.
Child Vowel Harmony

baby	[bibi], [bɑbɑ], [bæbæɪ]
hammer	[hæʰmæ]
tractor	[ʔsætæ]

Note: Superscript "h" indicates aspiration.
Source: Adapted from L Menn. *Pattern, Control, and Contrast in Beginning Speech: A Case Study in the Development of Word Form and Word Function.* Bloomington, IN: Indiana University Linguistics Club, 1978a.

CONSONANT-VOWEL ASSIMILATION.   When consonant-vowel assimilation occurs, a consonant's features change to make it more like an adjacent vowel or vice versa. Hyman (1975) provided a hypothetical example in which the palatal [ʃ] is found before the palatal (front) vowels [i] and [e], whereas alveolar [s] is found before the back vowels [u], [o], and [a]. Although [s] is more front than [ʃ], it is more distant from the actual place of production of [i], which is the palate. Palatal [ʃ] and [i] are ideally suited to each other with respect to place of articulation, and so they are the sounds that co-occur. When these ideal conditions are not met, [s] occurs. This is shown in Table 2-6.

Consonant-vowel assimilation results in the palatalization of many alveolars in English also, especially in casual speech. The palatal place of articulation of such consonants as [j, r, ʃ] and such vowels as [i, u] spreads to the preceding consonant, causing this consonant to become palatal as well. Examples are given in Table 2-7.

Hyman (1975) also provided another example from a language called *Feʔfeʔ-Bamileke* (a Bantu language spoken in Africa). In this language, the vowels [ɑ] and [a] (which are not contrastive in most dialects of American English) are affected by the consonant that follows. Briefly, [ɑ] is made with the tongue farther back, as is [k], so these occur together. The vowel [a] and the consonant [t] are produced with the tongue farther forward. The tongue is not involved in the articulation of [p] (even though it is, in a sense, a front consonant), and in this language, this

vowel patterns before [p] in the same manner as it does before [k], as illustrated in Table 2-8.

These examples are a good reminder that phonotactic patterns are based on human articulatory (and auditory) limitations and preferences and that such abstract phonological labels as *front consonant* and *front vowel* can be dangerous if their articulatory bases are forgotten. In this last case, expecting the two front consonants ([t, p]) to behave similarly could yield confusion. The appropriate generalization is rather that [a] occurs before tongue-tip ([coronal]) consonants and [ɑ] occurs before other consonants.

Child Phonology

REDUPLICATION, CONSONANT HARMONY, AND VOWEL HARMONY.   All of these types of assimilation and reduplication are found frequently in children's phonologies. They occur as original creations and, depending on the language, words that children learn from baby talk. Some examples of one child's reduplication, consonant harmony, and vowel harmony provided by Menn[6] (1978a) are shown in Tables 2-9 through 2-11.

Notice that, in this child's phonology, consonant harmony applied to all places of articulation. Describing his productions as segmental substitution patterns would require the claim that he both **fronts** (moves velar conso-

---

[6]Menn's transcriptions have been changed slightly to conform more closely to IPA.

TABLE 2-11.
Child Reduplication

down	[doʊdoʊ]
around	[wæwæ]
handle	[hɑhɑ]

Source: Adapted from L Menn. *Pattern, Control, and Contrast in Beginning Speech: A Case Study in the Development of Word Form and Word Function.* Bloomington, IN: Indiana University Linguistics Club, 1978a.

nants forward to both alveolar and labial placements) and **backs** (moves alveolar consonants back to a velar placement). This pattern would sound very confusing, when in fact the child was following a very simple rule: Do not ever change place of articulation within the same word. (Note, however, that it is not possible to predict, on the basis of these data alone, the consonant that will be selected when two different places of articulation occur in the word.)

Schwartz et al. (1980) reported that reduplication appears to have two motivations in children's phonologies. In these researchers' study, many of the reduplicating children failed to produce nonreduplicated multisyllabic forms, indicating that reduplication may have been a means for them to increase the number of syllables in the word without having to increase its segmental difficulty. A few also appeared to be using reduplication as a strategy for avoiding the use of final consonants.

Stoel-Gammon (1996) illustrated that word position has an impact on the frequency and development of harmony. For example, velars are associated more strongly with final position; therefore, velar harmony is more likely to occur if the triggering velar is in this word position. The author stated that velars in initial position are more likely to be fronted (i.e., changed to alveolar) than to cause harmony. Her findings emphasize again the importance of considering the entire word in analyzing harmony patterns.

CONSONANT-VOWEL ASSIMILATION. Davis and MacNeilage (1990) and MacNeilage and Davis (1990) demonstrated a strong consonant-vowel interdependency for one child in the earlier stages of phonological development. This child showed a strong tendency to produce high front vowels (both correctly and in error) in the context of coronal (alveopalatal) consonants, high back vowels with velar consonants, and middle and low vowels ([ʌ, ə, ɑ]) with labial consonants. These tendencies have a strong articulatory basis. Both high front vowels and coronal consonants involve raising the tongue tip to the alveopalatal region. High back vowels and velar consonants are formed by bunching the posterior body of the tongue upward toward the velum. Neutral and low vowels and labial consonants are dependent on mandibular positioning only.

Vihman (1992) tested this hypothesis using babbled syllables (and some very early words) from children exposed to American English, French, Swedish, and Japanese. None of the associations found by Davis and MacNeilage (1990) and MacNeilage and Davis (1990) were universal in these children; however, the majority showed a positive association between labials and central vowels. Approximately half showed a positive association between alveolars and front

TABLE 2-12.
Amahl's Consonant-Vowel Assimilation

pedal	[bɛgu]
lazy	[de:di:]
beetle	[bi:gu]
horses	[ɔ:tid]
bottle	[bɔgu]
sometimes	[fʌmtɑɪmd]

Note: The colon represents increased segment duration.
Source: Adapted from NV Smith. *The Acquisition of Phonology: A Case Study.* Cambridge, MA: Cambridge University Press, 1973.

vowels, and two-thirds of the children who used both velars and back vowels showed a positive association. For each comparison, some children showed a negative association (e.g., a tendency to use labials with other vowels). Vihman (1992, p. 405) emphasized "the strong role played by the individual child" at this transition point between babble and words and suggested that stronger associations might be found in earlier babble. Tyler and Langsdale (1996) also reported fewer such associations in older children. Similarly, Lleó (1996) used data from Spanish-speaking children to illustrate that some children demonstrate frequent consonant-vowel interactions in early words, whereas others exhibit interactions among consonants only or among vowels only (e.g., consonant or vowel harmony).

This connection between vowels and consonants in some children is in keeping with Stoel-Gammon's earlier (1983) report that coronal consonants tend to be produced (both correctly and in error) with high front vowels. For instance, one child, "Daniel," produced *bubble, bottle, ball,* and *balloon* with an initial [b], but *bye-bye* as [dɑɪdɑɪ] and *baby* as [didi]. *Pee-pee, Big Bird,* and *beep-beep* also were produced with an initial [d] (as were words that begin with [d] in the adult form). Thus, the child used [d] whenever the vowel was a high front one, even if the target consonant was [b]. Occasionally, this type of pattern has been documented also in children with disorders. This author observed it in a child who had DVD and pronounced *baby* as either [didi] or [bɑbɑ]. She could not produce either [bi] or [dɑ] in any context (SL Velleman, 1994). Williams and Dinnsen (1987) also documented such a case in a child with a phonological disorder.

Smith (1973) illustrated a case of consonant-vowel assimilation later in phonological development. The child, Amahl, demonstrated vowelization of final /l/, a pattern common among English-speaking children. Typically, adult final /l/ is produced as [u] in the child's speech. In Amahl's case, alveolars became velar (i.e., back) before the resulting [u]s. This process, again, could appear to be **backing**. However, without considering the effect of the vowels, one could not explain the reason for the occurrence of this backing only before [u]. In other word-medial contexts, alveolars remained alveolar, as shown in Table 2-12.

Clearly, these alveolar consonants were affected by the place of articulation of following vowels. They became velar before the back vowel [u].[7] Stoel-Gammon (1996)

---

[7]Further complications occur in Amahl's case but are not considered here.

TABLE 2-13.
"W"'s Fricative Migration

fall	[af]
fine	[aɪmf]
school	[kus]
soup	[ups]
zoo	[uz]
sheep	[ips]
shoe	[us]

Source: Adapted from LB Leonard, KK McGregor. Unusual phonological patterns and their underlying representations: A case study. *Journal of Child Language* 1991;18:261–272.

provided data from other children also, demonstrating that vowel place of articulation may have an impact on velar harmony.

Distribution Requirements

Languages of the World
As discussed earlier, some languages have restrictions on the types of sounds that can occur in certain syllable or word positions. English, for example, does not allow word-initial [ŋ] or word-final *-pf*. Typically, these constraints are local (i.e., they affect one word or syllable position, or they affect the co-occurrence of adjacent sounds). They are not restrictions on the phonetic repertoire of the entire language but on the place and the manner in which specific phones function within the language. Further examples of these local restrictions are provided in Chapter 3.

Child Phonology
Often, children from any language background have their own distribution requirements that may be far more restrictive than those of the adult phonology. Some of these distribution requirements may affect the phonetics of a word in a local way (e.g., a constraint against stops in word-final position, or a constraint against [s] in consonant clusters, phonetic distribution requirements that will be discussed further in Chapter 3). Other child distribution requirements may have a more global effect on entire word shapes. This type of constraint, often termed a **word recipe** (Menn, 1978a), is far more common in child phonology than it is in the languages of the world.

Word recipes are phonotactic templates—that is, specific syllable or word patterns—which can come to dominate a child's repertoire. Any child-specific phonotactic pattern can be designated a word recipe. A typical pattern is for children to avoid even attempting all but certain word shapes for a time (Schwartz & Leonard, 1982) and then to expand their vocabulary by changing the shapes of other words to fit their preferred shape (Waterson, 1971; Menn, 1978a).

The examples of reduplication and consonant and vowel harmony given earlier illustrate the reduplication and assimilation strategies that some children use to make adult words fit their preferred production patterns. Migration, in which one element of the word is produced in a

TABLE 2-14.
"Shelli"'s Velar Metathesis

buggy	[gɑbi]
piggie	[kibi]
monkey	[kɑmi]
dog	[gɔd]

Source: Adapted from RA Berman. Natural phonological processes at the one-word stage. *Lingua* 1977;43:1–21.

TABLE 2-15.
"Si"'s Labial-Alveolar Metathesis

Gloss	Adult Model	Child Form
apple	manzana	[mənnɑ]
shoe	zapato	[pwɑt̯t̯'o]
soup	sopa	[p'wæt'ɑ]

Source: Adapted from MA Macken. Permitted complexity in phonological development: One child's acquisition of Spanish consonants. *Papers and Reports on Child Language Development* 1978;11:1–27.

different word position than in the adult model, is frequently used also to implement word recipes. One child reported by Leonard and McGregor (1991) consistently put initial fricative sounds in final position, even when this resulted in final consonant clusters. Some sample words illustrating this tendency are given in Table 2-13.

Such global distribution requirements also may be the source of the most extreme form of metathesis. Recall that metathesis refers to cases in which more than one element appears to migrate. More specifically, two elements seem to trade places. In the more extreme cases, even nonadjacent consonants or vowels trade places with each other. This **long-distance metathesis** can be found even in young typical children.

Berman (1977) described a child, "Shelli," who initially avoided words that didn't have either consonant harmony or a velar in initial position. Later, she rearranged her words by using metathesis to fit her velar-first pattern. Note in Table 2-14 that Shelli did not simply move the velar to the front (migration); the velar consonant actually traded places with the other consonant in the word.

The velar consonant always came first, regardless of its position in the adult word. Thus, Shelli provided an example of a word recipe that was in evidence first in the child's avoidance of other word types, then in a consonant metathesis pattern.

Macken's (1978) monolingual Spanish girl "Si" (Table 2-15) is another case in point. She preferred a labial-alveolar pattern.

"V" (Vihman, 1976) was learning Estonian as her mother tongue, with some exposure to English. Her phonology at 15 months was restricted such that words could contain two different vowels only if the first was lower than the second. This constraint is not found in adult Estonian; it was V's personal preference. For months she avoided the Estonian words for *mommy*, *daddy*, and *meat* because they did not fit her phonotactic template. Finally, at 15

TABLE 2-16.
"V"'s Vowel Metathesis

Gloss	Adult Model	Child Form
father	isa	[ɑsi]
mother	ema	[ɑmi] or [ɑni]
meat	liha	[ɑti]

Note: V substituted [t] for /l/ in her production of *liha* for other reasons.
Source: Adapted from MM Vihman. From prespeech to speech: On early phonology. *Papers and Reports on Child Language Development* 1976;12:230–244.

months, she began to use vowel metathesis to change these word shapes to fit her word recipe so as to expand her productive vocabulary, as the examples in Table 2-16 illustrate.

Phonotactic preferences such as these have been found among children learning various languages around the world. Distribution requirements are discussed again in Chapter 3, as they relate in important ways to the phonetic repertoires of a language or a child's phonology and to word and syllable shapes.

Suprasegmentals

Languages of the World
Although they are used very differently in various languages, suprasegmentals are a universal aspect of phonology. There are three important components of English prosody: intonation, rate, and stress. Intonation is the "melody" of the language. Different pitch patterns express grammatical meaning (e.g., statement versus question) and psychological meaning (emotional, group membership, etc.). They identify breaks between clauses, sentences, paragraphs, or topics. Rate, or tempo, primarily expresses emotional meaning (anger, boredom, etc.) and situational meaning (hurrying versus relaxing). Stress patterns in English serve in the following capacities:

- To differentiate among words (e.g., cóntrast versus contrást)
- To differentiate phrases versus compounds (*líght hóuse-work* [easy cleaning] versus *líghthouse wórk* [helping ships to avoid danger])
- To mark new or contradictory information in a sentence (So *you* are the one who gave him my phone number; I live on *Apple* Blossom Lane, not *Cherry* Blossom Lane.)

In addition, each word has at least one syllable that receives the primary stress or nuclear accent. In the American English phonetic tradition, this stress typically is written with a left-pointing accent mark, or *acute* accent mark: [síləbəl]. Other syllables may be marked with secondary stress if the word is long enough. Secondary stress is indicated with a right-pointing accent mark, or *grave* accent mark: [ìnstɪtúʃən]. In English, unaccented syllables often are reduced, with vowels losing their quality and

being pronounced as [ə] (e.g., [əráʊnd] for *around*). Sometimes, consonants are reduced as well, usually emerging as [ʔ] (e.g., [koʔ] for *coat*). An entire syllable may be reduced to a single resonant consonant (e.g., [bʌʔn̩] for *button*). Unstressed syllables may even be lost completely in fast speech, especially at the beginnings of words (e.g., [trɑnto] for *Toronto*) or before another unstressed syllable (e.g., [dʒɛnrəl] for *general*; Hammond, 1997). These reductions, which English speakers may regard as sloppy shortcuts, often are very difficult for speakers of other languages to learn.

The stress patterns in multisyllabic words in English typically alternate between strong (S; stressed/accented) syllables and weak (W; unstressed/unaccented or even reduced) syllables. Words with too many consecutive weak syllables (e.g., *indefátigable*) are difficult even for many native English speakers to say. **Trochaic** words, in which the strong syllable occurs first, are preferred in English over **iambic** words, in which the weak syllable precedes. In contrast, all French words are pronounced iambically, with the stress on the final syllable. Compare, for example, the English and French words for *photograph*:

English: [fóragræf][8]

French: [fotográf]

Additionally, English is a stress-timed language—the time from one strong syllable to the next is kept constant, regardless of the number of syllables between. Thus, speakers hurry through the sequences of two weak syllables that occur in some words. In a word such as *quà-si-pèr-i-o-dí-ci-ty*, the time between the first and second stresses, which are separated by only one weak syllable, is the same as the time between the second and third stresses, which are separated by two weak syllables.

French, on the other hand, is syllable-timed, such that each syllable gets equal time, regardless of its position in the word. To have reduced vowels in a syllable-timed language would be quite unusual; there is no reason to rush through any vowel, regardless of whether or not it is stressed.

These differences in stress patterns contribute, far more than most people consciously realize, to foreign accents in any language. The individual sound segments may be pronounced correctly but with alien-sounding rhythms that immediately mark one as a foreigner.

Well over half of the languages of the world use pitch more segmentally than does English. These languages are called **tone languages**. In such languages, the meaning of a word may depend on the pitch level or the pitch contour with which it is produced. The most famous example of this is the set of four Chinese words (Table 2-17) all pronounced segmentally as [ma], each with its own distinctive pitch pattern (tone). Entire sentences can be devised using these four words, such as *Mama ma ma*, or "Mother scolds [the] horse" (Crystal, 1987).

---

[8]Note that alveolars in English are **flapped** (become [ɾ]) when they occur between a stressed and an unstressed vowel.

TABLE 2-17.
Chinese Tone Minimal Pairs: [ma]

Tone	Meaning
high level	mother
high rising	hemp
low falling rising	horse
high falling	scold

Source: Adapted from D Crystal. *The Cambridge Encyclopedia of Language.* New York: Cambridge University Press, 1987.

In other languages, tone is used to signal grammatical contrasts—for example, present versus past tense in Bini, a West African language (Crystal, 1987).

Child Phonology

Studies of the acquisition of suprasegmentals have been limited, and some contradictory results have not yet been resolved. It appears that some aspects of prosody are acquired at a very young age. For example, Demuth (1995) reported acquisition of rule-based (predictable) tone by age 2 years, 1 month in the African language Sesotho. However, some children may decide that they are learning a tone language when they are not: They may produce each word with a certain pitch pattern associated specifically with that word, regardless of the context. This may occur both in children who are otherwise developing normally (Jaeger, 1997) and in children with communication disorders.

Studies also have demonstrated very early development of one durational effect: the lengthening of phrase-final syllables in comparison to nonfinal syllables. This tendency has been found to emerge as early as age 8 months in some studies of some languages and as late as 30 months in others (de Boysson-Bardies et al., 1981; Konopczynski, 1991; Levitt, 1991; Robb & Saxman, 1990; Snow & Stoel-Gammon, 1994). The reason for the wide range of reported ages is not yet clear. In one study of English-speaking babies in which two suprasegmental effects found in final syllables were studied separately, falling pitch contours were found to be acquired by age 18 months, whereas phrase-final lengthening did not appear until age 24 months or so (Snow & Stoel-Gammon, 1994).

The impact of stress patterns on syllable omission in early phonology also has been investigated. Most agree that children tend to omit initial, but not final, unstressed syllables in such primarily trochaic languages as English and Dutch (Allen & Hawkins, 1980; Demuth, 1996; Echols & Newport, 1992; Fikkert, 1994; Gerken, 1991, 1994a,b; Gerken & McIntosh, 1993; Kehoe, 1995, 1996, 1997; Kehoe & Stoel-Gammon, 1997a,b; Schwartz & Goffman, 1995). This practice is believed to be due primarily to a preference for trochaic—strong + weak (i.e., SW)—word forms. (See Hochberg, 1988, and Pater & Paradis, 1995, for opposing viewpoints.) However, cases of children who appear to have an iambic bias (i.e., who prefer stress to fall on the final syllable of the word, in a WS pattern) do exist (Archibald, 1995; Kehoe, 1997; Vihman et al., 1997). In any case, just as are adults (Hammond, 1997), most English-speaking children are more likely to show syllable omissions in words with a weak + strong (WS)

TABLE 2-18.
Children's Stress-Related Syllable Omissions 1

Pattern	Strong + Weak	Weak + Strong
Target word	tíger	giráffe
Child production	taɪgɚ	ræf

Source: Adapted from LA Gerkin. A metrical template account of children's weak syllable omissions from multisyllabic words. *Journal of Child Language* 1994a;21:565–584.

TABLE 2-19.
Children's Stress-Related Syllable Omissions 2

Pattern	Strong + Weak + Strong	Weak + Strong + Weak
Target word	dínosàur	banána
Child production	daɪsɑr	næenʌ

Source: Adapted from M Kehoe and C Stoel-Gammon. The acquisition of prosodic structure: An investigation of current accounts of children's prosodic development. *Language* 1997a;73:113–144.

syllable pattern than in words with the opposite pattern, as in Table 2-18.

Similarly, as Table 2-19 shows, the first syllable is more likely to be omitted in a WSW trisyllabic word than in an SWS trisyllabic word. If a syllable is omitted from an SWS word, it will be the weak syllable. For example, *dinosaur* will be pronounced as [dáɪsɑr] (Kehoe & Stoel-Gammon, 1997a).

Gerken (1991) demonstrated that this preference may have an impact at the sentence level as well: Weak words (e.g., articles, pronouns) may be more likely to be omitted when they are *followed* by a strong syllable within a phrase. They are retained when they are *preceded* by a strong syllable. Kehoe (1995, 1997), Kehoe and Stoel-Gammon (1997a,b), and Schwartz and Goffman (1995) have further illustrated the impact of segments on these stress patterns and the impact of these stress patterns on segmental accuracy. Kehoe and Stoel-Gammon (1997a,b) indicated that intervocalic syllables with sonorant onsets (e.g., *illustrátion*) are more likely to be omitted than are syllables with obstruent onsets (e.g., *còmputátion*).

A few studies of the production of suprasegmentals among children with speech-language disorders have identified deficits in the use of these features among language-impaired children (Hargrove & Sheran, 1989), children with NFPs (Shriberg et al., 1992), and children with DVD (Shriberg et al., 1992, 1997a,b,c), in addition to children with autism (Baltaxe, 1984) and hearing impairments (Rosenhouse, 1986).

Few assessment tools are available for speech-language pathologists who wish to explore these parameters clinically. However, Shriberg et al. (1992) reported the development of a tool, the Prosody-Voice Screening Profile, which will facilitate the screening of prosody and voice characteristics in a wide range of disorder groups from any language background. Recent findings with this tool, reported by Shriberg et al. (1997a,b,c), indicated that stress errors may differentiate one subgroup of children with DVD from children who are developing normally

TABLE 2-20.
English Phrase-Level Interactions

Phrase	Careful Production	Casual Production
next stop	[nek**st** stɑp]	[nɛkstɑp]
Did you eat yet?	[d**ɪd** ju it jɛt]	[dʒiʔjɛʔ]
What did you do?	[wʌt **dɪd** ju du]	[wʌdʒədu]

Note: Boldface indicates omitted portions of utterances.

TABLE 2-21.
French Liaison 1

French Phrase	Production	Gloss
les cars	[leɪ kɑr]	the busses
les arts	[leɪ**z** ɑr]	the arts

Note: Boldface indicates the liaison element.

TABLE 2-22.
French Liaison 2

French Phrase	Production	Gloss
les zéros	[leɪ **z**eʀo]	the zeroes
les héros	[leɪ ɛʀo]	the heroes
les herbes	[leɪ**z** ɛʀb]	the grasses
les ères	[leɪ**z** ɛʀ]	the eras

Note: Boldface indicates the liaison element.

TABLE 2-23.
"Ellen"'s Phrase-Level Reduplication

no	no
bottle	bɑbɑ
not bottle	bɑ bɑbɑ (with head shake "no")
out	ɑu
not out	ɑu ɑu (with head shake "no")
No Stephen	dɪ:: di (with head shake "no")
more	mɔ
more cheese	bi ti
dog	gʌg
dog booboo	bu bubu

Note: Boldface indicates harmonized words; the colon represents increased segment duration.

and from children with speech delay not attributed to dyspraxia.

Phrase-Level Interactions

Languages of the World

Many of the patterns described above also apply in phrases or sentences. The use of pitch and stress in phrases and sentences has just been described. Other phrase-level effects may occur, primarily in fast or casual speech. For example, in English, clusters created by adjoining two words often are simplified. As indicated earlier and shown in Table 2-20, sometimes entire words are collapsed to make production of the phrase easier.

Certain rules predict whether such reductions can occur. In some cases, reduction helps to distinguish one word or phrase from another:

night rate	[nɑɪt reɪt]	[nɑɪʔreɪʔ]
nitrate	[nɑɪtreɪt]	can't reduce

The French language entails a process called liaison, which allows segments that are otherwise inaudible to become audible in certain contexts. The beginning of the following word determines whether the end of the preceding word will be pronounced. For instance, the final *s* in *les* (plural of *the*) is silent except before vowels, as shown in Table 2-21.

In a sense, this final [z] is acting as the initial consonant for a word that does not have one. Interesting questions arise from the fact that some words spelled with an initial *h* are treated as vowel-initial, whereas others are treated as consonant-initial, although, as illustrated in Table 2-22, the [h] is never pronounced itself. The phrase *the heroes* appears to permit two vowels in a row, though the phrases *the grasses* and *the eras* do not.

Child Phonology

Just as adults learning a second language often despair that "the words all run together in this language," chil-

dren may have some initial perceptual difficulties in parsing their native languages due to phrase-level interactions. DePaolis (personal communication) reported that his 5-year-old son, Caleb, was confused as to the allegiance of the [st] in a final consonant cluster in the middle of a commonly reduced phrase: "Mommie, why do you call it the [nɛkstoɚ] neighbor?" he asked. "It's not a store."

With respect to production, investigators have shown that at least some children's phonologies are organized even beyond the word level, at the level of phrases. Donahue (1986) cited examples from a child whose consonant harmony processes applied across words. Some words that the child could produce correctly in single-word utterances underwent velar harmony in phrases, such as [gɑɪkeki] for *bye Katie*. Similar phrase-level harmony patterns may be found in disordered phonology, as in the case of a child (known to this author) who said, [mɑɪ mæʔ] for *my hat* but [dædi dæʔ] for *daddy's hat*.

Phrase-level reduplication also may occur, as in the case of "Ellen" (the subject of Chapter 6), a 27-month-old diagnosed with mild DVD whose production accuracy decreased when she combined words into phrases, as illustrated in Table 2-23.

Matthei (1989) reported on another child's phrase-level restrictions. This little girl's first two-word utterances never were longer than two syllables. When she combined two-syllable words with other words, as in *baby's book*, one syllable of the longer word was dropped: [bei bu].

Stemberger (1988) collected data on a child who exhibited liaison, moving word-final consonants to the initial consonant position of adjoining words if they began with vowels. Boldface and arrows in Table 2-24 indicate con-

TABLE 2-24.
Child Liaison

Phrase	Production
...get **up** and go...	[dɑ → tʌ → piːn doʊ]
My ar**m** is cold.	[maɪ ɑʊ → miː tʰoʊ]
Don't find **us**.	[dʌt fɑi → nʌː]

Note: Boldface indicates liaison elements; the colon represents increased segment duration.
Source: Adapted from JP Stemberger. Between-word processes in child phonology. *Journal of Child Language* 1988;15:39–61.

sonants that have moved from final position to initial position of the next word.

Cases such as these are used to support the hypothesis previously discussed: Initial consonants typically are preferred and sometimes are obligatory in young children's phonologies in English and other languages.

Perception-Based Patterns

Ease of perception and of production can influence phonotactic patterns. If the syllable and word shapes of a language are too similar, comprehension will suffer. The main difference between the two types of patterns is that perception-based patterns tend to render production slightly more difficult, whereas the reverse is true of production-based constraints. Assimilation renders segments more similar and thus easier to produce as a sequence, yet harder to discriminate.

Dissimilation renders segments more distinct from one another and thereby more difficult to produce but easier to discriminate. Although omission of one element of a cluster renders the cluster easier to produce, epenthesis of an extra element can render the cluster easier to perceive.

Languages of the World
Epenthesis is a common pattern in the languages of the world. For example, in American English, speakers tend to epenthesize stops in some nasal + fricative medial clusters. For instance, the medial cluster in *hamster* typically is pronounced as though it includes a [p] like the medial cluster in *campfire*, even though the former word actually does not contain a /p/. The epenthesized [p] emphasizes the labial nasal, rendering it easier to perceive.

Epenthesis of this sort illustrates the tension between ease of production and ease of perception. Ease of production is responsible for the opposite tendency, which is to omit nasals in medial clusters. In this process, a nasal trace is left on the preceding vowel, evident in many people's casual pronunciations of *sandwich* as [sæwɪtʃ]. When ease of production factors are paramount, omission occurs; when ease of perception factors are paramount, epenthesis occurs.

Sometimes such strategies can be idiosyncratic to one word or to one person or family. In this author's family, for example, epenthesis of [d] is used to distance—and thus emphasize—the two [n]s in the phrase "Put your nightgown on," yielding [pʊtʃɚ naɪʔgaʊnd an], although *night-gown* is pronounced with no final [d] before words beginning with consonants. (At least one other New England family exhibits the same pattern.)

Some cases of epenthesis can facilitate both perception and production. In English, for example, some morphemes have the potential for creating sequences that would be difficult to produce and to perceive. Consider the following examples:

bus + plural = *busses*, not *buss*; [bʌsəz], not [bʌss]

Max + possessive = *Max's*, pronounced [mæksəz], not [mækss]

kiss + third-person singular = *kisses*, not *kisss*; [kɪsəz], not [kɪss]

pat + past = *patted*, pronounced [pærəd], not [pætt]

In each of these cases, a vowel ([ə] or, in some dialects, [ɪ]) is epenthesized to spare the speaker's having to produce the same consonant twice in a row (ease of production) and to render the grammatical ending as clear as possible to the listener (ease of perception).

Dissimilation is another way of maintaining a perceptual distinction within a word. In such a case, neighboring segments become less similar so as to highlight each one. An example from the Japanese native Yamato vocabulary was provided by Mester and Itô (1989), Kenstowicz (1994), and Dinnsen (1997). In this language, two voiced obstruents (stops or fricatives) do not occur within the same morpheme. Thus, *futa* (lid), *fuda* (sign), and *buta* (pig) are words, but *buda* cannot be. Usually, the first consonant in the second half of a compound word becomes voiced. However, this voicing does not occur if it will result in two consecutive voiced obstruents. Thus, when *iro* (color) and *kami* (paper) are combined, the result is *irogami*. However, when *kami* (divine) and *kaze* (wind) are combined, the second [k] does not become voiced. The word is pronounced [kamikaze]. The [k] and [z] in the second half of the compound remain dissimilar.

Child Phonology
Being egocentric creatures with little listener awareness, children tend to exhibit production-based constraints almost exclusively. Some possible examples of ease of perception strategies can be found, however. For instance, Macken and Barton (1979) demonstrated that some English-speaking children have difficulty in learning to produce the voicing contrast (e.g., [p] versus [b]) even though they are aware of it. Their subjects appeared to go through a stage in which they were attempting unsuccessfully to make voiced sounds sound different from voiceless sounds. In these cases, an acoustic difference occurred between the children's voiced and voiceless consonant productions, but it was imperceptible to adult speakers of English. Some children in this stage may be attempting to render the voiced-voiceless contrast more marked for the benefit of listeners. For example, Fey and Gandour (1982) described a child (nicknamed "Lasan," which is *nasal* spelled backward) who epenthesized a nasal after final voiced stops to differentiate them more clearly from final voiceless stops. For ease of production, the nasal

TABLE 2-25.
"Lasan"'s Final Voicing Contrast

drop	[dɑpʰ]
light bulb	[jɑjtʰbɑbm]
eat	[itʰ]
Fred	[wɛdn]
what	[wɑtʰ]
bad	[bædn]
talk	[dɔkʰ]
bag	[bægŋ]

Note: Superscript "h" indicates aspiration.
Source: Adapted from M Fey, J Gandour. Rule discovery in phonology acquisition. *Journal of Child Language* 1982;9:74–75.

TABLE 2-26.
"Molly"'s Vocalic Offsets

around	[wɑnə]
Brian	[pɑnə]
down	[tænə]
clock	[kɑkkɪ]
teeth	[tɪtʰi̥]
peek	[pekxe]
squeak	[kʰʊkʰʌ]
tick	[tɪtʰə]

Note: Transcription simplified somewhat for the reader's ease of perception. The open circle indicates a voiceless vowel, and the superscript "h" indicates aspiration.
Source: Adapted from MM Vihman, SL Velleman. Phonological reorganization: A case study. *Language and Speech* 1989;32:149–170.

TABLE 2-27.
"J"'s Segmental/Phonotactic Trade-Off

Age	Production of Silla
2 yrs, 1 mo	[ʃːɑ]
2 yrs, 2 mos	[kɪjɑ], [tɪːjɑ]
2 yrs, 3 mos	[ʃɪːjɑ]

Note: The colon represents increased segment duration.
Source: Adapted from D Ingram. The role of the syllable in phonological development. In Bell A, Hooper J (eds). *Syllables and Segments.* Amsterdam: North-Holland Publishing, 1978, 143–155.

he used was homorganic (produced at the same place of articulation as the preceding stop). Note, in Table 2-25, the contrasts between the pairs of target final consonants (/p/ versus /b/, /t/ versus /d/, /k/ versus /g/).

Menn (1983) described a child who had a similar strategy. He used an epenthetic nasal *before* the final (target) voiced stop to mark the final voicing contrast. For instance, he produced *Bob* as [bɑmp].

In Vihman and Velleman's 1989 study, "Molly" added a vocalic offset to final obstruents and nasals, possibly (in part) also to highlight these final consonants for the benefit of listeners, as shown in Table 2-26.

Summary

Several types of phonotactic patterns may be found in the languages of the world and also in child phonology. They include constraints on the number of syllables, harmony, assimilation, reduplication, and distribution requirements. These patterns can apply at the syllable, word, or phrase level, and they can be motivated by ease of production or ease of perception.

PHONOTACTIC ISSUES SPECIFIC TO CHILD PHONOLOGY

Already, we have seen many of the similarities between adult phonologies and child phonologies with respect to phonotactic effects. In this section, some of the differences are discussed in more detail.

Evidence for Processing at the Syllable Level and Above

Some of Ingram's arguments (1978) in favor of analyzing early child phonology syllabically as opposed to segmentally apply primarily to child phonology. First, the development of many segments differs according to their placement within the syllable. For example, certain classes of sounds (e.g., velars, fricatives, and voiceless consonants) typically are acquired first in final position in English. Others (e.g., voiced stops) appear first initially. Such feature-specific distribution effects certainly are present in adult phonologies,

but they are static as opposed to developmental. Furthermore, in adult phonology, initial position always is primary. No features occur only in final position in any language (John McCarthy, personal communication).

Segmental complexity interacts with syllabic/word complexity during acquisition. As segmental complexity increases, syllabic/word complexity may decrease, and vice versa. Ingram (1978) cited an example from Macken (1976) to illustrate this point. The child in question (referred to simply as "J") temporarily sacrificed the segmental accuracy of the initial sibilant fricative [s] in *silla* (Spanish for *chair*) to increase the number of syllables to two. Table 2-27 illustrates that he was capable of producing a sibilant (albeit [ʃ] rather than [s], probably due to consonant-vowel interactions) at the beginning of the word, but not when he was also producing both syllables.

This finding demonstrates a trade-off within J's system between segmental complexity (producing a more articulatorily difficult phoneme, such as [s]), and word-shape complexity (producing two syllables). The latter was sacrificed temporarily to the former, then vice versa, before J finally was able to control both types of complexity at once. Similar examples of trade-offs between segmental and syllabic complexity are given previously in "Phrase-Level Interactions."

Word Recipes

As described previously, word recipes clearly demonstrate that young children's phonologies are word-based. These recipes determine the order of the elements within a word, often ignoring the pattern of the adult form of the word.

TABLE 2-28.
"Si"'s Word Recipe

Gloss	Adult Model	Child Form
shoe	za**pato**	[pwat̚t'o]
elephant	ele**fante**	[batte]
dress	ve**stido**	['bɪttɪ]
(name)	Fer**nando**	[manno, wanno, nanno]
ball	pe**lota**	['p'atda]
apple	man**zana**	[mənna]

Note: Boldface indicates preserved elements.
Source: Adapted from MA Macken. Permitted complexity in phonological development: One child's acquisition of Spanish consonants. *Papers and Reports on Child Language Development* 1978;11:1–27.

TABLE 2-29.
"Molly"'s Apparent Regression

Age	Production	Gloss
1 yr, 0 mos, 26 days	[baɪŋ]	bang
	[bʌʔ]	button
1 yr, 1 mo, 8 days	[bæni]	bang
1 yr, 1 mo, 15 days	[pɑnnə]	button
	[pɑnə]	Brian

Note: Transcriptions simplified somewhat.
Source: Adapted from MM Vihman, SL Velleman. Phonological reorganization: A case study. *Language and Speech* 1989;32:149–170.

Sometimes a segment or feature-based word recipe may interact with a prosodic word recipe, as in the case of Macken's Si (1978). As illustrated earlier, Si preferred a labial-alveolar word pattern. She tended also to omit one syllable per trisyllabic word. Macken commented that Si appeared to retain either the initial or the medial syllable, whichever contained the required labial consonant. However, Si appeared also to retain the vowel of the stressed syllable, which in Spanish typically is penultimate. If the actual outputs are considered, it appears that this child achieved both a trochaic (strong syllable + weak syllable) word form and a labial + alveolar feature pattern by careful selection of consonants and vowels from the initial two syllables of each word. Sometimes, the child's production simply resembled a copy of the last two syllables of the adult form of the word. At other times, however, the child's production was a combination of elements from the first and last syllables, as illustrated in Table 2-28. Thus, Si was able to achieve word recipes at two levels of her phonology at once: phonotactics and phonetics.

Apparent Regression

The establishment of these word-recipe patterns in children's phonology may make them appear to be regressing. Parents sometimes protest that their child used to say the words almost correctly but no longer does. As illustrated previously, Macken's J (1976) initially produced *silla* with a fricative but ceased doing so once he produced it as a two-syllable word. However, these patterns reflect the onset of phonological systematization. They demonstrate that the child is no longer memorizing words as wholes but is trying to discover the patterns and rules of the adult phonology. Therefore, word recipes are harbingers of phonological development, not of regression.

Vihman and Velleman (1989) provided another example of such apparent regression. As we have seen, Molly developed a preference for a final vowel on target nasal-final (and voiceless obstruent-final) words, possibly to highlight these final consonants perceptually. Before this word recipe emerged, each nasal-final word had its own idiosyncratic ending—some with vowels, some with final nasals, and some with nasalization of the vowel only (no final nasal consonant produced).

The occurrence of some words with accurate productions of final nasals indicates that articulatory limitations were not the basis for Molly's new pattern. She was perfectly capable of producing final nasals. However, final nasals did not fit within her emerging phonological system at that time, so she ceased to take advantage of her full articulatory capabilities. Her mother noted in her diary of Molly's vocabulary development that words that previously had been easy to distinguish were all pronounced in the same way once Molly began producing all nasal-final words with a final vowel. Specifically, the mother reported that *button, balloon, banana,* and *bunny,* each of which had had its own unique phonetic shape previously, now were produced as [bʌn:ə] or [bɑn:ə]. Phonetic and acoustic analysis revealed also that *bang* and *button* became more similar to each other and to other words (such as *Brian*) and less like the adult model, once the word recipe illustrated in Table 2-29 had taken hold.

Thus, the onset of a phonological system, with its own phonotactic (and other) rules, may appear to cause regressions from the child's prior phonologically random—but sometimes quite phonetically accurate—productions. Parents who notice such changes should be reassured that systematization usually is a major first step on the road to adult phonology. It should be hailed as progress, not regression.

"Illegal" Phonotactic Patterns

Word recipes are nonadultlike restrictive phonotactic patterns. Most often, however, the patterns on which children choose to focus as their favorites are allowable phonotactic sequences in the adult language. The most common violations of phonotactic restrictions noted in child phonology involve distribution requirements. Despite an English restriction on *pw-* clusters, for instance, many children produce such clusters in their attempts to reproduce adult *pl-* and *pr-* clusters ("Let's [pweɪ pwínsɛs]"). Similarly, the English language restricts nonlow lax vowels ([ɪ, ɛ, ʊ]) in word-final position. Yet, many children who omit final consonants violate this restriction by pronouncing such words as *bed* and *good* as CVs [bɛ], [gʊ]. (For further discussion of this restriction, see Chapter 3.)

Additionally, as indicated previously, some children may use nonadultlike prosody for a certain period. For example, a child learning an intonation language may nonetheless associate a certain pitch pattern with each word, as though learning a tone language.

Summary

Some phonotactic factors specific to child phonology include development of segments by word position, interactions between segmental and syllabic complexity, the use of word recipes, apparent regressions, and the use of illegal phonotactic patterns.

ASSESSMENT

Phonotactic Factors to Be Considered in Assessment

The aspects of phonotactic patterns that must be considered in assessing a child's phonology include the following:

1. Syllable and word shapes produced by the child, including constraints on the allowable number of syllables per word, open versus closed syllables, and clusters in various word positions
2. Word-level patterns, such as harmony, assimilation, and reduplication patterns and, less commonly, dissimilation and epenthesis
3. Distribution requirements
4. Word recipes, including apparent regressions
5. Phrase-level effects: occurrences of any of the foregoing elements in phrases
6. Prosodic factors, such as deletion of unstressed syllables

All of these patterns are of primary importance in assessing children's phonology, especially if the child is young or his or her phonology is markedly delayed. It is vital to consider the patterns together as well as separately. Children who have only cluster constraints are much freer phonotactically than are those who also are restricted to one syllable per word. Children without cluster constraints but whose distribution requirements do not allow initial fricatives will not acquire #s- clusters (such as *sp-, sn-, sl-*) until they overcome this distribution requirement. (For further information, see Chapter 3; Chin & Dinnsen, 1992; McLeod et al., 1997.)

The reader may well feel overwhelmed by the length of this list; nightmare visions of extremely detailed, time-consuming phonological analyses may be appearing. However, all of these patterns can be reduced to a single question: Does the child have an appropriate number of phonotactic options, given his or her current communication needs?

If the phonotactic patterns observed are too restricted and are resulting in many homonyms or are forcing a child to supplement words with gestures, facial expressions, and sound effects, the client's phonology is non-functional. The clinician's job, in that case, is to expand these phonotactic possibilities so that more differentiation between words will be possible. If speech-language pathologists understand phonotactic patterns and the manner in which they can work to restrict or expand children's phonological possibilities, they have the information needed to facilitate phonological development in such cases. In the next section, specific procedures for assessing children's phonotactic systems are presented.

Assessment Tools

Two levels of analysis for phonotactic assessment exist: basic word and syllable shapes and syllable- and word-level effects. Often, the former level is not addressed at all by clinicians or by popular assessment tools. Many assessment tools available include syllable- and word-level effects within their analyses of phonological patterns, but often without differentiating these phonotactic patterns (e.g., reduplication, syllable deletion, assimilation) from segment-level patterns (e.g., backing, stopping). Nonetheless, it is important that the clinician differentiate. True alveolar backing (i.e., backing of all alveolars to velar), for example, should be treated differently from velar assimilation (i.e., backing of alveolars to velar only when there is a velar elsewhere in the word). The former is a phonetic or phonemic pattern, whereas the latter is phonotactic.

If quantitative data (standard scores, percentiles, etc.) or age norms are not needed, many phonotactic factors can be assessed fairly simply using a speech sample obtained variously from spontaneous speech, from the administration of a standard articulation or process test, or (preferably), from both. Then, worksheets can be used to determine *qualitatively* the phonotactic patterns used by the child. Any immature or deviant patterns identified can be *quantified* more thoroughly later to set baselines in therapy.

Word and Syllable Shapes

Informal assessment of the syllable and word shapes produced by children from any language background, including constraints on the number of allowable syllables per word, open versus closed syllables, and clusters in various word positions, is simplified by using a list of potential syllable and word shapes and cluster types, such as that provided in Form 2-1: Phonotactic Repertoire: Word and Syllable Shapes. This form, or a similar list that can be self-generated, can be used in three possible ways:

- Quantitatively, indicating percent occurrences for each type
- With approximate frequencies indicated, using such terms as *predominant, frequent, occasional, rare,* and *absent*
- By simply checking off each type that does occur

The very simplest option for using this form is merely to check off any pattern that is observed. An only slightly more time-consuming—but far more reliable—check-off rule would be to check off all forms or types that occur at least three times (or, if the speech sample is small, twice) in a

Phonotactic Repertoire: Word and Syllable Shapes

Name: Age:
Date: Examiner:
Source of sample: Size of sample:

Note: C = consonant
       V = vowel
       # = word boundary
       Predominant: 61–100%
       Frequent: 41–60%
       Occasional: 16–40%
       Rare: 1–15%

	% or ✓	Frequency estimate: Circle appropriate word.				

Syllable types[a]

Incomplete

C alone	_____	Predominant	Frequent	Occasional	Rare	Absent
V, Vʔ, ʔV	_____	Predominant	Frequent	Occasional	Rare	Absent
Open						
CV, CVʔ	_____	Predominant	Frequent	Occasional	Rare	Absent
Closed						
VC, ʔVC	_____	Predominant	Frequent	Occasional	Rare	Absent
CVC[b]	_____	Predominant	Frequent	Occasional	Rare	Absent

Clusters[c]

Initial

#CC-	_____	Predominant	Frequent	Occasional	Rare	Absent
#CCC-	_____	Predominant	Frequent	Occasional	Rare	Absent
Final						
-CC#	_____	Predominant	Frequent	Occasional	Rare	Absent
-CCC#	_____	Predominant	Frequent	Occasional	Rare	Absent
Medial						
-CC-	_____	Predominant	Frequent	Occasional	Rare	Absent
-CCC-	_____	Predominant	Frequent	Occasional	Rare	Absent

Word shapes[c]

# of syllables

1	_____	Predominant	Frequent	Occasional	Rare	Absent
2	_____	Predominant	Frequent	Occasional	Rare	Absent
3	_____	Predominant	Frequent	Occasional	Rare	Absent
4+	_____	Predominant	Frequent	Occasional	Rare	Absent

[a]Out of all syllables.
[b]Includes CCVC, CVCC, etc.
[c]Out of all words.

Maximum # of syllables produced in any word: _____

Notes:

FORM 2-1.
Phonotactic repertoire: word and syllable shapes.

child's sample. This reduces the listener error to some extent. Transcribers do tend to "fill in the blanks" sometimes, mentally assuming that missing elements actually were there in the process of interpreting disordered speech. However, if the speech-language pathologist transcribes the same element or pattern three times within one speech sample, chances are fairly good that it actually did occur.

If the speech-language pathologist prefers to indicate the approximate frequencies of occurrence of each type of syllable or word shape, the adjectives listed can be circled for this purpose. This method is more precise than the check-off approach yet is less time-consuming than counting and calculating frequencies. Although this option does *not* require counting and calculating, the clinician undoubtedly will estimate mentally the approximate frequencies to select among the adjective choices. For this purpose, the approximate frequencies that correspond to each adjective choice are the following[9]:

- Predominant: 61–100%
- Frequent: 41–60%
- Occasional: 16–40%
- Rare: 1–15%
- Absent: 0%

This approach reduces the clinician's burden from counting every instance of a pattern and figuring its exact percentage of occurrence to rating the approximate frequencies on a five-point scale. However, some people initially feel insecure about making such estimates. Using the exact counting method a few times typically increases their confidence.

The most reliable—and also the most time-consuming—approach to this worksheet is to count each instance of each pattern and to divide the total by the total number of potential occurrences of that pattern. It is important that percentages be based on the total number of instances of that type of element. For example, the percentage of CV syllables produced by a child should be computed by dividing the number of CV syllables produced by the total number of syllables (not words) produced. Similarly, the number of words with consonant cluster (CC) onsets is divided by the total number of word onsets (i.e., the total number of words) to identify the percentage of occurrence of initial consonant clusters.

Note that for these analyses, the (presumed) target forms of the words are not considered. Only a child's actual productions are analyzed. In other words, this is an independent phonotactic analysis and can therefore be used regardless of the target language. As a result, for example, *total number of syllables* refers to the total number of syllables produced by a child, regardless of the total number that would have been produced by an adult saying the same words. The clinician may wish to do a relational analysis—comparing a child's actual productions to his or her targets—at some later point. However, for the purpose of determining whether a child's phonotactic system is functional, analyzing what is actually being produced is far more useful.

---

[9]The individual clinician is, of course, free to use different frequencies if these appear inappropriate. However, consistency (always using the same frequencies within your own clinical practice) is vital.

TABLE 2-30.
Data from Molly at Age 13 Months

bɑ	box
pɑpʰ, pɑpʌp, pəp	burp
pɑnə	button
tʌŋ, dæn, dɑŋ::, ʔedɑɪn, dɑʊnə, dænə, tjæŋ	down
gʊgʊk, gʊgɣ, gɔgʌ, gɔgɔ, gʊgʌ, kʊgʊgʌ, kʊkʌ	good girl
hæʔ, hæʰ	hat
ætʰ, hæt, hætʰ, hæt̬, hæ	hot
hɑnʌ, hʌni, ænɪ, ænə	round
æp, ɔp̥	up

:: = lengthening (e.g., [ŋ::] is a long drawn-out velar nasal); [̥] = voicelessness (e.g., [ə̥] is a voiceless schwa); [ɣ] = a uvular trill such as babies make when they coo. Note: Transcriptions simplified somewhat.
Source: Adapted from MM Vihman, SL Velleman. Phonological reorganization: A case study. *Language and Speech* 1989;32:149–170.

The relevant formulas can be written as follows:

$$\frac{\text{\# of CV syllables}}{\text{total \# of syllables produced}} \times 100 = \% \text{ CV syllables}$$

$$\frac{\text{\# of initial CC}}{\text{total \# of words produced}} \times 100 = \% \text{ \#CC}$$

$$\frac{\text{\# of monosyllabic words}}{\text{total \# of words produced}} \times 100 = \% \text{ one-syllable words}$$

To take a very simple example, if a child produced 100 syllables and 50 of them were of the form CV, that child's percentage occurrence of CV syllables would be 50%. One question that arises often is that of counting or not counting multiple identical productions of the same word. This decision is left to the individual speech-language pathologist. Definite advantages arise in counting every occurrence (**token**) of each word, in that this strategy increases the amount of data that can be analyzed. Furthermore, it is important to note whether a child often produces multiple identical productions of the same word. However, if one word is produced several times in a very unusual manner (i.e., in a way that is not otherwise typical of a particular child), including every production will bias the analysis in an inappropriate direction. In any case, it is important to be consistent. If each production is counted for one analysis, the same approach normally should be used for all analyses of that child's sample.

Consider some sample word and syllable shape data and how the data would be entered on the form at each level. The data in Table 2-30, from Molly at age 13 months (Vihman & Velleman, 1989), can be used for this purpose. Example 2-1 illustrates the use of Form 2-1 to identify Molly's syllable types, clusters, and word shapes.

This analysis yields the following:

- *Syllable types*: Molly produced mostly open syllables (e.g., the syllables in such words as [bɑ], [pɑnə], [gɔgʌ], [hætə]), but CVCs (e.g., [tʌŋ], the second syllable of [gʊgʊk], and [hætʰ]) also occurred occasionally. VCs (e.g., [ætʰ]) are relatively rare.

Phonotactic Repertoire: Word and Syllable Shapes

Name: *Molly*
Date: *2/18/93*
Source of sample: *Spontaneous speech*

Age: *13 months*
Examiner: *SLV*
Size of sample: *32 word tokens*

Note: C = consonant
V = vowel
\# = word boundary
Predominant: 61–100%
Frequent: 41–60%
Occasional: 16–40%
Rare: 1–15%

	% or ✓	Frequency estimate: Circle appropriate word				

Syllable types[a]

	% or ✓					
Incomplete						
C alone	0%	~~Predominant~~	~~Frequent~~	~~Occasional~~	~~Rare~~	Absent
V, VʔʔV	6%	~~Predominant~~	~~Frequent~~	~~Occasional~~	Rare	~~Absent~~
Open						
CV, CVʔ	71%	Predominant	~~Frequent~~	~~Occasional~~	~~Rare~~	~~Absent~~
Closed						
VC, ʔVC	6%	~~Predominant~~	~~Frequent~~	~~Occasional~~	Rare	~~Absent~~
CVC[b]	23%	~~Predominant~~	~~Frequent~~	Occasional	~~Rare~~	~~Absent~~

Clusters[c]

	% or ✓					
Initial						
#CC-	3%	~~Predominant~~	~~Frequent~~	~~Occasional~~	Rare	~~Absent~~
#CCC-	0%	~~Predominant~~	~~Frequent~~	~~Occasional~~	~~Rare~~	Absent
Final						
-CC#	0%	~~Predominant~~	~~Frequent~~	~~Occasional~~	~~Rare~~	Absent
-CCC#	0%	~~Predominant~~	~~Frequent~~	~~Occasional~~	~~Rare~~	Absent
Medial						
-CC-	0%	~~Predominant~~	~~Frequent~~	~~Occasional~~	~~Rare~~	Absent
-CCC-	0%	~~Predominant~~	~~Frequent~~	~~Occasional~~	~~Rare~~	Absent

Word shapes[c]

	% or ✓					
# of syllables						
1	44%	~~Predominant~~	Frequent	~~Occasional~~	~~Rare~~	~~Absent~~
2	53%	~~Predominant~~	Frequent	~~Occasional~~	~~Rare~~	~~Absent~~
3	3%	~~Predominant~~	~~Frequent~~	~~Occasional~~	Rare	~~Absent~~
4+	0%	~~Predominant~~	~~Frequent~~	~~Occasional~~	~~Rare~~	Absent

[a]Out of all syllables.
[b]Includes CCVC, CVCC, etc.
[c]Out of all words.

Maximum # of syllables produced in any word: __*3*__

Notes: *Only #CC was tj- (palatalized [t]). Not consistent in # of syllables in attempts at same word (e.g., good girl = 2 or 3 syllables; down = 1 or 2 syllables). Also not consistent in closing syllables (e.g., hot = [hæ] and [hæt]).*

EXAMPLE 2-1.
Phonotactic repertoire: word and syllable shapes.

- *Clusters*: The only cluster that we can identify is the initial *tj-* in one production of *down* ([tjæŋ]).
- *Word shapes*: Molly produced both one- and two-syllable words quite frequently, with only one three-syllable production occurring in a single token of *good girl* ([kʊgʊgʌ]).

Making all three levels of analysis available on a single form allows the clinician to become comfortable with the form and the concepts it represents without becoming bogged down in counting and calculating percentages. As time permits, more specific data can be gathered *on the same form* as baselines for children who are to be seen in therapy. With practice, scoring the approximate frequency ratings will become almost as easy and quick as simply checking off those patterns that occur. Eventually, the clinician will find that the form has become a mental checklist, and these choices can be made on-line while conversing with a child.

Relational analysis, or comparing a child's phonotactic repertoire to that of the adult language, is not difficult to perform mentally after a worksheet such as Form 2-1 has been completed. English has multisyllabic words and consonant clusters in initial, medial, and final positions and in both open and closed syllables. Any English-learning child who lacks these exhibits nonadult phonology. However, a clinician may wish to make specific comparisons to establish how children match their productions to the adult's (presumed target) word shapes. For instance, some children may produce a closed syllable (of any type) only when the adult syllable ends with a voiceless stop. This is an indication that such children are aware of and able to produce syllable closure, at least in some instances. It identifies an area of phonological knowledge and skill that can be used as a base in therapy. These issues of relational analysis and correspondences between child and adult forms will be dealt with in more detail in Chapter 5.

Syllable- or Word-Level Patterns

Syllable- or word-level patterns, such as harmony, assimilation, and reduplication, can be screened also by using a similar simple worksheet. Again, because this is an independent analysis, the child's language environment is irrelevant to this form.

It is important to note that reduplication cannot occur unless children produce words of more than one syllable. The same is true of vowel harmony. To identify reduplication, it is necessary to know only whether children's multisyllabic words contain the same syllable two or more times, as compared to a variety of distinct syllables. The frequency of multisyllabic words with distinct syllables is compared with the frequency of such words with reduplicated syllables. To identify harmony in multisyllabic words, it is necessary to know whether the children's multisyllabic words contain the same consonant or vowel two or more times consecutively, as compared to a variety of distinct consonants and vowels. For harmony, words in which both (or more) consonants or both (or more) vowels are identical (or nearly identical) are counted. More specifically, the frequencies of words with distinct versus harmonized vowels and the frequency of words with distinct versus harmonized consonants are determined. Note that no word is counted as both reduplicated and har-

monized. If both consonants and vowels are harmonized, the word is counted as reduplicated only.

Form 2-2, Phonotactic Repertoire: Reduplicaton and Harmony, facilitates these analyses. Again, the simplest way to use this form is merely to check off those types of reduplication or harmony that do occur (three times or more) in a child's speech. Alternatively, the therapist can indicate an approximate frequency of occurrence of each type (*predominant, frequent, occasional, rare,* or *absent*). For more precision, the occurrence of reduplication (or harmony) can be quantified exactly by counting the total number of multisyllabic words and dividing this into the number of reduplicated (or harmonized) words:

$$\frac{\text{\# of reduplicated words}}{\text{total \# of multisyllabic words}} \times 100 = \% \text{ reduplication}$$

$$\frac{\text{\# of harmonized C words}}{\text{total \# of words with 2 or more Cs}} \times 100 = \% \text{ C harmony}$$

$$\frac{\text{\# of harmonized V words}}{\text{total \# of words with 2 or more Vs}} \times 100 = \% \text{ V harmony}$$

Note that only multisyllabic words are used to calculate the frequency of reduplication. Similarly, only words with two or more consonants are used to calculate the frequency of consonant harmony (e.g., *uppy* [ʌpi] would not count, as it contains only one consonant despite being bisyllabic). For parallel reasons, only words with two or more vowels are used to calculate the frequency of vowel harmony.

Unlike reduplication and vowel harmony, consonant harmony can occur in monosyllables (e.g., [gɔg] for *dog*, [bup] for *soup*) as well as multisyllabic words (e.g., [gɔgi] for *doggie*, [bʌpeɪp] for *cupcake*). To identify harmony in monosyllabic words, it is necessary to know only whether two different consonants occur within the same word. Again, words in which both consonants are identical are counted. For this calculation, the denominator is the total number of **CVC** words. A space for indicating the frequency of harmonized consonants in monosyllabic words is included toward the bottom of the form.

Using Form 2-2, we can determine the prevalence of reduplication and harmony in Molly's speech at 13 months, as shown in Example 2-2. Note that at least two syllables must be identical for the word to be considered reduplicated. If any pair of vowels in a multisyllabic word is harmonized in the child's production (regardless of whether they are the same in the adult word), the word is categorized as an example of vowel harmony. Vowels that differ only in tenseness (e.g., [i] versus [ɪ], [u] versus [ʊ]) may be considered identical for these purposes, especially for children whose phonologies are quite immature or deviant. Consonants may be considered identical if they differ in voicing only, as most young children and children with a severe NFP do not have control of voicing. Furthermore, transcription of voicing contrasts is notoriously unreliable. Therefore, the first two syllables of [kʊgʊgʌ] are considered to contain essentially identical consonants, and the production is classified as reduplicated.

Phonotactic Repertoire: Reduplication and Harmony

Name: Age:
Date: Examiner:
Source of sample: Size of sample:

Note: C = consonant
       V = vowel
       Reduplication = same syllable repeated in word (*baba*, *deedee*, *gogo*, etc.)
       Harmony = same C repeated (*goggie*, *tootie*, etc.) or same V repeated (*daba*, *boogoo*, etc.)
       Predominant: 61–100%
       Frequent: 41–60%
       Occasional: 16–40%
       Rare: 1–15%

	% or ✓	Frequency estimate: Circle appropriate word.				

Words of two syllables or more[a]

Reduplicated syllables	_____	Predominant	Frequent	Occasional	Rare	Absent
Harmonized vowels	_____	Predominant	Frequent	Occasional	Rare	Absent
Harmonized consonants	_____	Predominant	Frequent	Occasional	Rare	Absent

Monosyllabic CVC words[b]

Harmonized consonants	_____	Predominant	Frequent	Occasional	Rare	Absent

[a]Out of all **multisyllabic** words.
[b]Out of all **monosyllabic** CVC words.

Notes:

FORM 2-2.
Phonotactic repertoire: reduplication and harmony.

Phonotactic Repertoire: Reduplication and Harmony

Name: *Molly*   Age: *13 months*
Date: *2/18/93*   Examiner: *SLV*
Source of sample: *Spontaneous speech*   Size of sample: *32 word tokens*

Note: C = consonant
        V = vowel
        Reduplication = same syllable repeated in word (*baba, deedee, gogo*, etc.)
        Harmony = same C repeated (*goggie, tootie*, etc.) or same V repeated (*daba, boogoo*, etc.)
        Predominant: 61–100%
        Frequent: 41–60%
        Occasional: 16–40%
        Rare: 1–15%

	% or ✓	Frequency estimate: Circle appropriate word.

Words of two syllables or more[a]: *total of 18; 15 CVCV*

Reduplicated syllables	*16% (3/18)*	~~Predominant~~	~~Frequent~~	☐ Occasional	~~Rare~~	~~Absent~~
Harmonized vowels	*0% (0/18)*	~~Predominant~~	~~Frequent~~	~~Occasional~~	~~Rare~~	☐ Absent
Harmonized consonants	*33% (5/15)*	~~Predominant~~	~~Frequent~~	☐ Occasional	~~Rare~~	~~Absent~~

Monosyllabic CVC words[b]: *total of 8*

Harmonized consonants	*25% (2/8)*	~~Predominant~~	~~Frequent~~	☐ Occasional	~~Rare~~	~~Absent~~

---

[a]Out of all **multisyllabic** words.
[b]Out of all **monosyllabic** CVC words.

Notes:

EXAMPLE 2-2.
Phonotactic repertoire: reduplication and harmony.

The analysis of Molly's words at 13 months via Example 2-2 yields the following results:

- *Words of two syllables or more*: Most of Molly's words contained syllables that differed in some way; only 16% were reduplicated. The vowels almost always differed. The consonants were identical (harmonized) 33% of the time.
- *Monosyllables*: When two consonants were produced within the same one-syllable word, they were different 75% of the time (harmonized 25% of the time).

Thus, we can conclude that Molly had better control of vowel contrasts within a word than of consonant contrasts and that her ability to produce consonant contrasts was slightly better within monosyllabic words. Because Molly produced predominantly open syllables, in two-syllable words the consonants typically were both in syllable-initial position (e.g., [hætə]). When the word is a monosyllable, the two consonants in the word must be in syllable-initial and syllable-final position, respectively (e.g., [hætʰ]). (As there is only one syllable, both consonants cannot occupy syllable-initial position.) Therefore, Molly appeared to be better at distinguishing consonants in different syllable positions than in similar syllable positions. This common finding mirrors the harmony patterns in adult languages.

Consonant-Vowel Dependencies

Assimilation and *dissimilation*, which refer to the process whereby adjacent elements become more or less alike, respectively, typically include effects of vowels on consonants or vice versa in young or moderately to severely phonologically delayed children from any language background. These effects are assessed by looking for consonant-vowel dependencies (i.e., by determining whether certain consonants are restricted to co-occurrence with certain vowels or vice versa). Form 2-3 addresses this issue. This form can be used qualitatively simply by indicating with an X or ✔ those combinations that do occur, or quantitatively by tallying the frequency with which each combination occurs. Given that syllable-initial consonants are more likely to be affected by following vowels than are syllable-final consonants by preceding vowels, and that many children with moderate to severe disorders produce primarily open syllables, syllable-final consonants typically are not considered. However, vowel-consonant sequences could be tabulated as well by using another copy of the same form, if the clinician believed that it were relevant to a child's speech. Note also that strictly adjacent consonants and vowels are most likely to affect each other. Therefore, in the case of a cluster, it is the consonant that is beside the vowel being considered that should be examined. For example, the word *play* pronounced as [pleɪ] would be counted in the [l] + [e] box, not in the [p] + [e] or in the [l] + [ɪ] box.

On this form, percentages refer to the percentage of each type of consonant that co-occurs with each vowel type. Thus, for example, the number of syllables that fall within the labial stop + high front vowel square is divided by the total number of syllables that begin with a labial stop. In other words, percentages are calculated for each

row. If this form is used to assess Molly's word productions (see Table 2-30), the results are as shown in Example 2-3.

- Almost all consonants co-occur with the neutral mid-central vowels [ə] and [ʌ] (a common finding).
- Only coronal (alveopalatal) consonants (which require relatively front positioning of the tongue) and glottals (which do not involve the tongue) co-occur with front vowels. This arrangement makes sense; vowels and consonants that require anterior positioning of the tongue occur together so that Molly does not have to move her tongue very much as she transitions from consonant to vowel. Glottals do not require tongue positioning at all, so they do not interfere with the production of front vowels.
- Labial and velar consonants co-occur with back vowels: labials with low back vowels and velars with high back vowels. Physiologically, these patterns also make sense. The transition from a labial consonant into a low back vowel requires only the opening of the jaw. Both velars and mid to high back vowels require the back of the tongue to be raised toward the velum so that, again, minimal tongue movement is required.

Thus, Molly appears to have some consonant-vowel preferences. It is important to note, however, that these restrictions are not absolute in her case. Molly does produce some [dɑ] syllables, demonstrating that she is able and willing to combine tongue and mandible movement for certain productions. Coronal consonants appear to be most flexible in their co-occurrence patterns. Furthermore, it must be kept in mind that the language to which a child is exposed may be responsible for some biases in consonant-vowel co-occurrences. Given the physiological bases for some of Molly's preferences, it would be no surprise to find languages with some of the same tendencies. Also, one could not, of course, expect to find every possible combination of consonant and vowel in a small sample such as this. Therefore, general patterns rather than co-occurrences of specific consonants with specific vowels are of interest here.

Filling out these forms would have been even faster and simpler if the frequencies had been estimated rather than calculated for percentages. Of course, this procedure is far less precise than is using percentages, and both are far less precise than are the types of in-depth analyses suggested by Ingram (1981) and Grunwell (1985). However, the worksheets allow the speech-language pathologist quickly to identify possible areas of concern that can be explored in greater depth if needed to establish baselines for treatment. For Molly, if she were older and therefore phonologically delayed rather than simply young, possible intervention targets would include infrequent closed syllables, rare consonant clusters, frequent consonant harmony, and consonant-vowel dependencies.

Epenthesis must be addressed later. We cannot judge whether something extra has been added to a word without comparing the actual production to the target word, which will be the goal in the relational analyses discussed in Chapter 5. For the moment, the child's presumed **tar-**

Phonotactic Repertoire: Consonant-Vowel Dependencies

Name: Age:
Date: Examiner:
Source of sample: Size of sample:

Indicate (✓ or %) combinations that do occur:

C type	V type						
	High front (i, ɪ)	Mid front (e, ɛ)	Low front (æ)	Mid central (ə, ʌ)	High back (u, ʊ)	Mid back (o, ɔ)	Low back (ɑ)
Stops							
Labial (b, p)							
Alveolar (d, t)							
Velar (k, g)							
Nasals							
Labial (m)							
Alveolar (n)							
Glides							
Labial (w)							
Palatal (j)							
Liquids							
Alveolar (l)							
Palatal (r)							
Fricatives							
Labial (f, v)							
Interdental (θ, ð)							
Alveolar (s, z)							
Palatal (ʃ, ʒ)							
Affricates (tʃ, dʒ)							
Glottals (h, ʔ)							
Other							

Notes:

FORM 2-3.
Phonotactic repertoire: consonant-vowel dependencies.

Phonotactic Repertoire: Consonant-Vowel Dependencies

Name: *Molly*   Age: *13 months*
Date: *2/18/93*   Examiner: *SLV*
Source of Sample: *Spontaneous speech*   Size of sample: *32 word tokens*

Indicate (✓ or %) combinations that do occur:

C type	V type High front (i, ɪ)	Mid front (e, ɛ)	Low front (æ)	Mid central (ə, ʌ)	High back (u, ʊ)	Mid back (o, ɔ)	Low back (ɑ)
Stops							
Labial (b, p)				50%			50%
Alveolar (d, t)			29%	29%			42%
Velar (k, g)				28%	50%	22%	
Nasals							
Labial (m)							
Alveolar (n)	50%			50%			
Glides							
Labial (w)							
Palatal (j)			100% (1 example)				
Liquids							
Alveolar (l)							
Palatal (r)							
Fricatives							
Labial (f, v)							
Interdental (θ, ð)							
Alveolar (s, z)							
Palatal (ʃ, ʒ)							
Affricates (tʃ, dʒ)							
Glottals (h, ʔ)		ʔ 100% (1 example)	75%	12.5%			12.5%
Other							

Notes: *Mid central vowels co-occur with everything. Only alveolars, palatals (both anterior tongue positions) and glottals (no tongue involved) co-occur with front vowels. Mid to high back vowels (tongue back and high) co-occur only with velars. Some alveolar + [ɑ] syllables break the pattern.*

EXAMPLE 2-3.
Phonotactic repertoire: consonant-vowel dependencies.

get words are not being considered phonologically on our do-it-yourself forms, so epenthesis cannot be identified.

Stress Patterns
The area of production of multisyllabic words is important to explore for older or less phonologically delayed English-speaking children. The main question to be addressed is whether the child produces a variety of stress patterns or is limited, due to phonological deficits, to producing only a few. For example, a child might be segmentally accurate but be unable to produce words with nontrochaic (i.e., other than strong-weak) stress patterns. Form 2-4 is available for use in documenting children's stress patterns. On this form, examples of multisyllabic words produced by the children and exemplifying various stress patterns should be listed. The example words given on the form are intended only to help the speech-language pathologist to categorize the words the children have produced. The client should not necessarily be required to repeat those particular words.[10] For example, the production by English-speaking school-age children of words that fit only within the SW and SWSW categories would be cause for concern. If some examples of WS, WSW, and similar patterns were found in addition to earlier-developing trochaic patterns (e.g., SW and SWSW), the children most likely would not have a deficit in stress pattern production. It is important to remember that the English language demonstrates a preference for trochaic (SW) words, so the proportion of iambic (WS) forms should not be expected to approach even 50%.

A second stress form (Form 2-5) facilitates relational analysis of stress patterns. For each stress pattern, the clinician should list words that the children attempt with that pattern, indicating whether the word is produced correctly, with weak syllable(s) omitted, with strong syllable(s) omitted, or with other outputs (e.g., coalescence of two syllables into one). Once again, the examples in parentheses are intended to facilitate the speech-language pathologist's recognition of varied stress patterns only. The children should not necessarily be required to attempt these particular words.

PLANNING FOR INTERVENTION

General Guidelines

The main goal in phonotactic intervention is to expand children's phonotactic capabilities. The clinician should not strive for segmental accuracy per se. For example, if a child who produces only open syllables can be taught to close those syllables, the actual consonants that he or she uses to do so are of secondary importance. To determine a starting point, consider the list of a child's current

---

[10]Lists of words with various stress patterns are provided in Appendix B as models for determining the target stress patterns of words that the child happens to produce. These lists could be used also for probing various stress patterns in a relational analysis using Form 2-5.

phonotactic patterns that have been generated through using Forms 2-1 through 2-5. Presumably, the available patterns are insufficient for effective communication. Various considerations dictate the choice of patterns to target first, but the primary question to ask is: What is preventing this child from producing phonotactically varied words? What syllable or word-level restrictions are most limiting for this child?

Additional questions include the following:

1. Are any other patterns beginning to emerge in this child's speech? If, for instance, the child typically is restricted to CV word shapes but occasionally says "mama" rather than simply "ma," the speech-language pathologist may be able to capitalize on this alternate word shape by introducing other two-syllable reduplicated CVCV words (*dada, yo-yo, boo-boo, bye-bye, pee-pee, no-no*, etc.).

2. What new pattern would buy the child the most in terms of communicative effectiveness? If, for example, the child is restricted to CV word shapes and therefore has many CV homonyms (e.g., [mɑ] for *mom, mad, mine, moo, milk, money*; [bɑ] for *bottle, bye-bye, bike, bath, back, ball*), either adding final consonants or adding second syllables (as described previously) would be helpful in differentiating the child's words. Usually, homonyms are an important clue to determining communicative effectiveness, as will be discussed at greater length in Chapter 4. (Increasing such children's differentiation of vowels would be very helpful also, but that is a topic for the next chapter.)

3. What patterns occur first developmentally? All else being equal, two-syllable words or final consonants usually would be targeted before, for instance, consonant clusters.

4. Regarding motivation, which words does the child seem to need? What does the child want to express that he or she cannot? If, for example, the child needs to be able to express emotions, perhaps such CVCs as *mad, sad*, and *bad* could be targeted. If a child has many siblings who pick on him or her verbally, a CVCV insult reply such as *Dummy!* could be helpful (Judith Johnston, personal communication).

The Phonotactics of Developmental Verbal Dyspraxia

DVD appears to differ from other phonological delays and disorders in that it is more specifically a phonotactic disorder. Although children with DVD certainly do have trouble producing various segments in isolation and in words, their major difficulty lies in putting these segments together into a smooth, coherent syllable—that is, their problem lies not as much in hitting the targets as in getting from one target to the next. As such, the problem calls for special attention to be paid to their phonotactic constraints and possibilities. However, it is important to note that the options available for children with DVD are the same as for other children with simple phonologies.

Stress Patterns: Independent Analysis

Name: Age:
Date: Examiner:
Source of sample: Size of sample:

For each stress pattern, list words that the child produces with that pattern, whether or not they are correct. Examples in parentheses are intended to facilitate the speech-language pathologist's recognition of varied stress patterns only. The child should not necessarily be required to attempt these words.

Note: S = strong syllable
        W = weak syllable

Target stress pattern	Examples from child
SW (e.g., mónkey)	
WS (e.g., giráffe)	
ŚWS̀ (e.g., télephòne)	
SWW/ŚS̀W (e.g., hámburger)	
WSW (e.g., spaghétti)	
WWS/S̀WŚ (e.g., kàngaróo)	
ŚWS̀W (e.g., cáterpìllar)	
WŚWS̀/S̀ŚWW (e.g., rhìnóceros)	
WWSW/S̀WŚW (e.g., dìsappóinted)	
Other 4-syllable words (SWWS, WSWS, WSSW)	
5+ syllables	

FORM 2-4.
Stress patterns: independent analysis.

Stress Patterns: Relational Analysis

Name: Age:
Date: Examiner:
Source of sample: Size of sample:

For each stress pattern, list words that the child attempts with that pattern, indicating whether the word is produced correctly, with weak syllable(s) omitted, with strong syllables omitted, or with other outputs (e.g., coalescence of two syllables into one). Examples in parentheses are intended to facilitate the speech-language pathologist's recognition of varied stress patterns only. The child should not necessarily be required to attempt these particular words.

Note: S = strong syllable
        W = weak syllable

Target stress pattern	Correct	W omitted	S omitted	Other
SW (e.g., mónkey)				
WS (e.g., giráffe)				
ŚWS̀ (e.g., télephòne)				
SWW/ŚS̀W (e.g., hámburger)				
WSW (e.g., spaghétti)				
WWS/S̀WŚ (e.g., kàngaróo)				
ŚWS̀W (e.g., cáterpìllar)				
WŚWS̀/S̀ŚWW (e.g., rhìnóceros)				
WWSW/S̀WŚW (e.g., dìsappóinted)				
Other 4-syllable words (SWWS, WSWS, WSSW)				
5+ syllables				

FORM 2-5.
Stress patterns: relational analysis.

In a study of two children with DVD, SL Velleman (1994) identified phonotactic simplifications that are not unknown in other children but that were more extreme in these subjects. When first evaluated, one child ("Marina," age 3 years, 11 months) reduced the complexity of the syllables she produced by relying on certain CV combinations. She did not combine alveolars with back rounded vowels nor labials with high front vowels. Alveolars preferentially combined with vowels produced in the same region, such as [i]. Labials preferentially combined with vowels that did not require tongue-tip articulation, such as [ɑ]. Thus, she could not be stimulated to produce such syllables as [du], [do], or [bi], [mi]. Sometimes, her word for *baby* was produced as [didi] and, at other times, as [bɑbɑ]. Marina, then, was able to combine consonants and vowels into simple CV syllables only when a minimum of movement was required from consonant to vowel.

"Holly," age 2 years, 4 months, provided an interesting contrast. She relied to an unusual extent on nonsyllabic isolated consonants and isolated vowels. Some examples of her words are given in Table 2-31. A disturbing number of Holly's words consisted of either consonants alone or vowels alone; she appeared to have difficulty in building complete syllables. The few CV syllables that she produced were undifferentiated and were overused for a wide variety of words. For example, [bɛ, bijə, bɪʊ] were used interchangeably for *bunny, bear, bird, baby, bell, pig,* and *Bert* (i.e., all nouns beginning with bilabial stops). Similarly, [dɪ, deɪ, di, dɛ, dɑ, dʌ] were used interchangeably as deictics.

These types of patterns are not unknown in other children, but they may be more pervasive or persistent in children with DVD. Shriberg et al. (1997a,b,c) demonstrated that approximately 50% of children with suspected developmental apraxia of speech—but not a matched group of children with speech delay—exhibited a pattern of inappropriate word stress. In an ongoing study, Velleman and Shriberg (in preparation) have demonstrated that a subgroup of English-speaking children with suspected developmental apraxia demonstrated the same types of difficulty with noncanonical stress patterns (e.g., such iambic patterns as WSW) as do very young normal children and also young children with generic phonological delays and disorders. As indicated earlier in this chapter, children in all three groups tended to omit weak syllables in nonfavored positions, such as the first weak syllable in a WSW word. However, even two 14-year-olds in this subgroup of children with dyspraxia did not seem to have reached a point at which they were able to produce these stress patterns, as other children do. It appeared as though as they got older or more phonologically mature, they did cease to omit such syllables, as did the other groups. However, instead of producing stress correctly, some of the children with DVD resolved their stress difficulties by overstressing these same weak syllables. The result was a monostress speaking pattern, which yielded the robotlike speech typical of many older children with dyspraxia.

For these reasons, a focus on phonotactic factors, especially stress, is even more critical among children who are suspected of having DVD.

TABLE 2-31.
"Holly"'s Limited Syllable Shapes

[m:]	food, eat
[tʰ, tˢ]	tree, kitty, coffee, and other nonlabial nouns
[ʃ]	sleep
[n]	in
[φ]	elephant (voiceless bilabial fricative)
[ɑʊ]	out
[o]	open
[ɑ:]	all gone

Note: Superscript "h" indicates aspiration; the colon indicates increased segment duration; [tˢ] is an alveolar affricate.
Source: Adapted from SL Velleman. The interation of phonetics and phonology in developmental verbal dyspraxia: Two case studies. *Clinics in Communication Disorders* 1994;4:67–68.

RECENT PHONOTACTIC CONCEPTS FROM LINGUISTIC THEORY

Nonlinear phonology was an attempt to address the growing body of evidence of the primacy of the syllable and the word in the adult phonologies of the languages of the world. Given the pervasiveness of syllable- and word-level effects in child phonology, such as those that have just been described, this model is particularly appropriate for describing phonological development. Although the rule systems used by nonlinear phonologists have now been replaced by a newer system known as optimality theory (see Chapter 5), the elements and structures of nonlinear phonology remain popular and relevant.

Myriad subtle theoretical differences exist in various approaches to nonlinear phonology, but all divide words into syllables. Syllables are subdivided further into an onset (the initial consonant) and a rhyme (the remainder of the syllable, including a vowel or diphthong and often a final consonant). Using this hierarchical approach, phonologists can make predictions about the way in which different portions of syllables will act and interact with one another. These predictions actually hold true for all or most languages of the world.

For the speech-language pathologist, differentiating syllable positions in this way makes it easier to describe the syllable-level patterns listed by Ingram (1978) for child phonology. Specifically, syllable-initial consonants (**onsets**) might behave differently from syllable-final consonants (**codas**). Certain types of phonemes may be acquired sooner in some positions (e.g., coda) than in others (e.g., onset). Including a syllable level in the theoretical phonological hierarchy makes it easier to refer to some phonological processes, such as cluster reduction and final consonant omission, which function primarily to simplify syllables. Similarly, the inclusion of a phonological word level facilitates the description of other processes, such as unstressed syllable deletion and reduplication, which operate only on entire words. The fact that all these levels are connected hierarchically to one another and to the segments (either directly or indirectly) via other levels makes it easier to illustrate the interactions between segmental complexity (the difficulty

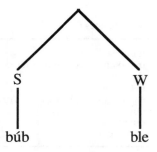

FIGURE 2-1.
Trochaic (strong [S] and weak [W] syllable) foot: *bubble*.

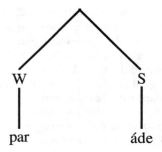

FIGURE 2-2.
Iambic (weak [W] and strong [S]) foot: *parade*.

and variety of sounds within the word) and syllabic complexity (the shape of the syllable). This outcome is important, as segment-syllable interactions may trigger such processes as assimilation.

Nonlinear phonology can be subdivided into subdisciplines in a variety of ways; many of these subdisciplines overlap with one another. The aspects of the theory that are most relevant to phonotactics are metrical and autosegmental phonology.

Metrical Phonology

Metrical phonology deals with the stress patterns of sentences, phrases, words, and syllables. The critical element for stress patterns is a unit composed (almost always) of two syllables—typically, one strong and one weak—called the **foot**. Recall that strong syllables are stressed and weak syllables are not. Furthermore, syllables that include more segments (i.e., CVC and CVV syllables) are usually strong.

The English stress pattern is an alternation between strong and weak syllables, usually with the strong syllable going first in a trochaic pattern. In some words, a foot may consist of one strong and two weak syllables, exemplified in the word *syllable*: SWW. A foot must contain exactly one strong syllable and may contain no, one, or two weak syllables:

$$\begin{bmatrix} S & W \\ \textbf{su} & per \end{bmatrix} \quad \begin{bmatrix} S & W \\ \textbf{ca} & li \end{bmatrix} \quad \begin{bmatrix} S & W \\ \textbf{fra} & gi \end{bmatrix} \quad \begin{bmatrix} S & W \\ \textbf{lis} & tic \end{bmatrix}$$

$$\begin{bmatrix} S & W \\ \textbf{ex} & pi \end{bmatrix} \quad \begin{bmatrix} S & W \\ \textbf{a} & li \end{bmatrix} \quad \begin{bmatrix} S & W \\ \textbf{do} & cious \end{bmatrix}$$

Within words or phrases, feet also can be identified as strong or weak, as can words. Thus, instead of marking a vowel as +stress or −stress, as was done previously, trees are drawn to illustrate the strong versus weak (more versus less stressed) portions of the unit being analyzed. Trees are used because the cumulative pattern of strong and weak stresses at each level, from the syllable up, determines the ultimate stress pattern of the entire utterance. For instance, a stressed syllable within a stressed word would be

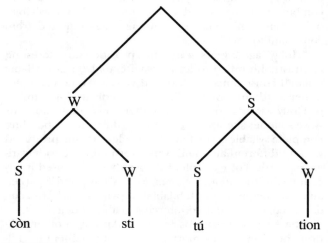

FIGURE 2-3.
Metrical tree for *constitution*: Both syllables and feet are labeled as strong or weak.

stronger than a stressed syllable within an unstressed word. Thus, the tree structure helps us to predict the point at which the stress will fall.

Those who remember the trees from a syntax class may find that they look familiar in some respects. As in syntax, the trees actually are upside down, with the trunk at the top and the branches hanging down. (Perhaps they should be called *root systems* instead of trees!) In the word *bubble*, for example, the first syllable is strong, and the second is weak, so the tree would be drawn as in Figure 2-1.

As discussed earlier, a foot with this type of stress pattern is labeled by using a term from poetry, **trochee**. Feet with the other main type of stress pattern are called **iambs**. In an iamb, the first syllable is weak and the second is strong, as in *parade* (Figure 2-2).[11]

Feet are combined at one of multiple levels within the tree into phrases or multisyllabic words, such as *constitution* (Figure 2-3). Note that the syllable that is both strong itself and within a strong foot—*tu*—has the primary stress in the

---

[11]Linguists show very little interest in audiologists' favorite stress pattern, the spondee.

X

(x .) (x .)

con sti tu tion

FIGURE 2-4.
Metrical grid for *constitution*.

TABLE 2-32.
Morphologic Effects on Stress in English

eccéntric	èccentrícity
eléctric	èlectrícity
sénile	senílity
periódic	pèriodícity

word. The *sti* gets the least emphasis, as it is a weak syllable within a weak foot. In fact, in fast speech the vowel in this syllable barely is pronounced: [kɑ̀nstºtúʃən]. Another alternative to illustrating a cumulative stress relationship of this sort is a diagram in which Xs represent stress, dots represent unstressed syllables, and parentheses represent feet. This type of diagram is called a **metrical grid** (Figure 2-4). The syllable marked by two Xs is the most strongly stressed. In all respects that are of concern here, a metrical grid of this type is equivalent to the tree in Figure 2-3. (See Goldsmith, 1990, and Hayes, 1995, for further details about metrical grids.)

The concepts of metrical phonology are most important for studying the development of prosody. As discussed previously, in trochaic languages such as English and Dutch, very young children and children with DVD may have difficulty with iambic word shapes. Such children tend to omit initial, but not final, unstressed syllables in these languages (Fikkert, 1994; Gerken, 1991; Gerken & McIntosh, 1993; Kehoe, 1995, 1997; Kehoe & Stoel-Gammon, 1997a,b; Schwartz & Goffman, 1995). This tendency is believed to be due to a language-based preference for trochaic word forms. English-speaking children are more likely to demonstrate difficulty in words with a weak + strong syllable pattern (e.g., *banána* or *giráffe*) than in words with the opposite (preferred) pattern (e.g., *mónkey* or *ápple*). Such children may omit initial unstressed syllables or, in the case of children with DVD, overstress syllables that should be weak. In either case, the natural rhythm of English prosody is disturbed by these changes, and the child's speech will not sound appropriate.

Many aspects of word stress are related also to morphology, such as the change in stress that occurs with the addition of *-ion* to *discríminate* to get *discrìminátion*. The penultimate (next-to-last) syllable of *discrimination* must be stressed to preserve the strong-weak syllable alternation. The second syllable (-*crim*-) preserves its status as a strong syllable, although it receives secondary stress only once -*ion* is added. Even more complicated effects may occur when a two-syllable affix is added. Consider the pairs of words in Table 2-32.

The main stress in the word moves "right," occurring just before the -*ity* ending. Why does this happen? To account for such a pattern, linguists hypothesize that the strong-weak stress pattern in English is applied (subconsciously) from right to left—that is, to stress an unfamiliar word, speakers of American English typically calculate from the end of the word to the front. Also, certain affixes, such as -*ity*, have fixed stress patterns that do not change from word to word. In this case, -*ity* is a sequence of two weak syllables; neither of its syllables ever are stressed. Given that the word *periodicity*, for example, will end in two weak syllables, a strong syllable must precede them. Thus far, then, the word will be as follows: *periodícity*. In the word *periodic*, the *o* is strong. However, it cannot be strong in *periodicity*, as that would put two strongs together and would destroy the alternating rhythm. Therefore, the *o*—and the *i* that precedes it—will be weak. Given that *per* precedes two weak syllables, it too must be strong. The final result, then, is *pèriodícity* (with the main stress on the second *i* and a secondary stress on the *e*).

Normally developing older children are usually able to use their (subconscious) knowledge of the English metrical system to discern the stress patterns of unfamiliar multisyllabic words. Children with current NFPs or histories of phonological delay or disorder may not have these insights unless they are taught directly about them.

The same principles that apply to stress patterns in words seem to apply to stress patterns in phrases and sentences as well. For instance, a stressed word within a stressed phrase (such as the word *king's* in the sentence, "I didn't know he stole *the **king's** jewels*") will be a stressed syllable within a stressed foot (composed of *the* + *king's*) within a stressed phrase (*the king's jewels*, due to the speaker's choice of emphasis) within the sentence, and therefore will receive more emphasis than would a stressed word within an unstressed phrase (such as *king's* in the sentence, "*I didn't **know** he stole the king's jewels*") and far more than an unstressed word within an unstressed phrase (such as the word *the* in that same sentence.) For these reasons, metrical phonology is applied also to many questions in morphology and syntax.

Autosegmental Phonology

Autosegmental phonology is based on the premise that some of the features that may affect sound segments actually are autonomous from them in some ways. An often-drawn analogy is the notes and words in a song. Although one usually couples a particular note to a particular word or syllable, the note and the syllable can be dissociated under certain circumstances, such as by singing "la, la, la" instead of the words, humming, changing the words, or reciting the words without singing. Furthermore, sometimes one syllable is sung over two different notes or two syllables are sung on the same note, so the syllables and the notes do not have to be matched up one to one.

The tones in tone languages behave very much as do the notes in a song. One tone may be held over two sylla-

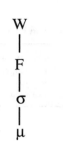

FIGURE 2-5.
Prosodic hierarchy.

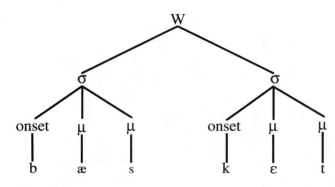

FIGURE 2-7.
Autosegmental form of *basket*.

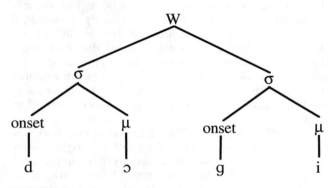

FIGURE 2-6.
Autosegmental form of *doggie*.

bles, or two tones may apply to the same syllable. Tone languages were the first application of autosegmental phonology. However, the same principles may apply also to other features that we usually consider to be more segmental. The units on autosegmental trees can include the following elements[12]:

• **"Prosodic" word**: represented by W.
• **Foot**: represented by F; composed of two to three syllables, which are strong or weak, as in metrical phonology.
• **Syllable**: represented by σ. Again, there are two basic types: **Heavy** syllables have one or more elements after the (optional) onset, such as a vowel plus a final consonant in the syllable (e.g., [kæt, tostɚ, ɚθ]) or another vowel that forms a diphthong with the first (e.g., [kɑʊ, bɔɪlɚ]). The final consonant of the syllable (if any) is the coda. **Light** syllables have only one vowel and no final consonant (e.g., [lɔ, pʌpi] etc.). Like heavy syllables, they may or may not have an onset.
    The first consonant of the syllable (if any) is called the **onset**. Everything after the onset is further divided into moras.
• **Mora**: represented by μ; minimal prosodic unit; building block of the syllable.

The term *mora* applies to a vowel or to a consonant that is not in onset position in the syllable. A mora is a measure of the weight of the syllable. A syllable with only one vowel and no final consonant is light—just one mora. A syllable with a diphthong, especially if it also has a final consonant, is heavy and would be considered to be two or more moras in most languages. (Note that syllable weight is a language-specific variable. A syllable considered light in one language might be considered heavy in another.) Thus, in English, a CV syllable has one onset and one mora (e.g., p + ɑ); a CVV or CVC syllable has an onset and two moras (e.g., p + ɑ + r; p + æ + d; b + ɔ + ɪ).[13] In other words, a light syllable is one that includes only one mora (usually a vowel following the onset consonant), whereas a heavy syllable has two (usually two vowels—a diphthong—or a vowel plus a consonant, following the onset consonant). The hierarchy is shown in Figure 2-5.

In other words, words are subdivided into feet, which are subdivided into syllables, which are subdivided into onsets and moras. Feet are not really relevant unless the word is multisyllabic, a less common finding in English among children who are fairly young or very phonologically disordered. The child may have merged foot and word levels in a metrical representation (Demuth, 1996). Thus, *doggie* could appear as shown in Figure 2-6, and *basket* could be as shown in Figure 2-7.

Harmony or assimilation patterns may be represented as two segments sharing a feature. In very early phonologies or very delayed phonologies in various languages, sound features often are **autosegmentalized** (Goldsmith, 1979). This means that the feature (such as [labial]) applies to more than just one sound segment. It is attached at a spot higher in the phonological tree than would be expected in adult phonology. Children who pronounce *bottle* as [bɑbɑ], for instance, may not be representing the two consonants separately in their phonology; the entire word may be marked as [labial] instead of the individual consonants being so marked. This is illustrated in Figure 2-8: The [labial] feature is

---

[12]I assume the relevance of onsets, codas, and moras here—in a sense, merging ideas from onset-rhyme and moraic theory—as each of the three units appears to play a role in some languages. This has been done before (e.g., by Stonham, 1990).

[13]Some question whether English diphthongs (as in the words *pay*, *buy*, *boy*, and *wow*) should count as one mora or two.

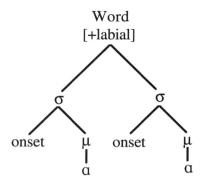

FIGURE 2-8.
Autosegmentalized [labial] in *bottle*—[bɑbɑ].

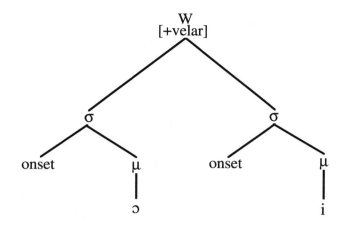

FIGURE 2-9.
Autosegmentalized [velar] in *doggie*—[gɔgi].

specified at the word level, because such children never produce two different consonants in the same word. It appears that, for them, the entire word is variously labial, coronal, or velar. Contrast within the word is not a possibility.[14]

Similarly, when a child says [gɔgi] instead of *doggie*, [gægɛk] instead of *basket*, and [ɛg gigɚ] instead of *egg beater*, the feature [velar] is applying to all consonants in all syllables of the word or phrase, not just to one segment. Formerly, this pattern was difficult to describe as a phonological rule, but now rules do not have to be linear. A tree illustrates that the [+velar] feature is autosegmental—that is, it is attached not just to one consonant but to the entire word. Now, *doggie* would be represented as in Figure 2-9 and *egg beater* would be as shown in Figure 2-10.

Of course, this account ignores the presence of vowels in words such as *bottle*. If the entire word were labial, it would be pronounced [bobo] (because the labiality would make the vowels rounded). To account for the fact that some consonant rules seem to ignore intervening vowels and vice versa, phonologists (e.g., Besnier, 1987; McCarthy, 1989; Menn, 1978b) have proposed that, in phonotactically simple phonologies, different **planes**, or **tiers**, are available for representing consonants versus vowels. This separation of consonants from vowels is referred to as **planar segregation**. Planar segregation separates these two fundamental segment types so that, for example, consonants do not get in the way of patterns of interaction among vowels, and vice versa. This practice makes sense, as consonants are more likely to affect each other (e.g., in consonant harmony) than to affect vowels, and the reverse also is true. Thus, in the first example just presented, the child who said [bɑbɑ] for *bottle* actually demonstrated both vowel harmony and consonant harmony, but the vowels did not affect the consonants or vice versa. So, in fact, her production of *bottle* should be represented as in Figure 2-11, with two sets of

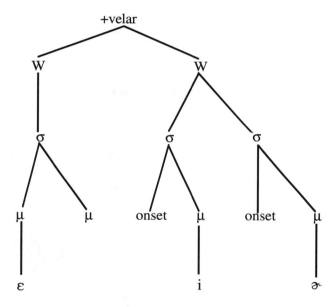

FIGURE 2-10.
Autosegmentalized [velar] in *egg beater*—[ɛg gigɚ].

autosegmental features: one for the consonants and one for the vowels.

However, sometimes vowels and consonants do affect each other. At later stages in phonological development, these planes or tiers may come together (McCarthy, 1989), at which point the vowels and consonants can interact and trigger such patterns as consonant-vowel assimilation. Levelt (1992) provided several interesting examples of such interactions from Dutch children. One child ("Elke"), for instance, attempted to produce the Dutch word *schoen* (shoe), pronounced by adults as [sχun].[15] Elke's pronunciation was [pum]. Why did she produce both the initial and final consonants as labial?

---

[14]Note that, at this phonological stage, voicing typically is not under the child's control. Therefore, the voicing distinction between [p] and [b] is being ignored here.

[15][χ], *chi*, is a voiceless uvular fricative.

C tier

[+labial]

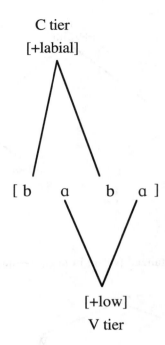

[b ɑ b ɑ]

[+low]

V tier

FIGURE 2-11.
Planar segregation of consonants and vowels on separate tiers.

Word

[+labial]

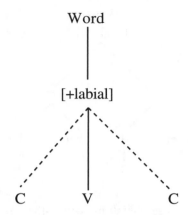

C   V   C

FIGURE 2-12.
Spreading of labialization from a round vowel to nearby consonants. (Adapted from C Levelt. Consonant harmony: A reanalysis in terms of vowel-consonant interaction. Presented to Boston University Conference on Child Language Development, Boston, October 1992.)

None of the target consonants in this word are labial; from whence arose this place of articulation? Levelt claimed that it must have been spread from the vowel, which is [round] or [labial].[16] Figure 2-12 illustrates the onset and coda consonants of *schoen*, which are linked with [labial].

Lleó (1996) illustrated that Spanish-speaking children tend to demonstrate either planar segregation (e.g., consonant harmony) or consonant-vowel interactions, which cannot occur if consonants and vowels are on separate levels. It is not known whether these two patterns typically both occur in sequence during development or whether it is more common for each child to do one or the other but not both.

In some languages, words are broken up, as in such secret languages as Pig Latin, or when swear words are inserted into the middle of the word ("That tele-f#@$ing-phone is ringing again!"). In other cases, morphemes that

have social meanings only (such as the *-ie* added in English baby talk to yield *horsie, piggie,* etc.) are added to words. Phonologists have found that it is easier to describe these processes by referring to the units of nonlinear phonology (feet, syllables, or moras and sometimes onsets) than by referring to specific segments or numbers of segments (McCarthy, 1991; McCarthy & Prince, 1986, 1990). Findings such as these help to confirm the psychological reality of the nonlinear elements.

Implications for Nonlinear Phonology Intervention

All of these figures and new terminology may seem overwhelming at first sight. It is important to remember that neither the pictures nor the jargon are critical to the nonlinear perspective and that the perspective can be summed up in a few simple statements: Phonology operates at several interconnecting, interdependent levels, from the feature all the way up to the phrase (and beyond). Thus, the phonological representation of a certain syllable or word has both breadth (adjacent elements at the same level) and depth (elements at each level associated with elements at the next level up or down). Those levels above the segment level correspond to what may be termed the phonotactic and prosodic systems.

Bernhardt (1992a) stressed the importance of the theoretical notion that prosody (e.g., stress patterns), phonotactics (word and syllable shapes), and segments are represented on different levels in nonlinear phonological representations. This theory implies that each of these aspects of the phonology may be impaired or delayed independently. In other words, children might have prosodic, phonotactic, or segmental difficulties that differ in severity. Furthermore, such children might have diffi-

---

[16]Note that, again, data from real people remind us that our technical labels for things should stem from and always refer back to human speech production and perception capabilities. Traditionally such consonants as [b, m, p] have been termed [labial], whereas such vowels as [u, o] were termed [round], despite the fact that all share dependence on the approximation of the lips. Cases such as these have caused phonologists to reanalyze their feature categories to make them correspond more closely to actually observed patterns of speech production. In many current approaches, vowels and consonants now share the same features to facilitate descriptions of just this sort of phenomenon. This reanalysis process is at the heart of the aspect of nonlinear phonology that is termed **feature geometry**. See Chapter 3 for details.

culty specifically making associations from one level to the next (Bernhardt, 1990, 1992b). This type of difficulty is seen in children with dyspraxia, for example. They may be able to produce consonants in isolation but not combine them into syllables. Alternatively, they might be able to produce syllables, but not combine them into words (Velleman & Strand, 1994).

Interactions between levels also may be critical. Fikkert (1994), for example, claimed that Dutch children's use of final consonants may be influenced by the weight (contents) of the syllable. If the syllable includes a long vowel or diphthong (i.e., two vowel moras), the child is less likely to use a final consonant, as that syllable is already heavy. A short, simple vowel has a higher probability of being followed by a final consonant, as the vowel portion (**nucleus**) provides only one mora, and the syllable can thus accept a second, consonantal, mora.

For these reasons, each level must be assessed individually and in its interactions with other levels. Independent phonological goals should be established as needed. Bernhardt's clinical studies of nonlinear phonological intervention (e.g., Bernhardt, 1990, 1992b) have substantiated these ideas.

Bernhardt (1992b) provided one specific example of the application of nonlinear phonology. In this case, Bernhardt chose separate prosodic and segmental goals, in keeping with her belief that different tiers are addressed separately. Thus, one goal was the production of two consonant slots in initial position. Although par-ticular clusters (composed of consonants already within the child's singleton repertoire) were modeled, the goal was not the correct production of those particular consonant clusters. Rather, Bernhardt hoped to increase the child's ability to produce initial two-element clusters in general. This goal was, in fact, met. Not only did the child increase correct productions of those particular clusters, but use of other initial clusters also increased. Furthermore, the child's use of a default cluster (*fw-*), which had served as a replacement for several other clusters, decreased markedly. This case study testifies to the benefits of considering the phonotactic level separately from the segmental or phonetic level in setting goals.

Summary

Important concepts from nonlinear phonology allow us to provide more elegant, comprehensive descriptions of familiar child phonological patterns. **Autosegmentalization** occurs when a feature applies to a whole syllable or word, rather than to a single segment, resulting in harmony or assimilation. **Planar segregation** separates consonants from vowels so that they can interact independently when consonant or vowel harmony occur. In general, nonlinear phonology encourages the clinician to consider all the levels within a phonology, assessing and treating each individually and in interaction with each other.

CHAPTER THREE

Phones and Features

Traditionally, speech sounds have been regarded as the basic building blocks for speech. Most phonologists and speech scientists now recognize that speech probably is processed most often at the syllable level or above and that the **transitions** between the brief steady states that humans recognize as consonants and vowels are at least as important to the actual processes of perception and production as are the relatively steady-state segments themselves. Recent theories of speech production have claimed that articulatory gestures form the basis for phonetic development from infancy onward and that speech sounds (phones or phonemes) and features emerge from gestural regularities (Goodell & Studdert-Kennedy, 1991; Kent, 1997; Lindblom, 1992; Studdert-Kennedy & Goodell, 1992; see also under Gestural Phonology).

However, the fact remains that, at a conscious level, it is easier to think of speech as a stream of consecutive sounds, like beads on a string. What speakers perceive as a misproduction of a particular consonant may in fact be a miscoordination of the transition from a preceding vowel into that consonant or from that consonant into the following vowel, but our perception that something was awry at the consonantal level is nonetheless valuable information. Children who have difficulty with oral-motor timing or spatial coordination will be perceived as being unable to produce certain sound segments or types of sound segments of their native language. Therefore, it is still appropriate to analyze the sound segments within children's sound repertoires. However, care must be taken to remember that these sounds are not used in isolation, and that contextual factors (word position, syllable shape, stress patterns, the influence of other sounds within the word, rate, semantic and syntactic context, etc.) are extremely important to consider.

The same sounds may function in different ways in different languages. Those sounds that are in contrast with each other (i.e., that differentiate words; see Chapter 4) within a language are termed **phonemes**; others that occur but not contrastively are called **allophones**. These phonological functions of sounds are discussed in Chapter 4. For the moment, this contrastive function of speech sounds will be ignored. This chapter focuses on the major sets of sounds and phonetic features that tend to occur within any language.

SOUND CLASSES

Sounds are grouped into sets by their articulatory, auditory, and phonological characteristics. These characteristics are called **features**. Many feature classification systems have been proposed. The most recent approach to classification of features, feature geometry, is discussed at the end of this chapter. However, as the purpose here is not to take a theoretical stand on any particular classification system, the feature terminology of Chomsky and Halle's *The Sound Pattern of English* (1968), which is most familiar to most speech-language pathologists, will be used whenever possible, and other terms will be defined as needed. Definitions of many sound classes are given within this chapter. A key to the International Phonetic Alphabet (IPA) and diacritic symbols used in this book is provided as Appendix C; see also Tables 3-1 through 3-4.

The primary feature distinctions that must be made within any classification scheme are those that differentiate among consonants, vowels, and those sounds (such as glides, nasals, and liquids) that have some of the characteristics of both consonants and vowels. The feature [consonantal] differentiates consonants ([+consonantal]) from vowels ([−consonantal]). The feature [sonorant] differentiates resonant sounds ([+sonorant]), such as liquids, nasals, and so on, from nonresonant sounds ([−sonorant]), such as stops and fricatives. The other major feature distinctions that are made are those of place of articulation (back, high, etc.), manner of articulation (continuant, nasal, etc.), and voice (voiced or voiceless).

One goal of any theoretical proposal about phonological features must be that the proposed feature system make it easy to generalize about the production (or perception) of the sounds described by the feature system. For this reason, for example, the evidence for consonant-vowel interactions presented in Chapter 2 has motivated some phonologists to propose that the same features should be used for consonants and vowels (e.g., [b] and [u] both classified as [+labial]; Levelt, 1996). Furthermore, when the commonalties among the sounds (or the features of sounds) that are lacking in a child's phonetic repertoire are considered, it should be possible to determine the types of articulatory postures or movements or the types of gestural coordination that are difficult or unknown to the child. For example, chil-

TABLE 3-1.
Feature Specifications for American English Consonants

	p	b	f	v	m	t	d	θ	ð	n	s	z	tʃ	dʒ	ʃ	ʒ	k	g	ŋ	r	l	h	w	j
Syllabic	−	−	−	−	−	−	−	−	−	−	−	−	−	−	−	−	−	−	−	−	−	−	−	−
Consonantal	+	+	+	+	+	+	+	+	+	+	+	+	+	+	+	+	+	+	+	+	+	+	−	−
Sonorant	−	−	−	−	+	−	−	−	−	+	−	−	−	−	−	−	−	−	+	+	+	−	+	+
Nasal	−	−	−	−	+	−	−	−	−	+	−	−	−	−	−	−	−	−	+	−	−	−	−	−
Continuant	−	−	+	+	−	−	−	+	+	−	+	+	−	−	+	+	−	−	−	+	+	+	+	+
Anterior	+	+	+	+	+	+	+	+	+	+	+	+	−	−	−	−	−	−	−	−	+	−	+	−
Coronal	−	−	−	−	−	+	+	+	+	+	+	+	+	+	+	+	−	−	−	+	+	−	−	+
Voice	−	+	−	+	+	−	+	−	+	+	−	+	−	+	−	+	−	+	+	+	+	−	+	+

Source: Adapted from N Chomsky, M Halle. *The Sound Pattern of English*. New York: Harper & Row, 1968.

TABLE 3-2.
Feature Specifications for American English Vowels

	i	ɪ	e	ɛ	æ	ə/ʌ	u	ʊ	o	ɔ	ɑ
Syllabic	+	+	+	+	+	+	+	+	+	+	+
Consonantal	−	−	−	−	−	−	−	−	−	−	−
Tense	+	−	+	−	−	−	+	−	+	−	−
High	+	+	−	−	−	−	+	+	−	−	−
Low	−	−	−	−	+	−	−	−	−	−	+
Front	+	+	+	+	+	−	−	−	−	−	−
Back	−	−	−	−	−	−	+	+	+	+	+
Round	−	−	−	−	−	−	+	+	+	+	−

Source: Adapted from N Chomsky, M Halle. *The Sound Pattern of English.* New York: Harper & Row, 1968.

TABLE 3-3.
American English Consonants by Place and Manner of Articulation

		Bilabial	Labiodental	Interdental	Alveolar	Palatal	Velar	Glottal
Stops	vd	b			d		g	
	vl	p			t		k	ʔ
Nasals		m			n		ŋ	
Glides		w				j		
Fricatives	vd		v	ð	z	ʒ		
	vl		f	θ	s	ʃ		h
Affricates	vd					dʒ		
	vl					tʃ		
Liquids					l	r		

vd = voiced; vl = voiceless.

dren who produce no fricatives may not have the control required to approximate two oral structures (e.g., the tongue and the alveolar ridge, the teeth and lower lip) in such a way as to leave enough of a groove for the air flow to pass through, yet only enough of a groove that the air becomes turbulent (yielding the frication sound). If they stop fricatives (e.g., say [p] for /f/), they are going too far and creating contact rather than frication between the two articulators. If they glide them (e.g., say [w] for /f/), they are not approximating closely enough, allowing the air to flow too freely. These articulatory considerations are the motivation for gestural phonology, described in the theoretical portion at the end of the chapter.

Whatever feature system is used, sounds that are articulated similarly—either in place or manner of articulation or in voicing—tend to behave in similar ways within any phonology. No clinician is surprised to find that a child who stops one fricative stops others, that a child who glides /l/ also glides /r/, or that a child who voices initial /p/ and /t/ also voices initial /k/. This basic insight lies behind theories of phonological rules, processes, or constraints. Knowledge of the features relevant to the sound repertoire of a particular language enables us to recognize such patterns even if they do not have a popularized name. Many process tests or process analyses do not include consideration of nasalization or frication, for example, yet some children do nasalize certain speech sounds (e.g., fricatives) or fricate others (e.g., stops). If this is a pattern exhibited by a client, it will have to be addressed in therapy. The clinician can address the pat-

TABLE 3-4.
American English Vowels by Place and Manner of Articulation

	Front	Central	Back
High			
Tense	i		u
Lax	ɪ		ʊ
Mid			
Tense	e		o
Lax	ɛ		ɔ
Low		ʌ,e	
	æ		ɑ

Source: Adapted from N Chomsky, M Halle. *The Sound Pattern of English.* New York: Harper & Row, 1968.

tern much more efficiently by focusing on the entire class of sounds affected than by teaching each affected speech sound one by one. However, to do so, the speech-language pathologist must first recognize the pattern as such. These issues are discussed in greater depth in Chapter 5.

EASE OF PERCEPTION AND PRODUCTION

The IPA includes well over 100 sounds used by various languages throughout the world. Each language selects some subset of those sounds for use in its words. These subsets are by no means random. Two major forces work together to determine a subset of possible sounds that will be functional for the language: our old friends ease of perception and ease of production.

Ease of perception requires that the set of sounds chosen be easily perceptible and different enough from each other that the listener can identify the sound intended by the speaker. This is why [θ] is not a popular sound among the languages of the world; it has very low acoustic energy and is therefore difficult to hear. Although [f] also is difficult to perceive auditorily, it has the benefit of easy visual identification and is therefore more common than [θ].

Other sounds may be easy enough to hear but auditorily too close to each other to be discriminated easily. English, for instance, includes the auditorily salient alveolar ([s]) and palatoalveolar ([ʃ]) voiceless fricatives and the less salient interdental ([θ]). Already this set of voiceless coronal (alveopalatal) fricatives is quite large. Sometimes, listening conditions (e.g., telephone) or speaking conditions (e.g., drunkenness) make these three difficult to differentiate. Some languages include a retroflex voiceless fricative, which is made in a manner similar to [s] but with the tongue-tip curled back; other languages include a lateral voiceless fricative, which also is made in a manner similar to [s] but with a flatter tongue, rendering the frication noise more slushy sounding. These languages do not include the English fricative sounds as well; too much confusion would result. Similarly, if such sounds were to be added to the English sound repertoire, ease of perception could be compromised seriously. Speakers would confuse these other fricatives quite often with [s], [ʃ], or [θ].[1]

Ease of production requires that most of the sounds in the language be fairly easy to produce in an appropriate number of combinations with each other to create a reasonably sized, pronounceable vocabulary. Stops and nasals, for example, are among the simplest to produce and to combine; therefore, they are very common in the languages of the world. It is known from data on order of acquisition that some sounds, such as the English retroflex [r], are more difficult to make accurately. Such sounds are used less commonly by languages of the world. Other sounds may be easy to produce but difficult to combine into syllables. Raspberries (lingualabial trills), for example, are not hard to produce, but try substituting them in words that contain the [b] or [p] sound—not very efficient! (Try saying "ru*bb*er *baby buggy bumpers*" three times with raspberries in place of *b* and *p*, then see how long it takes to untangle your tongue!) Your tongue and jaw have to protrude so far to make a good juicy raspberry that it takes much too long to get them back into an appropriate position for making a vowel.

Ease of perception and ease of production compete with each other in many cases. For instance, [s] is one of the trickiest sounds to produce accurately. This is known not only from acquisition data but also from studies of speakers who become deafened adventitiously, whose trigeminal nerves are anesthetized (Borden & Harris,

1994), who are drunk (Lester & Skousen, 1974), or who are subjected to delayed auditory feedback (Smith, 1962). Under all these conditions, [s] is one of the first sounds to be distorted in production, yet it is very popular among the languages of the world because it is such a high-intensity sound that it is very easy to perceive, even at a distance. The fact that English includes both [θ] and [ʃ] in addition to [s] places a heavier burden on its speakers. We have to produce [s] very accurately so that it is not misperceived as either of these close neighbors. Yet, Velleman (1988) demonstrated that children who misproduce [s] typically can discriminate it perceptually from their substitution sound ([θ], [ʃ], etc.). In contrast, children who misproduce [θ] often do not appear to be aware of distinctions between this sound and its substitutes ([f], [s̪], etc.).

Ease of perception and ease of production, then, exert a major influence on the sound repertoires of a language. In this chapter, the effects of such factors on phonetic repertoires are considered. Phonetic universals, markedness and defaults, sound systems, and distribution requirements are discussed with respect to their effects on phonetic repertoires. In each case, generalizations about the languages of the world are followed by an explanation of the way in which these generalizations are reflected in normal and disordered child phonology. Suggestions and worksheets for easy assessment and implications for setting goals are provided. Finally, a brief overview of feature geometry is presented.

PHONETIC UNIVERSALS

Languages of the World

Human ease of perception and ease of production together yield phonetic universals: statements that can be made about tendencies within the sound systems of all languages; they are assumed to result from human physiological restrictions. Universals have been collected or described by Greenberg (1978); Lindblom et al. (1993); Maddieson (1984); and Maddieson and Precoda (1989). Such universals are important to an understanding of child phonology because all children are affected by human physiological restrictions in very important ways, especially in early and very disordered phonologies. Sounds that are preferred universally typically are acquired early; those that are rare among the languages of the world usually are acquired later (Locke, 1983), although the language that the child is learning can influence this (de Boysson-Bardies & Vihman, 1991; de Boysson-Bardies et al., 1992; Vihman, 1996). The universals that are most relevant to phonological development in English are given here (from Maddieson, 1984, unless otherwise specified).[2]

---

[1]In fact, we do use a retroflex voiceless fricative immediately before [r] in such words as *shrub*. However, this sound never contrasts with [s] or [ʃ]; they do not occur immediately before [r]. Thus, confusion is avoided.

[2]Note that Maddieson actually is reporting on sounds presumed to be phonemes in these languages. In this chapter, the phone-phoneme distinction is ignored. Possibly, the data reported here would differ very slightly if all phones had been counted (allophones as well as phonemes), but the differences in proportions of occurrence likely would be very small.

Vowels

Vowels are speech sounds "formed without a significant constriction of the oral and pharyngeal cavities, and that serve as a syllable nucleus" (Shriberg & Kent, 1995, p. 64). The following universals apply:

1. All languages have at least three vowels.
2. The most common number of vowels in a language is five.
3. As discussed later in this chapter, 86% of languages have vowel systems with vowels that are articulatorily evenly spaced (i.e., their places of articulation are distributed evenly throughout the oral cavity). Another 10% have nearly even spacing.
4. Some two-thirds of the languages in the world have diphthongs. Of these, perhaps 75% have [ɑɪ] (or something similar), and 65% have [ɑʊ] (or something similar; Ladefoged & Maddieson, 1996).

Stops

Stops are consonants that are "formed by a complete closure of the vocal tract, so that airflow ceases temporarily and air pressure builds up behind the point of closure" (Shriberg & Kent, 1995, p. 64). The following universals apply:

1. All languages have stops.
2. If a language has two stop series, the two will differ in voicing (as do the two English series [p, t, k] and [b, d, g]). It is important to note in this connection that what English speakers tend to consider as voiced stops actually are voiceless unaspirated. Among the languages in the world, there are three types of voicing. In a language with two stop series, each of those two series is likely to fall in a different one of the three categories:
   a. **Voiceless aspirated**: long lag between consonant release and beginning of voicing, so that we perceive a puff of air being released with the consonant, as in English word-initial [p, t, k] in the words *pea*, *tea*, and *key*: [pʰi], [tʰi], [kʰi].
   b. **Voiceless unaspirated**: short or no lag between consonant release and beginning of voicing, exemplified by English so-called voiced consonants, such as those in the words *boo*, *do*, *goo*, which usually are transcribed by English speakers as [bu], [du], [gu]. The same sounds also occur as English voiceless stops in *s*-clusters, such as *speed*, *steep*, and *ski*, usually ethnocentrically transcribed as [spid], [stip], [ski]. English speakers typically transcribe these two sets of sounds differently because they are associated with different phonemes, but in fact they are acoustically the same.
   c. **Voiced or prevoiced**: voicing begins before consonant release. Typically, this does not occur in English except in the oral communication of deaf speakers. It is a voicing option used by many other languages, such as Spanish and French, however.
3. Most languages (98%) include stops at bilabial, dental or alveolar, and velar places of articulation.

4. If a language has [p], it has [k], and if it has [k], it has [t] (dental or alveolar voiceless stop). In other words, [t] is most common, followed by [k] and then [p].
5. If a language has [g], it has [d] (dental or alveolar voiced stop), and if it has [d], it has [b]. In other words, [b] is most common, followed by [d] and then [g]. (Note that the order of this **implicational universal** is different with respect to place of articulation from the order for the voiceless stop series.)

Nasals

Nasals are consonants "produced with a complete oral closure (like a stop) but with an open velopharynx, so that voicing energy travels out through the nose" (Shriberg & Kent, 1995, p. 65). The following universals apply:

1. Most languages (97%) have at least one nasal.
2. Most nasals (93%) are voiced (as are English nasals).
3. If a language has any nasals at all, it will have [n].
4. If a language has a nasal at a certain place of articulation, it will have an obstruent (stop, affricate, or fricative) at that same place of articulation (e.g., [m] and [b]; [n] and [d]).

Liquids

Liquids are "vowel-like consonant[s] in which voicing energy passes through a vocal tract that is constricted only somewhat more than for vowels. The shape and location of the constriction is a critical defining property, being distinctive for a given type of liquid." (Shriberg & Kent, 1995, p. 65). The following universals apply:

1. Most languages (96%) have at least one liquid.
2. Languages with only one liquid most often (99%) have a lateral liquid (such as [l]).
3. Languages with two or more liquids usually (86%) include one lateral (such as [l]) and one nonlateral (such as [r]).

Fricatives

A fricative is a "sound ... produced with a narrow constriction through which air escapes with a continuous noise" (Shriberg & Kent, 1995, p. 65). The following universals apply:

1. Some 93% of languages have at least one fricative.
2. If a language has only one fricative, it is [s] (dental or alveolar voiceless sibilant).
3. If a language has only two fricatives, it is most likely to have [s] and [f], although other pairs also occur. Languages with only two fricatives avoid pairs that differ in voicing only (e.g., [s], [z]).
4. The most common fricatives are [s], [f], and [ʃ].
5. Voiced fricatives are far less common than are voiceless; languages with any voiced fricatives usually have an entire set of voiced-voiceless fricative pairs. In other words, if a language has any voiced fricatives at

TABLE 3-5.
Sound Classes Used by 24-Month-Olds

	Initial Position		Final Position	
Sound Class	50%	90%	50%	90%
Stop	b, d, g, t, k	b, d	p, t, k	t
Nasal	m, n		n	
Fricative	f, s		s	
Liquid/glide	w, h		r	

Source: Adapted from C Stoel-Gammon. Phonological skills of 2-year-olds. *Language Speech and Hearing Services in the Schools* 1987;18:323–329.

all, it will have as many or more voiceless fricatives as voiced ones. If any voiced-voiceless pair in the language is incomplete, it is likely to be [ʃ]–[ʒ] (as was the case for American English until exposure to French led to the introduction of [ʒ] in a small set of words).

Glides
Glides are sounds with "a vocal tract constriction somewhat narrower than that for vowels but less severe than that for stops and fricatives ... characterized by a gliding motion of the articulators from a partly constricted state to a more open state for the following vowel" (Shriberg & Kent, 1995, p. 66). The following universals apply:

1. Some 86% of languages have at least one glide.
2. Languages with only one glide are more likely to have [j].
3. Most languages (71%) that have [w] also have [j].

Child Phonetic Inventories

Stoel-Gammon (1987) reported that the consonants used by at least 50% of 33 American English–speaking 24-month-olds were stops, nasals, fricatives, glides, and liquids. Those phones that were present in 90% of the children's inventories were [b, d] in initial position and [t] in final position. In general, a wider variety of phones occurred in initial position than in final position. Stoel-Gammon's specific findings are listed in Table 3-5.

Those sounds that are used most commonly in the languages of the world tend to be those that children babble and use in their first words most often, according to Locke (1983). Presumably, in these sounds, the balance between ease of perception and ease of production is maintained most easily, although ease of production clearly is given more weight by children, and ease of perception is relatively more important to adults. These same sounds also tend to be those that are produced correctly by the majority of 2-year-olds, as illustrated by data drawn from Maddieson (1984) and Locke (1983),[3] presented in Table 3-6.

Note that all the child data are derived from children who are being raised in English environments. Children from other environments may show slightly different patterns, as the language that the child hears has been shown to affect the child's phonetic repertoire from the late babbling period onward (de Boysson-Bardies et al., 1992; de Boysson-Bardies & Vihman, 1991; Vihman, 1996).

Despite the obvious difficulty for children, the frequency of sibilants (e.g., [s]) in the languages of the world likely is due to their relatively high perceptual salience. Conversely, the relative infrequency of [h] in languages, despite its obvious ease of production (i.e., frequent use in babble), is probably due to its lower salience. Given that stops are quite frequent in languages of the world, in babble and in early words, it is unexpected to see a somewhat low percentage of stops correct at 2 years of age. This incidence may be attributable to within-class errors (fronting, backing, etc.). It cannot be determined from Locke's data whether a stop substituted for another stop (e.g., [t] for /k/) was considered correct or incorrect.

Dinnsen (1992) has used a similar type of analysis to identify a hierarchy of phonetic repertoires among English-speaking children with functional phonological disorders. He claims that such children's phonetic repertoires will fall into one of several levels and that remediation can be expected to facilitate the child's transition from one level to the next, more phonetically elaborated level. The levels that he proposes are as follows:

- Level A: vowels, glides, voiced stops, nasals, glottals
- Level B: level A sounds + voicing contrast for stops
- Level C: level B sounds + some fricatives or affricates
- Level D: level C sounds + one liquid consonant (lateral [l], nonlateral [r])
- Level E: level D sounds + more liquids *or* more obstruents (e.g., fricatives or affricates)

These levels are in keeping with the adult and child universals described earlier: All languages have stops and vowels, 97% have nasals, and 86% have glides; sibilants and liquids are relatively frequent among adult languages but are not as frequent in babble or early words. Similarly, sibilants most often are produced incorrectly by normally developing 2-year-olds, so it should not be surprising that stops, vowels, nasals, and glides are present in even the simplest of phonetic repertoires among phonologically delayed children or that liquids and sibilants are not. The early addition of a

---

[3]Data on percentages of languages with stops, nasals, liquids, glides, and [h] are derived from Maddieson (1984). All other data are drawn from Locke (1983). Locke's data on universal patterns reportedly are based on Ruhlen (1976); his data on relative frequency of sounds in babbling of 11- to 12-month-olds exposed to English are based on Irwin (1947), Fisichelli (1950), Pierce and Hanna (1974); his data on relative frequency of phones in initial position in early words from 10 children ages 16–22 months are based on Leonard et al. (1980); and his data on correct production of consonants by 2-year-olds are based on Prather et al. (1975).

TABLE 3-6.
Correspondences Between Sound Use in Babble and Languages

Sound Class	Percent of Languages	Percent of Babble	Percent Use in Early Words	Percent Correct (Age 2)
Stops	100	43	100	81.7
Nasals	99.6	9.2	100	93.3
Liquids	95.9	1.22	0	90.9
Glides	86	17	60	87.5
Sibilants	90.6	1.6	50	33.5
Other fricatives	73	1.8	30	31.3
[h]	63	23.7	50	86

Source: Adapted from I Maddieson. *Patterns of Sounds.* Cambridge: Cambridge University Press, 1984; and J Locke. *Phonological Acquisition and Change.* New York: Academic Press, 1983.

TABLE 3-7.
Stoel-Gammon Data/Dinnsen Levels

Age (mos)	Number of Subjects	Dinnsen Level(s)	Phone Classes
15	7	Pre-A	Voiced stops, h
18	19	A	Voiced stops, nasals, glide w, h
21	32	A	Voiced stops, nasals, glide w, h
24	33	C	Voiced and voiceless stops, nasals, glides, fricatives

Source: Adapted from DA Dinnsen. Variation in developing and fully-developed phonologies. In Ferguson CA, Menn L, Stoel-Gammon C (eds). *Phonological Development: Models, Research, Implications.* Timonium, MD: York, 1992,191–210; and C Stoel-Gammon. Phonetic inventories, 15–24 months: A longitudinal study. *Journal of Speech and Hearing Research* 1985;28:505–512.

voicing contrast for stops also is not surprising in light of the fact that many languages use this type of contrast as they expand their stop series.

Among the languages of the world, Dinnsen (1992) reported that no known language has a level A phonetic inventory. One might think that too few phonological contrasts would be possible with such a small set of sounds. In fact, however, some languages contain even *fewer* consonant sound classes than those listed in level A. According to Dinnsen, for example, a dialect of Salish (a Native American language spoken in the Puget Sound area of Washington state) lacks all sonorant consonants, including nasals. He proposes the existence of a level even simpler than level A including only obstruent consonant sounds.

Stoel-Gammon (1985) reported on phonetic inventories for 34 normally developing children from 15 to 24 months of age. The initial-consonant inventories she reported for consonants produced by at least 50% of these children at each age fall into Dinnsen's categories as indicated in Table 3-7.

Thus, the children in the early phonological period (at 15 months) were pre–level A, and children at 18 and 21 months produced level A sounds. Rapid changes apparently occurred between 21 and 24 months, with 2-year-olds producing a far wider range of level C sounds. When Stoel-Gammon divided the children further into groups according to their ages of onset of word use, she found that those children who talked relatively early (first words by 15 months) had larger phonetic inventories (i.e., were at higher levels) at each time period than did the children who talked later (at 18 months) or very late (at 21

months). Thus, a large phonetic inventory was predictive of earlier lexical acquisition. These differences did diminish somewhat with age.

Note that these data are not strictly in keeping with other universals that were reported earlier. For instance, languages with only one glide are more likely to have [j], and most languages (71%) that have [w] also have [j]. Yet, the majority of these children produced [w] but not [j].

Dinnsen (1992) reported that all the phonetic inventories of 40 young children with moderate to severe nonfunctional phonologies (NFPs) could be assigned uniquely to one of the five distinct levels of complexity listed previously. In addition, regardless of whether every element at a given level was addressed in treatment, no child progressed beyond that level without acquiring all the phonetic features within that level. For example, several children acquired a liquid consonant along the way as they progressed from level C to level E without treatment on liquid sounds.

Gierut et al. (1994) confirmed that the phonetic repertoires of children with NFP can be assigned uniquely to Dinnsen's four levels. They reported further that no relationship between age and phonetic level existed in their group of 30 subjects.

It is important to note that this schema of levels may be less appropriate for children with extremely small lexicons (e.g., 10–20 words); they may evidence apparent anomalies (Dinnsen, 1992). Such anomalies are noted in longitudinal data from "Timmy," a child whom Dinnsen would categorize as being in level B at 15 months (on the basis of data presented by Vihman et al., 1986; Timmy's phonology was described more thoroughly by Vihman et al.,

1994). From 11 to 14 months, Timmy used only two syllable types: <bɑ>[4] (for *ball, block, box,* and imitations of *basket, bell, boat, book, button*) and <kɑ> (for *kitty, quack-quack, car, duck, key*). Although [b] is a voiced stop, [k] is voiceless and therefore would not be expected (by Dinnsen, 1992) before the introduction of nasals and glides. However, the presence of [b] but not [p], and [k] but not [g], in Timmy's pattern does fit within known tendencies of the languages of the world with respect to voiced and voiceless stops: Usually, when one or two gaps are found in a voiced or voiceless stop series, [p] and [g] are the missing element(s) (Gamkrelidze, 1975). Also, Timmy did exhibit some voicing variation, such that <bɑ> occasionally was less voiced, and <kɑ> occasionally was more so. Thus, the voicing distinction really had not been mastered. Timmy added one glide to his repertoire at 14 months ([j], again in keeping with phonetic universals), bringing himself closer to level A status. His repertoire then expanded rapidly thereafter. By the end of his fifteenth month, he actually had all the features that typify level C: voiced and voiceless stops, nasals, a glide ([j]; [w] did not emerge until 16½ months), a bilabial fricative ([β]), and a palatal affricate ([ɟ]).

Summary

Speech sounds are categorized into classes according to their articulatory and auditory characteristics and their phonological functions. Ease of perception and ease of production often are contradictory forces that determine the sounds and sound classes that are preferred by the languages of the world and are used less commonly phonologically. Those sounds and sound classes that are preferred universally also tend to occur more frequently in children's babbling and early words and to be produced correctly early on in phonological development. However, ease of perception has more of an influence on adult phonologies than on children's phonologies. The latter tend to be determined by production factors far more than by listeners' needs.

MARKEDNESS AND DEFAULTS

Languages of the World

Any patterns that are present but uncommon in the languages of the world (or in a specific language) are termed **marked**. For instance, 75% of the languages of the world use either subject-verb-object or subject-object-verb word order in sentences. These word order choices therefore are considered to be **unmarked**. Object-first word orders are the least common. According to Crystal (1987), these orders— object-subject-verb (OSV) and object-verb-subject (OVS)— were thought until recently to be totally nonexistent. They

are considered to be very marked. Crystal suggested that the oddity of OSV word order (to speakers of all but a very few languages) is exploited in the 1983 movie, "Return of the Jedi" (20th Century Fox, 1983). The character Yoda's "alienness" is emphasized through the use of marked OSV word order in such sentences as "Your father he is" and "When nine hundred years you reach, look as good you will not."

The notion of markedness can be applied also to the semantics of a particular language, using the term *unmarked* to refer to the more general or expected element of a pair. For example, we use *tall*, not *short*, when we ask about a person's height, unless we are insulting the listener intentionally: "How short are you?" Therefore, *tall* is considered to be the unmarked and *short* the marked element of this pair of opposites. Similarly, *dog* is a more general term than is *bitch*, although in a sense they are also opposites (the word *dog* is used to refer specifically to male dogs and also to all dogs). Thus, *dog* is considered to be the unmarked term and *bitch* the marked term of the pair. This distinction can be written in semantic features by saying that [+female] (or [−male]) is a marked feature for dogs. The choice of adjective (female or male) really does not matter. It is not necessary that the minus feature always be the marked (or the unmarked) one, for example.

Often, semantic markedness is affected by culture. In Switzerland, for instance, the phrase *un verre* (a glass), when ordered in a restaurant, automatically means a glass of the local white wine. Wine is the unmarked beverage in that country and [+white] (or [−red]) is the unmarked color of that beverage. In Texas, a restaurant order for *tea* automatically refers to *iced* tea (even at breakfast in January), whereas in Massachusetts, it is assumed to mean *hot* tea (even at dinner on a hot humid night in August). In Texas, [+cold] (or [−hot]) would be the unmarked value for tea; in Massachusetts, it would be [−cold] (or [+hot]).

Morphological forms can also be marked. In English morphology, adding *-s* is the usual (unmarked) way to indicate plural. Therefore, voicing changes (e.g., *elf–elves*) and vowel changes (*woman–women*) are considered to be marked morphological patterns (Crystal, 1991).

Speech sounds and features can also be marked or unmarked. Such interdental fricatives as [θ] and [ð], for example, are rare in the languages of the world, due to their low perceptual salience, and are therefore considered to be marked phones. In contrast, [s] is extremely common and is therefore in the universally unmarked category. In feature terms, [+alveolar] is less marked than is [+interdental].

The markedness of sounds also can be language specific. For instance, many languages have a **default** vowel that tends to be used whenever a vowel needs to be epenthesized. In French, [ə] is used in songs and poetry, in hyperformal speech, and in some contexts to separate two consonants. For example, *Arc de Triomphe* may be pronounced as [aʀkə də tʀiɔ̃f] (Hyman, 1975) to separate the [k] and [d] sounds or even (if someone is being very snobbish) as [aʀkə də tʀiɔ̃fə]. In Japanese, [u] is the default vowel. It is used via epenthesis to break up disfavored consonant clusters (as seen in Chapter 2) and also to avoid ending words with certain types of (non-nasal) consonants.

---

[4]Angled brackets are used because, within this <bɑ> category, voicing did vary.

This [u]-epenthesis is demonstrated in the examples of English loan words given in Table 3-8 (Hyman, 1975).

These defaults—preferred, unmarked items—are just like the semantic defaults (e.g., *short, dog, tea*) that speakers of any language use in our everyday lives. Defaults of this sort assumed a more important role in the theory of non-linear phonology; this topic is discussed in more detail in Chapter 4.

As is described later, certain sets (and types of sets) of speech sounds are very common universally, whereas other combinations are considered to be marked. Also, the degree to which a specific sound fits within the set of sounds of a particular language can determine whether that sound is considered to be marked in that language. In a language with only one fricative, for example, frication would be marked.

Features of sounds also have marked and unmarked **values**. For instance, for fricatives the feature [+voice] is marked, whereas [–voice] is unmarked. This distinction reflects the fact that voiced fricatives are less common than are their voiceless counterparts. Therefore, *plus* voice ([+voice]), the less common value, is the marked value of the feature. As already indicated, languages with only one liquid tend to have a lateral liquid (such as [l]). Thus, *minus* is the marked (less common) value of the feature [lateral]. Similarly, the glide [j] is [–anterior] because of its place of articulation behind the alveolar ridge and [+coronal] because it is produced with the blade of the tongue. As indicated earlier, [j] is more common universally than is the labiovelar glide [w]. The latter is [+anterior, –coronal], which means that it is produced forward of the alveolar ridge, and the tongue blade is not used. Therefore, minus is the unmarked (more common) value for [anterior] for glides, and plus is the unmarked value for [coronal] for glides. In fact, theories of feature geometry indicate that [+coronal] is the universally unmarked place of articulation feature for all types of consonants.

Children's Markedness and Defaults

Timmy's early phonology is a perfect example of defaults in child phonology (Vihman et al., 1994). Although he produced his first words between 12 and 14 months, it was not until 16 months that any word contained any vowel other than [ɑ]. Furthermore, even when [i] finally appeared at 16 months and [u] at 16½ months, their uses were restricted to certain words and certain phonotactic contexts. For Timmy, then, [ɑ] was a default vowel.

Another child, "Alice" (also described by Vihman, 1992, and Vihman et al., 1994) provides an example of a less expected default. Alice produced many palatals in her babble and in her early words. Although she quickly began producing a wider variety of consonant and vowel sounds, many of her words continued to be at least occasionally produced with a palatal or palatalized consonant or with a palatal vowel ([ɪ] or [i]). At 14 months, for instance, she produced *daddy* in several different forms, including [jæɪji] and [tɑɪdi]. Thus, Alice's unmarked feature for both consonants and vowels could be said to be [+palatal].

TABLE 3-8.
Japanese Default Vowel

English Word	Japanese Pronunciation
paprika	[papurika]
public	[paburikku]
pulse	[parusu]

Source: Adapted from LH Hyman. *Phonology: Theory and Analysis*. New York: Holt, Rinehart and Winston, 1975.

(Note that another possible interpretation of Alice's pattern is given later in the chapter.)

Summary

Certain linguistic structures, including speech sounds, are preferred and therefore are considered to be *unmarked*. Sounds may be either universally marked (or unmarked) or marked within a certain linguistic system. Thus, particular languages have default—highly preferred—sounds, as do particular children's phonologies.

SOUND SYSTEMS

Languages of the World

Consonant Inventories
Many of the phonetic universals given previously referred to sounds that tend to pattern similarly within a language (i.e., to classes of sounds). Sound classes share features; the sounds that share certain features tend to behave in similar ways within a given language. Sound **systems** of languages are not random; usually, they are quite predictable.

Inventories in the languages of the world range from 6 to 95 consonants in size. The average number of consonants per language is 22.8 (Crystal, 1987). Rice and Avery (1995) stated that small consonant inventories, in particular, tend to be very similar, including mostly the least marked segments. As the phonetic inventories of some languages expand over time, different languages may elaborate different aspects of the initial repertoire. Each language tends to use the new sound features that it has adopted in as many combinations with other features as possible, making maximum use of the available features (Lindblom et al., 1993). The set of stops used in English, which follows the universals given earlier for stops in that it includes a voicing contrast and three places of articulation, is a case in point, as shown in Table 3-9.

This table contains no holes; every stop place of articulation is used in combination with both values of the feature [voice]. The set of English fricatives, shown in Table 3-10, is similar.

Word shapes that follow the rules of the language but just do not happen to occur (e.g., *blick* in English) are called **lexical accidental gaps** (Hyman, 1975). A similar term—**phonological accidental gaps**—can be used for holes in sound

TABLE 3-9.
English Stops

	Labial	Alveolar	Velar
Voiced	b	d	g
Voiceless	p	t	k

TABLE 3-10.
English Fricatives

	Labiodental	Interdental	Alveolar	Palatal
Voiced	v	ð	z	ʒ
Voiceless	f	θ	s	ʃ

TABLE 3-11.
Swiss German Vowels

	Front Rounded		Back Rounded	
High	ü			u
Mid		ö	o	
Low		?	ɔ	

Note: Boldface question mark indicates the accidental gap in these dialects.
Source: Adapted from T Bynon. *Historical Linguistics.* Cambridge: Cambridge University Press, 1977.

classes. Accidental gaps that occur in sound systems are believed to be easier to fill in (i.e., to learn or to borrow from another language) than are sounds that do not fit an existing pattern. For example, [ʒ] has not been used in English for long, as illustrated by the small number of words that incorporate this sound and by the exotic sound of some of them (*garage, mirage, rouge, Zsa Zsa*, etc.). In fact, some American dialects still have not added this sound to their systems and, therefore, speakers of these dialects pronounce *garage*, for instance, as [gərɑdʒ] instead of [gərɑʒ]. This sound was added to the English sound repertoire through contact with other languages (especially French; Bynon, 1977). It was relatively easy for English to add [ʒ] to its repertoire because this sound represented an accidental gap. English already had an almost-full set of voiced and voiceless fricatives, including a voiceless palatal ([ʃ]). Adding a voiced palatal to complete the series of voiced fricatives was far more natural than it would be to add a voiced palatal fricative to a language with no other voiced fricatives (or no other palatal fricatives) at all.

This latter type of case, in which an entire sound class is missing, is called a **systematic gap**. The word-level parallel is the set of words that do not occur in a language because they violate its phonological rules (such as *bnick* in English; Hyman, 1975).

In another case of sound borrowing, English has loaned [ŋ] to French to fill in an accidental gap in its system (perhaps in repayment of the [ʒ] loan). Previously, both the nasals [m] and [n] were present in French, as were the velars [g] and [k], but the velar nasal [ŋ] was absent. Then, this sound was borrowed from English in words such as *dancing* and *smoking*, which are now French nouns corresponding to *dance hall* and *smoking jacket* in American English (Bynon, 1977).[5] Languages do resist additions to their sound repertoires but usually are far less resistant if the sound in question is an accidental gap rather than a systematic gap. Lindblom et al. (1993) have hypothesized that an economical phonological system

with no gaps is learned more quickly than is a disorganized collection of sounds.

Vowel Inventories
Like consonant inventories, vowel inventories also may be more receptive to new members that will make them more symmetrical. In the German dialect spoken in northeastern Switzerland, for example, both back and front rounded vowels occur, but the dialect contains one accidental gap, marked by a question mark in Table 3-11. This accidental gap—a low front rounded vowel—has been filled in some dialects, such as that spoken in the town of Kesswil (Bynon, 1977).[6]

Vowel systems are patterned so commonly that predictions can be made about which specific vowels a language will have on the basis of the number of vowels it has. For instance, most languages with only three vowels have exactly those three vowels that make up the so-called vowel triangle: [i, ɑ, u]. These three vowels are quite distinctive with respect to perception and articulation, yet do not require extreme effort to produce. Because of their articulatory positions toward the extremes of the vowel space, they often are labeled **corner vowels**. Like the sink, stove, and refrigerator of the much-acclaimed "kitchen work triangle," each is easy to reach, yet does not interfere with any other's function. In addition, Stevens (1972, 1989) proposed that the acoustic qualities of these vowels are less affected by slight changes in articulation than are the acoustic qualities of more central vowels. Thus, speakers can articulate more sloppily when producing these corner vowels and still be understood clearly.

However, languages with three-vowel systems make up less than 6% of the languages of the world. The most common vowel system contains five vowels; approximately 21% of the world's languages have opted for such a system (Maddieson, 1984). These five vowels almost always are spaced in such a way as to maximize articulatory and perceptual distinctiveness, leaving as few gaps as possible. The most common configuration for a five-vowel system also is a triangle. More than 90% of the five-vowel systems studied by Maddieson and Precoda (1989) had the set of vowels illustrated in Table 3-12.

---

[5]For example, "Il va au dancing" means "He is going to the dance hall"; "Il met son smoking" means "He puts on his smoking jacket"; the words *parking* and *camping* have been adapted in similar ways.

[6]Note that [o] is not produced quite as far back as is [u], and [ö] not quite as far forward as is [ü], and so on; hence, the staggered pattern within each column.

TABLE 3-12.
Five-Vowel System

	Front	Central	Back
High	i		u
Mid		e	o
Low		a	

Source: Adapted from I Maddieson, K Precoda. Updating UPSID. *Journal of the Acoustic Society of America* 1989;86:S19.

Note that although [e] is considered to be a [front] vowel, it is not articulated as far front as [i]; similarly, [o] is not articulated as far back as [u]. Thus, these vowels do fall into a rough triangle shape in terms of their production locations within the oral cavity.

The English vowel system includes far more elements, but it also forms a slightly flattened triangular shape, as shown previously in Table 3-4. In English, the nonlow (i.e., high and mid) vowels pattern together, and the low vowels pattern together. For example, all the nonlow front vowels are unrounded, and they occur in tense-lax pairs (i.e., [i]–[ɪ] and [e]–[ɛ]). All the nonlow back vowels are rounded, and they also occur in tense-lax pairs (i.e., [u]–[ʊ] and [o]–[ɔ].) None of the low vowels is either rounded or paired.

Summary
Sound systems are not random collections of sounds that are easy to articulate or perceive. Each language tends to maximize the use of the features that it has selected by incorporating sounds with all possible combinations of those features. Combinations that could but do not happen to occur in that language's phonology are called *accidental gaps* and are more likely to be borrowed from other languages. Entire sound classes that are not present in a particular phonology are termed *systematic gaps* and are far less subject to borrowing.

Child Phonology

Consonant Inventories
Stoel-Gammon (1985) studied the phonetic inventories of children from 9 to 24 months and reported on the development of those inventories from the onset of words (which ranged from 15 to 24 months) to age 2. As indicated previously, her subjects' inventories generally followed the developmental progression proposed by Dinnsen (1992). It is interesting to look at the detail of her subjects' consonant development over time (Table 3-13). This table illustrates that the subjects did not simply acquire individual sounds in a random order; their consonant repertoires appeared to develop in a patterned manner.

Although these children had many systematic gaps to fill, they appeared to do so in a patterned manner that took advantage of accidental gaps whenever possible. Note, for instance, that when nasals first appeared, they occurred at the places of articulation that already had been used for

TABLE 3-13.
Phonetic Inventories: 9–24 Months

	Labial	Alveolar	Velar	Glottal
15 mos				
Stop (voiced)	b	d		
Fricative				h
18 mos				
Stop (voiced)	b	d		
Nasal	m	n		
Glide	w			
Fricative				h
21 mos				
Stop				
(voiced)	b	d		
(voiceless)		t		
Nasal	m	n		
Glide	w			
Fricative				h
24 mos				
Stop				
(voiced)	b	d	g	
(voiceless)		t	k	
Nasal	m	n		
Glide	w			
Fricative	f	s		h

Source: Adapted from C Stoel-Gammon. Phonetic inventories, 15–24 months: A longitudinal study. *Journal of Speech and Hearing Research* 1985;28:505–512.

voiced stops, as did fricatives later.[7] Similarly, when the velar place of articulation was introduced, both voiced and voiceless features (already in use for [d] and [t]) were applied.

Grunwell (1985) proposed a stage model of phonetic development that also demonstrates this concept of a patterned phonetic repertoire in which most (if not all) features available at each stage are used fully. Added phones share some of the features of the old phones and, as new features are added, the new combinatorial possibilities are exploited. Table 3-14 (adapted from her Developmental Assessment worksheet) illustrates this filling of the phonetic repertoire. (Note that sounds in parentheses are considered to be emerging.)

Although these and other phonologists (e.g., Robb & Bleile, 1994) report slightly different patterns of acquisition for the phonetic repertoire of English, they agree on the notion that children acquire sounds in a patterned manner, not randomly. Also, within Dinnsen's 1992 hierarchy of levels of phonetic development, it is important to note that the first task appears to be that of filling one systematic gap at a time (voiced stops, then fricatives or affricates, then liquids, etc.). By the time they reach level E, however, children (in Dinnsen's view) are dealing primarily with accidental gaps: adding more liquids, fricatives, or affricates to a system that already includes some members of each of these classes.

How does one child's acquisition pattern compare to these reports based on larger groups of children? Did Timmy, the child mentioned earlier (and in Vihman et al.,

---

[7]Technically, [f] is labiodental but, as no strictly labial fricative exists in English, these two places of articulation are considered together.

TABLE 3-14.
Development of Phonetic Inventories

Stage	Age (yrs; mos)		Labial	Alveolar	Velar	Glottal
				Phonetic Repertoire		
II	1;6–2;0					
		Stop				
		(voiced)	b	d		
		(voiceless)	p	t		
		Nasal	m	n		
		Glide	w			
III	2;0–2;6					
		Stop				
		(voiced)	b	d	(g)	
		(voiceless)	p	t	(k)	
		Nasal	m	n	(ŋ)	
		Glide	w			
		Fricative/affricate				
		(voiceless)				(h)
IV	2;6–3;0					
		Stop				
		(voiced)	b	d	g	
		(voiceless)	p	t	k	
		Nasal	m	n	ŋ	
		Glide	w	j		
		Fricative/affricate				
		(voiceless)	f	s		(h)
		Liquid		(l)		
V	3;0–3;6					
		Stop				
		(voiced)	b	d	g	
		(voiceless)	p	t	k	
		Nasal	m	n	ŋ	
		Glide	w	j		
		Fricative/affricate				
		(voiceless)	f	s	ʃ,tʃ	(h)
		Liquid		l		
VI	3;6–4;6					
		Stop				
		(voiced)	b	d	g	
		(voiceless)	p	t	k	
		Nasal	m	n	ŋ	
		Glide	w	j		
		Fricative/affricate				
		(voiced)	v	z	dʒ	
		(voiceless)	f	s	ʃ,tʃ	h
		Liquid		l	(r)	
VII	4;6+					
		Stop				
		(voiced)	b	d	g	
		(voiceless)	p	t	k	
		Nasal	m	n	ŋ	
		Glide	w	j		
		Fricative/affricate				
		(voiced)	v ð	z	(ʒ), dʒ	
		(voiceless)	f θ	s	ʃ,tʃ	h
		Liquid		l r		

Source: Adapted from P Grunwell. *Phonological Assessment of Child Speech (PACS)*. San Diego: College Hill, 1985.

1986, 1994), acquire the sounds of English in a patterned manner? The developmental progression given in Table 3-15 illustrates his somewhat random-looking initial phonetic repertoire and its gradual patterned expansion into a system that exploited more fully the possible combinations of available features.

Although Timmy seemed to start out somewhat randomly, from 15 months on, new sounds appeared to be added in sets. At 15 months, two systematic gaps were filled: two palatals ([j] and [ɨ]) were added; [ɨ] also shared the approximant class with the new bilabial [β]. At 15½ months, an accidental gap was filled: The existing features [labial] and [nasal] were combined to yield [m]. At 16 months, the existing features [alveolar] and [–voice] were combined to fill an accidental gap with [t]. Further, at 16½ months, the accidental gap formed by the combination of the [glide] and the [labial] features was filled with [w].

Vowel Inventories

Some studies have shown that the vowel repertoires to which children have been exposed have exerted an influence on the babble vowel space by age 10 months (de Boysson-Bardies et al., 1986). As children enter the period of word production, their vowel inventories, like their consonant inventories, tend to grow in a patterned manner, mirroring the shapes of adult vowel systems. Timmy's vowel repertoire, for example, developed into a predictable three-vowel system. His only vowel was [ɑ] in all words from 12 to 15½ months. Finally, at 16 months, he produced some words with [i] and, at 16½ months, he also added [u]. Thus, just as in the majority of languages that have three-vowel systems, Timmy's early three-vowel system at 16 months included the three corner vowels, [ɑ, i, u].

Otomo and Stoel-Gammon (1992) stated (on the basis of a review of the literature) that these three unmarked (i.e., universally preferred) corner vowels often are acquired early in children who are developing normally. Their own study of the acquisition of the English unrounded vowels (/i, ɪ, e, ɛ, æ, ɑ/) of six normally developing children from ages 22 to 30 months confirmed the early development of [i] and [ɑ]. (The rounded vowel /u/ was not studied.)

Stoel-Gammon and Herrington (1990) compared the vowel systems of two children with NFPs to those of another group of children who were developing normally. All of these children, like the children discussed previously, showed earlier acquisition and higher accuracy rates for corner vowels. However, the authors also reported early acquisition and high accuracy for [o] for both groups of children. Their findings indicated that unstressed vowels (e.g., [ə]) caused difficulty for children with NFPs but not for children with normally developing phonologies. This possibility is currently under investigation by Velleman and Shriberg (in preparation) for children with developmental verbal dyspraxia (DVD).

Pollock and Keiser (1990) also studied the vowel errors of 15 children with NFP. Among their subjects, /i, u, ɔ/ most often were produced correctly (more than 95% of the time). The vowels /ɑ/ and /o/ also had high accuracy rates (in excess of 90%). These investigators additionally performed analyses of the children's productions of diphthongs and rhotic vowels—vowels that are colored by a following [r] (e.g., bird, [bɚd]; store, [stoɚ]). These vowel types are far less common among the languages of the world (and therefore considered to be marked) and were especially difficult for the children with NFPs to produce accurately.

In a follow-up study, Pollock and Hall (1991) studied the vowel productions of five children between ages 8 and 11 who had received diagnoses of DVD. These children also exhibited particular difficulty with the marked rhotic vowels and diphthongs. Among the less marked vowels, /ɑ/ most often was produced correctly (100%), with accuracy rates also above 90% for /i, o, ɔ, ʌ/.

In a similar study of younger children (ages 2–7 years), Velleman et al. (1991) compared a group of phonologically delayed and disordered children with many characteristics of DVD versus a group of children

TABLE 3-15.
"Timmy"'s Phonetic Repertoire

Age (mos)		*Labial*	*Alveolar*	*Velar*	*Glottal*
		Phonetic Repertoire			
9–10	Stop	b			
11–13	Stop				
	Voiced	b			
	Voiceless			k	
14	Stop				
	Voiced	b			
	Voiceless			k	
	Glide			j	
15	Stop				
	Voiced	b			
	Voiceless			k	
	Nasal		n		
	Glide			j	
	Approximant				
	Voiced	β		ʝ	
15½	Stop				
	Voiced	b			
	Voiceless			k	
	Nasal	m	n		
	Glide			j	
	Approximant				
	Voiced	β		ʝ	
16	Stop				
	Voiced	b			
	Voiceless		t	k	
	Nasal	m	n		
	Glide			j	
	Approximant				
	Voiced	β		ʝ	
16½	Stop				
	Voiced	b			
	Voiceless		t	k	
	Nasal	m	n		
	Glide	w		j	
	Approximant				
	Voiced	β		ʝ	

Source: Adapted from MM Vihman, SL Velleman, L McCune. How abstract is child phonology? Towards an integration of linguistic and psychological approaches. In Yavas M (ed). *First and Second Language Phonology*. San Diego: Singular, 1994, 9–44.

who were also delayed or disordered phonologically but with few such characteristics. In keeping with the Pollock studies, they also reported particularly high error rates on rhotic vowels (except for the simplest rhotic, [ɚ]) and on diphthongs for all the children. No errors were reported for /i/; few were reported for /ʌ, ɚ, u, ɑ/. Furthermore, [ɑ] was the vowel that served most often as a substitute for incorrect vowels. The children with many (more than 14) characteristics of DVD had higher vowel error rates (as measured by vowel deviations on the *Assessment of Phonological Processes, Revised* [APP-R]; Hodson, 1986), but their actual *patterns* of errors did not differ substantially from those of the children with functional phonological delay or disorder.

Summary

Like those of adult languages, children's sound systems are not random collections of sounds that are easy to articulate or perceive. Each child's system tends to maximize the use of the features that already are available by incorporating sounds with all possible combinations of those features. When a new feature (e.g., [nasal] or [velar]) is learned, the entire class of sounds associated with that feature (in combination with existing features) typically is learned at once. In other words, the child tends spontaneously to fill all accidental gaps created by the addition of a new feature.

Children's early vowel systems tend to mirror the simplest vowel systems of the languages of the world. The corner vowels [i, u, ɑ] that usually occur in languages with simple three-vowel systems typically are produced earlier and more accurately by young children, children with NFPs, and children with DVD. Other back vowels (e.g., [o, ɔ]) also appear to be acquired sooner than are front vowels ([e, ɛ]) by all these groups of English-speaking children.

DISTRIBUTION REQUIREMENTS

Languages of the World

Most languages have rules about the phones or types of phones that can occur in various positions in the word, especially syllable-initial and syllable-final position. In English, for instance, [ŋ] does not occur in syllable-initial position. Furthermore, the language restricts the vowels that can occur in open syllables word-finally. English [ɪ], [ɛ], and [ʊ] are not permitted in word-final position, whereas [i] (*knee*), [e] (*neigh*), [u] (*new*), [o] (*no*), [ɔ] (*gnaw*), and [ɑ] (*spa*) are permitted. The low front vowel [æ] is borderline; it occurs mostly in slang, colloquial, and baby-talk contexts, such as *yeah* for *yes*, *nah* for *no*, *dada* for *daddy*, and the like. Monty Python took advantage of the restriction on word-final [ɪ] in "Monty Python and the Holy Grail" (Columbia Pictures Home Entertainment, 1974). The Knights of Nih terrorize people by saying [nɪ] to them, which is funny (or terrifying?) because it is not a phonotactically permissible word in English.[8] Later in the movie, the knights switch to saying, "[ɛkɪ ɛkɪ ɛkɪ ɛkɪ fkɔŋ zupɔɪŋ]," which includes both word-final [ɪ] and the nonpermissible initial cluster #fk-.

Beckman (1995, 1996) illustrated that certain features may be more protected from loss in certain positions of words. In Shona (a Bantu language spoken in Zimbabwe), for example, high vowels are protected from vowel harmony in initial position only (Beckman, 1995). In Tamil, coronal sonorants are protected from assimilation only in initial position (Beckman, 1996). Beckman (1995) suggested that, in other languages, privileged positions (in which harmony will not occur) may include final syllables, stressed syllables, or long vowels.

Additionally, constraints may limit the consonants that can co-occur. For example, skw- is allowed in English, but

spw- and stw- are not. In fact, one of the most commonly cited examples of cluster constraints (i.e., distribution requirements that affect clusters) in English is that of initial triple-consonant clusters. If three consonants occur in sequence at the beginning of a word in English, the first must be [s], the second must be a voiceless stop ([p, t, k]), and the third must be a liquid or a glide ([r, l, j, w]). Actually, the rule is even more specific than that, as restrictions limit the liquids and glides that can follow certain voiceless stops in such a cluster. Akmajian et al. (1984) pointed out that if the second consonant is [t], the third must be [r], as #stl- and #stw- are not permitted; in some dialects, #stj- is allowed, as in British *stew*. This particular part of the rule is especially interesting for three reasons. First, #tw- is permitted at the beginning of a word, but #stw- is not; *twin* is allowed, but *stwin* is not. Second, this -stw- cluster is permitted in medial position where two morphemes adjoin, as in *westward*. Finally, many children appear to violate this restriction by producing #stw- clusters (e.g., in [stwɪŋ] for *string*). Whether the first two factors may influence children to assume at some point in their phonological development that #stw- should be an approved cluster is an open question. (See Chapter 4 for a discussion of whether these substitutions of [w] for /r/ are actually target /w/s within the child's phonological system.)

Other languages have very different phonotactic constraints (distribution requirements) for initial consonant clusters. Spanish, for example, does not allow initial [s] + stop clusters but does allow them in medial position. For that reason, Spanish speakers tend to epenthesize a vowel before these clusters when they speak English, making the clusters medial instead of initial. This tendency leads to such stereotypical productions as "I a-speak a-Spanish" ([ɑɪ əspik əspænɪʃ]; Hyman, 1975). German, on the other hand, allows types of clusters different from those of English, such as the ʃw- and -pf clusters (as in *Schwarzkopf*) mentioned in Chapter 2. Americans tend to simplify these clusters to make saying them more comfortable.

Clusters similar to allowed clusters often make their way into our language, but they still sound odd and may be more likely to be adopted with humorous meanings. This may account, for instance, for the Yiddish words that have and have not been assimilated into American culture. In standard English, for instance, [ʃ] is not allowed in an initial cluster with either the sonorant [m] or the obstruent [v], but it (or a very similar retroflex fricative) is allowed before the sonorant [r], as in *shrub*. Sm- is allowed in initial position, but sv- is not. Thus, ʃm- is similar to allowed clusters (ʃr- and sm-), but ʃv- is somewhat more distant.[9] This distinction may explain, at least in part, why such words as *shmooze* and *schmaltzy* have been adopted into colloquial English, whereas other words, such as *shver* (difficult), *shviger* (mother-in-law), and *shvitz* (sweat) have not. Many Yiddish words with similar borderline clusters and humorous meanings have been adopted into American slang (e.g., *schlock, shlemiel, shlep, shnook, shnoz*). The *shm-* cluster also has been adopted as a marker of sarcasm, as in "Clus-

---

[8]The vowel [ɪ] may be permissible word-finally in one of the dialects of British English. This possibility does not alter its marginal status within the language as a whole. Depending on the view that other British English speakers have of the speakers of this particular dialect, their use of this sound may even confirm to others its marginal status.

[9]English has borrowed a few Greek words that begin with *sf* ("sph"), but only three are in general use: *sphere, sphincter, sphinx*.

TABLE 3-16.
Child Voicing Constraints

pig	[bɪt]
big	[bɪt]
fork	[bɔt]
Bob	[bap]
soup	[dup]
talk	[dɔt]
dog	[dat]
cot	[dat]
cup	[dəp]
shed	[dɛt]

Source: Adapted from P Grunwell. *Clinical Phonology.* Rockville, MD: Aspen, 1982.

TABLE 3-17.
"Molly"'s Final Nasal Constraint

button	[paⁿnə]
down	[taŋə], [daʊnə]
round	[hanʌ]
Brian	[panə], [pani]
hand	[hanɛ]

Source: Adapted from MM Vihman, SL Velleman. Phonological reorganization: A case study. *Language and Speech* 1989;32:149–170.

ter, shmuster!" Words with clusters that are farther out and words that are not humorous are rejected (e.g., *shtuss, shtarker, shmaktes, shlaff;* see Naiman, 1981, for definitions and a humorous introduction to Yiddish English).

Dialects within the same language may differ also in the clusters that they allow. Some Southerners, for example, avoid the -*kl* cluster and may use various strategies to simplify it. The best-known instance is the pronunciation of *nuclear* as [nukjələ-] rather than [nuklijə-] in some dialects. Some speakers of African-American English dialects avoid -*sk-* and tend to metathesize (reverse the order of) the [s] and the [k] to yield a preferable cluster, as in [æks] for *ask* and [bæksɪt] for *basket.*

Several phonologists have proposed that the order of consonants in clusters (and indeed, the positioning of all sounds within words) is dependent, at least in part, on a **sonority hierarchy.** Sonority is the "degree of opening of the vocal apparatus during production, or the relative amount of energy produced during the sound" (Goldsmith, 1990, p. 110). The most sonorant segments (i.e., vowels) occur in the middle of the syllable, with segments of decreasing sonority toward the edges, so that the least sonorant segments (i.e., stops) are at syllable boundaries. Sonority progresses from vowels, which are the most sonorant, through glides, liquids, nasals, fricatives, and affricates to stops, the least sonorant.

If clusters were bound by this hierarchy, such initial clusters as *pl-* and *sm-* and such final clusters as -*rk,* and -*nt* would be allowed, but such clusters as initial *lt-* or final -*pm* would not. In fact, these statements are true of English and many other languages. Unfortunately, [s] breaks the rules in English (and some other languages): Such clusters as initial *sk-* and final -*ks* should not occur, as [s] is more sonorous than is [k] and therefore should be closer to the middle of the syllable. However, the sonority hierarchy does explain many of the cluster patterns observed around the world (Goldsmith, 1990).

Child Phonology

Many authors have explored children's preferences for certain features in certain positions. Some, such as

Edwards (1996), Macken (1996), and Velleman (1996b), have stressed the importance of edges of words in this regard (i.e., these preferences tend to occur in either initial or final, not medial position). Default consonants, in contrast, tend to occur in medial position (Priestly, 1977; Stemberger, 1993; Velleman, 1996b).

Some very young or very disordered children may have very simple distribution constraints, such as allowing voiced consonants only in initial position and voiceless consonants only in final position. Grunwell (1982) provides an example (Table 3-16).

Another common pattern is for stops to occur in initial position, whereas fricatives occur in final position (Dinnsen, 1996a; Edwards, 1996; Farwell, 1976; Fikkert, 1994). Additionally, velars may occur in final but not initial position in some children's phonological systems (Ingram, 1974). Although they are by no means universal (Stoel-Gammon, 1985), constraints of these types are common in both normal and disordered child phonologies.

Some children have less common types of distribution requirements. As discussed earlier, Japanese has a constraint against certain types of (non-nasal) consonants in final position; epenthesis of [u] is used to fix loan words that end with such consonants (e.g., *public* is pronounced as [pabɯrikkɯ]; Hyman, 1975). "Molly," the child studied by Vihman and Velleman (1989), also had a restriction on final consonants from 13½ to 15 months. This restriction included a constraint against final nasals. Usually, she repaired such words by epenthesizing her own default neutral vowel, as the examples in Table 3-17 (slightly simplified) illustrate.[10]

Other global types of child distribution requirements have been studied more systematically by a few investigators, including Macken (1996) and Velleman (1996b). Such requirements are reflected in child word recipes, such as that of Berman's "Shelli" (1977), who used metathesis to make her words fit a velar-first pattern (e.g., [gabi] for *buggy,* [kibi] for *piggie,* and [god] for *dog;* discussed at length in Chapter 2).

In addition to their limits on the number of adjacent consonants and the locations of clusters, children may

---

[10]Fikkert (1994) suggested that this epenthesis of final vowels could be the child's way of achieving trochaic (strong syllable + weak syllable) word patterns. However, such bisyllabic words as *button* and *Brian* already have trochaic forms and, therefore, should not undergo this transformation as do the monosyllabic words. Therefore, Fikkert's analysis cannot account for all of Molly's pattern.

TABLE 3-18.
Acquisition of Clusters

Cluster Type	Approximate Age of Acquisition (yrs; mos)
Stop + [w]	4
Stop + [l], fl-	5;6
[s] + stop, nasal, glide, or liquid; stop + [r] and fr-	6
Three elements; θr-	7–9

Source: Adapted from AB Smit, L Hand, JJ Freilinger, et al. The Iowa articulation norms project and its Nebraska replication. *Journal of Hearing and Speech Disorders* 1990;55:779–798; and SB Chin, DA Dinnsen. Consonant clusters in disordered speech: Constraints and correspondence patterns. *Journal of Child Language* 1992;19:259–286.

also have restrictions on co-occurrences of particular consonants with each other. According to Grunwell (1981, 1997), initial obstruent + approximant clusters (e.g., *pl-, dr-, kw-*) are acquired between ages 2½ and 4 years. She indicated that initial consonant clusters composed of /s/ + another consonant are mastered slightly later, between 3 and 4 years. Other researchers (e.g., Chin & Dinnsen, 1992; Smit et al., 1990) have found that English word-initial clusters tend to be acquired on the timetable given in Table 3-18. Thus, the English clusters that violate the sonority hierarchy ([s] + stop) are not reported to be acquired later than other [s] clusters.

Correct production of consonant clusters does appear to be predicted by markedness in many English-speaking children, however. Bleile (1995) stated that the consonant acquired earliest (typically, the least marked) will remain when others are omitted. Both Ingram (1989) and Chin and Dinnsen (1992) suggested that the marked member of a two-element cluster is more likely to be omitted than is the unmarked member. Thus, English-speaking children tend to omit the first element, [s], in [s] + stop clusters (e.g., [dɑp] for *stop*; [dɛk] for *desk*). In contrast, they omit the second element, the liquid, in word-initial stop + liquid clusters (e.g., [gɑk] for *clock*). Although some English-speaking children may delete the unmarked member of a cluster while preserving the marked member, it is rare and brief, according to Ingram (1989). Individual children's consonant cluster repertoires will be determined by such phonotactic factors as the word position and the allowable number of consecutive consonants and by such phonetic factors as the specific consonants or consonant features available in the child's phonetic repertoire (Chin & Dinnsen, 1992; McLeod et al., 1997). Lleó and Prinz (1996), however, reported differences for different language groups as well. For target initial stop + sonorant consonant clusters, for example, German-speaking children preserve the stop, whereas Spanish-speaking children preserve the sonorant. The same holds true for medial obstruent + sonorant clusters. Thus, language-specific factors may override sonority or markedness.

Summary: The Acquisition of Phonetic Inventories

According to Lindblom et al. (1993), the order and process of phonetic development is affected by several factors, including ease of production and markedness, the language to which the child is being exposed, and the system on which the child has to build at any time. In the child's preexisting system, important aspects that may impact on further learning include the combinatorial possibilities of the elements (both features and phones) that the child already has learned.

IMPLICATIONS OF PHONETIC TENDENCIES FOR INTERVENTION

Why should speech-language pathologists care about phonetic tendencies among the adult languages of the world? First of all, those sounds that are most universal can be assumed to be easier to perceive or articulate (or both) than are those that are rare. Markedness has been shown to predict order of acquisition of vowels, singleton consonants, and consonant clusters, at least partially. Therefore, unmarked sounds and clusters can be assumed to be better targets for early remediation, and the phonologies of children who acquire marked sounds first (e.g., some children with dyspraxia) possibly may be considered deviant.

Second, as described previously, the kinds of sound repertoires that tend to occur in languages with consonant or vowel inventories smaller than those in English may occur in early stages of the development of English phonology. Systems of this sort should be cause for less concern than are systems that do not conform to universal tendencies.

Third, the tendency for all sound systems to be orderly—using the features that are relevant within the language to their maximum and being more receptive to new sounds that fill accidental rather than systematic gaps—is reflected in children's sound systems as well. Speech-language pathologists can capitalize on this tendency in choosing remediation targets. The clinician should work toward sound systems that are organized in keeping with universal phonetic tendencies. Intervention goals should be chosen to fill accidental gaps first, using all possible combinations of existing features within the child's system. Furthermore, children who lack the corner vowels [i, ɑ, u] or whose vowel systems are uneven (e.g., all low vowels, no back vowels) should be encouraged to fill out their vowel repertoires.

In 1982, Schwartz and Leonard demonstrated that children are more likely to attempt new words if the words share the phonological characteristics of their individual lexicons. The children more often tried to say these "in" words in imitation, and they learned to use them spontaneously in fewer sessions than it took for them to learn the "out" words that did not fit their own current systems. In 1987, Schwartz et al. extended this finding, demonstrating that words containing consonants that the child has attempted but never produced correctly are attempted and learned as reluctantly as out words that contain consonants

TABLE 3-19.
"Alice"'s Palatal Pattern

no	[njæ]
bottle	[bœjœ]
dolly	[dɑli]
elephant	[ʔɑɪ], [ʔɛni]
Bonnie	[bɑɲi]
Daddy	[tædi], [jæɪji]

Source: Adapted from MM Vihman, SL Velleman, L McCune. How abstract is child phonology? Towards an integration of linguistic and psychological approaches. In Yavas M (ed). *First and Second Language Phonology*. San Diego: Singular, 1994, 9–44.

TABLE 3-20.
"Emma"'s Labial-Alveolar Pattern

berry, bird, booster	[bu:di:]
pillow, playdough	[be:də]
elephant	[ɑbi:n]
airplane	[ɑpi:n]
tomato	[me:nə]
raisin	[we:di:]
happy birthday, cranberry, raspberry	[ɑbu:di:]

Source: Adapted from EW Goodell, M Studdert-Kennedy. Articulatory organization in early words: From syllable to phoneme. In de Boysson-Bardies B, de Schonen S, Jusczyk P, MacNeilage P, Morton J (eds). *Proceedings of XIIth International Congress of Phonetic Sciences, Vol. 4.* Aix-en-Provence, France: Université de Provence, 1991, 166–169; and M Studdert-Kennedy, EW Goodell. Gestures, features, and segments in early child speech. *Haskins Laboratories Status Report on Speech Research* 1992;SR-111/112:1–14.

that the child has never attempted. Only those words that contain sounds that the child already has produced successfully are attempted earlier and more successfully.

Unfortunately, this study has not been extended to examine words with in and out *features*. However, it seems likely that child phonologies will be more receptive to sounds that include only—or mostly—features that they already have mastered rather than sounds that include features that they have not produced successfully. The former type of sounds would fill accidental gaps, which is far easier to accomplish. Therefore, in determining remediation goals for children with limited sound repertoires, speech-language pathologists should identify the children's accidental gaps and attempt to plug them first. Addressing accidental gaps typically is far easier than attempting to add systematic gap elements, which do not fit within the child's existing system. Eventually, of course, systematic gaps also must be addressed. When systematic gaps are to be the goals, such developmental feature hierarchies as Dinnsen's (given earlier) should be used to select the sound class to be targeted.

A further concept that could be explored within this same framework would be to study in versus out **articulatory gestures**. For instance, if children already have a word containing a front-to-back articulation pattern (e.g., labial followed by velar consonants), would it be easier to teach them additional words with this front-to-back articulation pattern, even if the words do not contain exactly the same sounds or features? In other words, is it the sounds or features themselves that determine a word's in or out status, or is it the articulatory movement pattern that underlies the sequence of sounds or features?

One child studied by Vihman (1992) and Vihman et al. (1994) demonstrated an acquisition pattern that could be described either in terms of default features (see "Children's Markedness and Defaults") or in terms of articulatory gestures. This child, Alice, frequently used the palatal glide [j] between vowels in her babble. When she began to produce words, she incorporated palatalization into them (Table 3-19). With respect to consonants, she achieved palatalization by using [j] and other palatal and palatalized consonants (e.g., the palatal nasal [ɲ], as in *canyon*). With respect to vowels, Alice used nonlow front (palatal) vowels, such as [i] and [œ]. The latter is a rounded mid-front vowel that normally does not occur in English; it is a

vowel sound that Americans often make when they are imitating a Swedish accent. Alice's use of this sound, then, indicated that she was motivated more by her preferred patterns than by her listener's needs.

Note that these words are fairly different from each other in their actual phonetic forms; yet, all share a palatal nucleus. Thus, for this child at least, the organizational basis for word forms may not be either particular phones or features in the traditional sense but a palatal articulatory gesture.

In her babble, "Emma," another child who has been described by Goodell and Studdert-Kennedy (1991) and Studdert-Kennedy and Goodell (1992), exhibited a pattern of lip versus tongue closant alternations. Some babbles began with consonants and others with vowels, and vowel quality, nasality, utterance duration, and other features varied considerably from one vocalization to the next. However, all contained this lip-tongue-tip alternation pattern, as in the following examples:

[ɑbi:nɑbi:nɑbi:nɑbi:n]
[be:dəbe:dəbe:dəbe:də]

When she began producing words, Emma is reported to have learned a majority of words that fit the articulatory gestural pattern of her favorite babble and to have altered other words to fit this same pattern better (Table 3-20).

Notice that, like Alice's words, these words contained a variety of actual consonant and vowel features and sounds; the consistency lay in the general movement pattern of her mouth. For Emma, like Alice, word production may have been organized around an articulatory gesture rather than around features or sounds per se. Babble may be the source of such articulatory gestures; Jaeger (1997); Lindblom et al. (1993); Menn (1978a, 1983); and McCune and Vihman (1987) also noted babble subroutines, or **vocal motor schemes**, that form the basis for early word learning.

Whatever the basis for such patterns, it is clear that children's preferences have a strong impact on their developing lexicons. By tuning in to the child's system, often it is possible to make an educated guess about aspects of the system that may or may not be ready for change. By accepting the child's most fundamental constraints or preferences (e.g., word recipes), but pushing the limits of the aspects of the child's pattern that are more vulnerable (e.g., accidental gaps), change can be achieved.

In summary, studies have shown that children are more open to attempting to produce words that are consistent with their current phonetic systems than words that contain unknown sounds. However, it is important to remember that phonetic systems operate on several levels: Features, phones, and even more comprehensive articulatory gesture patterns may be key to determining what is in a particular child's system.

ASSESSMENT OF CHILDREN'S PHONETIC REPERTOIRES

Screening a child's production of speech sounds is quite easy using most traditional articulation tests. Assessment for intervention requires more care. To determine whether a particular sound truly has been mastered by the child, all possible word positions must be considered. This includes syllable-initial position within words (e.g., [d] in *window*), syllable-final position within words (e.g., [n] in *window*), true intervocalic position (e.g., [n] in *winnow*) and various possible positions within various possible clusters (including, for example, initial position in initial clusters, such as the [s] in *string*; medial position in medial clusters, such as the [s] in *hamster*; and final position in final clusters, such as the [s] in *flirts*), in addition to the more commonly studied initial and final word positions. The number of syllables and the stress pattern in the word also should be considered (e.g., the comparison between the two *na* syllables in *banana*). As discussed in Chapter 2, even the number of words and the intonation pattern of the utterance in which the word occurred could have an important effect. The effects of assimilation and the other whole-word phonotactic patterns also cannot be ignored; the influences of other phones within the word on the sound in question could be significant.

Obviously, such an in-depth analysis is totally prohibitive for most speech-language pathologists in terms of time. What can be done to derive a fairly representative overview of the child's phonetic repertoire without devoting one's life to the enterprise? The focus here is on independent analysis via do-it-yourself worksheets.

Consonant and Vowel Repertoires

Both articulation tests and process tests are designed for relational analysis of the child's consonant productions, comparing the presumed target sounds to the child's production. Most ignore the child's vowel repertoire. Some in-depth analyses provide appropriate means for assessing the child's consonant repertoire, but vowels typically are ignored there as well. Furthermore, in-depth analyses are quite time consuming. To get an idea of a child's phonetic repertoire more quickly, notations can be made on consonant and vowel inventories for English (Forms 3-1 and 3-2).

These forms can be used very simply by circling those sounds that the child was observed to produce during the assessment. Recall that this is independent analysis, so it does not matter whether the child's production is the same as the adult production. The question to be answered is "What speech sounds is this child capable of producing?" The question is not "Does this child produce speech sounds correctly?" The speech-language pathologist can determine the criterion for mastery, depending on the size of the sample and level of confidence in the data collected. Three occurrences in an assessment session (or set of sessions) in which the child produced at least 100 utterances, or two occurrences in at least 50 utterances if more cannot be obtained, are recommended as appropriate criteria. Those phones that never are produced should be crossed out. The others (which are neither circled nor crossed out) will be assumed to be emerging in the child's speech. If desired, the numbers of occurrences of each of these emerging sounds can be indicated with a raised numeral. (See Forms 3-1 and 3-2.)

Typically, only consonant singletons should be accounted for on this form. Consonants that occur in clusters will appear on a later form. Similarly, elements of diphthongs do not count in the single-vowel portion of the vowel form. Thus, for example, [ɔ] and [ɪ] would not be counted here if the child said, [ɔɪ]. Note also that [r] is not listed in final position on the consonant inventory as [ɚ] is considered by this author to be a rhotic *vowel* and therefore is listed on Form 3-2. This phone should be credited as a consonant in medial position only where it is a syllable onset (e.g., in the word *ma.roon*), not where it is vocalic (e.g., in the word *mur.der*).

In choosing goals based on these forms, it is important for the speech-language pathologist to remember the relevance of gaps and symmetry. The forms are laid out in a manner intended to facilitate identification of systems that are asymmetrical or that have gaps. A speech sample obtained through the administration of the APP-R (Hodson, 1986) to "Jonathan," a 5½-year-old with DVD, is used to demonstrate how these forms can be used for this purpose. This sample is given in Table 3-21 and used to generate Examples 3-1A and 3-2A.

This sample is small and is based on the APP-R words, which are slightly more heavily weighted to clusters. However, more singleton consonants are available for analysis from Jonathan's productions as he reduces most clusters. Trends observed in this analysis will be confirmed through less formal sampling procedures in therapy.

Recall that this is an *independent* analysis. In other words, Jonathan's consonant and vowel productions are not compared to the consonants and vowels of the target words. Errors are not the focus. Rather, the purpose is to identify those consonants and vowels that Jonathan actually does produce. This practice informs the clinician about the status of the boy's phonetic repertoire and about accidental and systematic gaps within his system. In this way, specific remediation goals can be identified.

Consonant Repertoire

Name: Age:
Date: Examiner:
Source of sample: Size of sample:

Note: Phones circled are mastered (i.e., occurred at least ___ times in that position in any context, whether correct or not). Phones marked with an X did not occur in any context.

	Labial	Interdental	Alveolar	Palatal	Velar	Glottal	Other/notes:
Initial							
Stops	b		d		g		
	p		t		k		
Nasals	m		n				
Glides	w			j			
Fricatives	v	ð	z	ʒ			
	f	θ	s	ʃ		h	
Affricates				tʃ, dʒ			
Liquids			l	r			
Medial							
Stops	b		d		g		
	p		t		k	ʔ	
Nasals	m		n		ŋ		
Glides	w			j			
Fricatives	v	ð	z	ʒ			
	f	θ	s	ʃ		h	
Affricates				tʃ, dʒ			
Liquids			l	r			
Final							
Stops	b		d		g		
	p		t		k	ʔ	
Nasals	m		n		ŋ		
Fricatives	v	ð	z	ʒ			
	f	θ	s	ʃ			
Affricates				tʃ, dʒ			
Liquids			l				

Note: [r] not listed in final position as [ɚ] is a rhotic **vowel**. Medially, [r] should be counted only where it is consonantal (e.g., *around*), not vocalic (e.g., *bird*).

FORM 3-1.
Consonant repertoire.

Vowel Repertoire

Name: Age:

Date: Examiner:

Source of sample: Size of sample:

Note: Phones circled are mastered (i.e., occurred at least _____ times in any context, whether correct or not). Phones marked with an X did not occur in any context.

	Front	Central	Back
Simple vowels			
High			
Tense	i		u
Lax	ɪ		ʊ
Mid			
Tense		e	o
Lax		ɛ	ɔ
Low		ʌ,ə	
	æ		ɑ

Diphthongs

ɔɪ

ɑɪ

ɑʊ

Rhotic vowels

  High

iɚ   uɚ

  Mid

ɛɚ   ɔɚ

  Low   ɚ

ɑɚ

FORM 3-2.
Vowel repertoire.

Consonant Repertoire

Name: *Jonathan*   Age: *5;6*
Date: *10/6/95*   Examiner: *SLV*
Source of sample: *APP-R*   Size of sample: *50 words*

Note: Phones circled are mastered (i.e., occurred at least ___3___ times in that position in any context, whether correct or not). Phones marked with an X did not occur in any context.

	Labial	Interdental	Alveolar	Palatal	Velar	Glottal	Other/Notes:
Initial							
Stops	ⓑ		ⓓ		ⓖ		
	X̶		X		X		
Nasals	ⓜ		n²				
Glides	ⓦ			ⓙ			
Fricatives	ⓥ	X̶	X	X			
	ⓕ	X̶	s¹	X		h²	
Affricates				X̶ʧ, X̶ʤ			
Liquids			X	X			
Medial							
Stops	ⓑ		ⓓ		g¹		
	X̶		X		X	ʔ¹	
Nasals	m¹		X		X̶		
Glides	X̶			j²			
Fricatives	v¹	X̶	X	X			
	ⓕ	X̶	X	X		X̶	
Affricates				X̶, X̶ʤ			
Liquids			X	X			
Final							
Stops	X̶		X̶		X̶		
	p²		ⓣ		ⓚ	X	
Nasals	m¹		X̶		X̶		
Fricatives	X̶	X̶	X	X			
	f²	X̶	ⓢ	ʃ²			
Affricates				X̶, X̶ʤ			
Liquids			X				

Note: [r] not listed in final position as [ɚ] is a rhotic **vowel**. Medially, [r] should be counted only where it is consonantal (*around*), not vocalic (*bird*). Superscript numbers represent numbers of occurrences of marked phones.

EXAMPLE 3-1A.
Consonant repertoire.

Vowel Repertoire

Name: *Jonathan*

Date: *10/6/95*

Source of sample: *APP-R*

Age: *5;6*

Examiner: *SLV*

Size of sample: *50 words*

Note: Phones circled are mastered (i.e., occurred at least ___3___ times in any context, whether correct or not). Phones marked with an X did not occur in any context.

	Front	Central	Back
Simple vowels			
High			
Tense	ⓘ		ⓤ
Lax	ⓘ		υ^1
Mid			
Tense	ⓔ		ⓞ
Lax	ⓔ		$\mathrm{\mathfrak{o}}^1$
Low		Ⓐ ,ⓔ	
	ⓐæ		ⓐ

Diphthongs

$\mathfrak{o}\mathrm{I}^1$

aI^1

$\mathrm{a\upsilon}^2$

Rhotic vowels

High			
	✗		✗
Mid			
	✗		✗
Low		✗	
			✗

Note: Superscript numbers indicate the numbers of occurrence of marked phones.

EXAMPLE 3-2A.
Vowel repertoire.

TABLE 3-21.
APP-R Data from "Jonathan," Age 5;6 Years

bæəs	basket	dã	nose
botʰ	boats	bes	page
dæ	candle	ɛbɪ	(air)plane
de	chair	wɪn	queen
gɑʊbɔɪʔætʰ	cowboy hat	wɑkʰ	rock
de	crayons	sæ dʌs	Santa Claus
bi	three	du dɑ	screwdriver
bæk	black	sdu	shoe
ji	green	wɑɪ	slide
jɑjo	yellow	nok	smoke
fɛbʊ	feather	nɛtʰ	snake
fɪʃ	fish	dʌp	soap
væ:	flower	bu	spoon
fɔk	fork	gɛ	square
dæ	glasses	s:tɑ	star
dʌf	glove	wi	string
gʌm	gum	wɛ:ə	sweater
hæ	hanger	dɛvɪdi	television
hɑs:	horse	ʌm	thumb
ɑs du	ice cubes	bɛbʌʃ	toothbrush
jʌp dʌt	jump rope	dʌkʰ	truck
vif	leaf	ve	vase
mæs	mask	wɑ	watch
mɑʊ	mouth	jɑjo	yoyo
mugi mætʰ	music box	jip	zipper

APP-R = *Assessment of Phonological Processes, Revised* (Hodson, 1986).

Clearly, Jonathan has a very limited repertoire of mastered consonants, although there are several more that he produces occasionally. No voiceless stops occur in initial or medial positions, and no voiced stops occur in final position. Very few fricatives are in evidence, especially voiced fricatives. Jonathan appears to have a preference for bilabials in initial and medial position but not in final position. These patterns highlight Jonathan's systematic gaps. Some of the accidental gap sounds appear to be emerging and could be encouraged through therapy: [n] and [s] in initial position, [p] and [f] in final position. Other gaps that Jonathan's speech-language pathologist might hope to fill include [z] in initial position. The systematic gap bilabials seem to be emerging together in final position. If [j] or [v] do indeed continue to develop in medial position, the clinician should be able to facilitate the accompanying glide [w] (as bilabial already is established for [b]) and the accompanying fricative [s] or [z] (as alveolar already is established for [d]). If [m] does continue to develop in final position, [n] and [ŋ] should not be far behind, given that the alveolar feature already is established for [t] and [s] and that the velar feature already is established for [k]. In general, it is encouraging that various nasals and fricatives appear to be emerging in all positions. These sound classes likely will become established without an extreme amount of effort.

Jonathan's repertoire of simple vowels is less limited. The infrequent occurrence of [ʊ] and [ɔ] in his speech may well be due to their scanty presence within the APP-R words (and within English in general). However, the APP-R does include an appropriate number of rhotic vowels, none of which were produced by this child. This represents a systematic gap in his vowel inventory.

TABLE 3-22.
Babble Sample from "Marvin" at 21 Months

ʃugɑgɑ
gɪgɪ
tʰɪtʰɪ
r::: (alveolar trill)
dɪdɪ
x:: (voiceless velar fricative)
ɪdɛwəwʊ
i:dʊjedʊɪdə
kədʌwe:
ɑʊkə
dɪʊkə
hɑɪdʊ
dʊɪ
dɑxəgɑʊgə
gəgədədə
β::: (voiced bilabial fricative)
æ::
kwɪkəkʰɪkə
kətʰɪtʰɪkətʰɪ
dʊkdʊkə
ktʃə
ɑɣɑɪgəgəgɑgə (ɣ: voiced velar fricative)
dʊkə
ɑdʊdʊkə

The same forms can be used also to examine the babble repertoires of prelinguistic children. This capability is exemplified in Examples 3-1B and 3-2B using a babble sample (given in Table 3-22) from "Marvin," a 21-month-old with hypotonia (low muscle tone). Note that essentially identical babble forms that Marvin produced several times are not listed repeatedly in the table. Also, given the smaller size of the sample, two occurrences are used as the criterion for mastery in this case. Further observation will be used to confirm these findings.

Marvin produces voiced and voiceless alveolar and velar stops in his babble, with the medial labiovelar glide [w]. No nasals and no other labials are noted; these limitations are somewhat unusual and should be monitored. Various non-English fricatives are used, especially as isolated consonants, a habit not uncommon in babble. The total lack of final consonants is not critical at this speech stage although, of course, it does constitute somewhat of a delay for Marvin's chronological age. When he begins to produce adult-based words, his phonetic repertoire will be expected to expand gradually to include more consonant types and his phonotactic repertoire to include more word shapes. For the moment, remediation efforts will focus on increasing Marvin's awareness and use of bilabials. This work will include efforts to increase his labial tone, tactile stimulation of the labial area, and modeling of attention-getting bilabial sounds (e.g., raspberries and bilabial trills), bV ([b] + vowel) syllables, and bilabial words. Efforts should be made also to increase his visual attention to others' mouths as they speak by having the speakers make interesting sounds, hold toys at mouth level, and wear bright lipstick (as appropriate).

Marvin's vowel repertoire is spread across the oral cavity, with all vowels—front, back, high, and low—occurring.

Consonant Repertoire

Name: *Marvin*   Age: *21 mos*
Date: *4/3/94*   Examiner: *SLV*
Source of sample: *babble sample* Size of sample: *50 babbles*

Note: Phones circled are mastered (i.e., occurred at least __2__ times in that position in any context, whether correct or not). Phones marked with an X did not occur in any context.

	Labial	Interdental	Alveolar	Palatal	Velar	Glottal	Other/Notes:
Initial							
Stops	X		ⓓ		ⓖ		*C's in*
	X		t¹		ⓚ		*isolation:*
Nasals	X		X				[r, x, β]
Glides	X			X			
Fricatives	X	X	X	X			
	X	X	X	ʃ¹		h¹	
Affricates				Xtʃ, Xdʒ			
Liquids			X	X			
Medial							
Stops	X		ⓓ		ⓖ		
	X		ⓣ		ⓚ	ⓥ	
Nasals	X		X		X		
Glides	ⓦ			j¹			
Fricatives	X	X	X	X			ɣ¹
	X	X	X	X	X		
Affricates				Xtʃ, Xdʒ			
Liquids			X	X			
Final							
Stops	X		X		X		*No final*
	X		X		X	X	*consonants*
Nasals	X		X		X		
Fricatives	X	X	X	X			
	X	X	X	X			
Affricates				Xtʃ, Xdʒ			
Liquids			X				

Note: [r] Not listed in final position, as [ɚ] is a rhotic **vowel**. Medially, [r] should be counted only where it is consonantal (*around*), not vocalic (*bird*).

EXAMPLE 3-1B.
Consonant repertoire.

Vowel Repertoire

Name: *Marvin*
Date: *4/3/94*
Source of sample: *babble sample*

Age: *21 mos*
Examiner: *SLV*
Size of sample: *50 babbles*

Note: Phones circled are mastered (i.e., occurred at least ____2____ times in that position in any context, whether correct or not). Phones marked with an X did not occur in any context.

	Front	Central	Back
Simple vowels			
High			
Tense	i^1		u^1
Lax	Ⓘ		Ⓤ
Mid			
Tense	✗		✗
Lax	Ⓔ		✗
Low		Ⓐ , ⓐ	
	æ^1		ⓐ

Diphthongs

	Front	Central	Back
		✗	
		Ⓐⓘ	
		Ⓐⓤ	

Rhotic vowels   *No rhotic vowels*

	Front	Central	Back
High			
Mid	✗˞		✗˞
	✗˞		✗˞
Low		✗	
		✗˞	

Note: Superscript numbers indicate the numbers of occurrence of marked phones.

EXAMPLE 3-2B.
Vowel repertoire.

TABLE 3-23.
APP-R and CELF-P Data from "Bryan," Age 3 Years, 11 Months

ɛɚpeɪnt	(air)plane
bots	boats
fwɪdz	bridge
bʌtɪnz	buttons
feɪənz	crayons
aɪsmɪnt	elephant
fwʌv	glove
fint	green
aɪs **kjubs**	ice cubes
sʌmt	jumped
wʌntʃ	lunch
mæsk	mask
owɪndʒ	orange
feɪfaʊnd	playground
su **swaɪbə**	screwdriver
sju	shoe
swaɪd	slide
fwɪŋki	slinky
smok	smoke
sneɪk, seɪnt	snake
spaɪdə	spider
spunt	spoon
swɛɚ	square
staɪ	star
swɪŋ	string
swɛdə	sweater
swɪŋ	swing
swi	three
taɪmz	times
ʃwʌk	truck
wapɪnt	wrapping
swɪpə	zipper

APP-R = *Assessment of Phonological Processes, Revised* (Hodson, 1986); CELF-P = *Clinical Evaluation of Language Fundamental–Preschool* (Wiig, Secord, & Semel, 1992).
Note: Clusters in initial and final position are in boldface.

The frequent occurrence of lax vowels and the infrequent occurrence of tense vowels probably is a result of his low oral muscle tone. Occasional diphthongs also are in evidence. Rhotic diphthongs are not expected at this age or this stage. In therapy, oral stimulation and motor activities will address his low oral tone. Tense vowels ([i, e, u, o]) will be modeled in play contexts (e.g., *Oh!* for surprising events, *Whee!* for sliding) in an attempt to stimulate his motivation and ability to achieve the labial and lingual muscle tone required for such vowels.

Consonant Clusters

Consonant clusters can be screened also by using similar forms (Forms 3-3 and 3-4). Clusters observed to occur should be indicated with a ✔, a number (representing number of occurrences), or a percentage (percentage of occurrences of all clusters produced). If a check system is used, requiring a minimum number of occurrences is preferable to checking all clusters that occur even once. However, given the number of clusters in the language and their reduced frequency of occurrence in comparison to singletons, lower criteria for mastery could be used (e.g., two occurrences per 100 utterances). Boxes representing

cluster combinations that do not occur are left blank. Obviously, in analyzing the phonology of a child who already has been determined to produce no clusters of any kind or even very few clusters (using Form 2-1; see Chapter 2), the clinician will not bother with Forms 3-3 and 3-4. For example, a speech-language pathologist would not waste time using these forms with either of the children just discussed, as neither has more than a few clusters.

"Bryan," age 3 years, 11 months and experiencing language and phonological delay, has several clusters, as shown in Table 3-23. In the table, his clusters are boldfaced to render them more easily identified. The types of clusters that he finds easiest to handle are clear when his APP-R data and words he produced during administration of the Clinical Evaluation of Language Fundamentals–Preschool (CELF-P; Wiig, Secord, & Semel, 1992) are transferred to Examples 3-3 and 3-4.

Of Bryan's 21 initial consonant clusters, 13 (62%) are fricative + glide, including two cluster types that typically do not occur in adult English (*fw-* and *ʃw-*). Three others are fricative + stop, and two are fricative + nasal. Clearly, Bryan prefers fricative-initial clusters. He is just beginning to branch from fricative + glide to stop + glide (one instance of *kj-*) and to three-element fricative + stop + glide clusters (one instance of *stw-*).

Of Bryan's 16 final clusters, almost half are -*nt*. Overall, 13 of 17 (76%) are nasal-initial. More than half of these nasal-initial clusters (8 of 13, or 62%) are nasal + stop, and the others are nasal + fricative or affricate. He has three stop + fricative clusters (including one instance of -*bs*, which normally does not occur in English) and one fricative plus stop cluster (-*sk*).

It is obvious that a clinician who has decided to expand Bryan's repertoire of consonant clusters should focus on the emerging initial types (stop + glide and fricative + stop + glide) and on increasing the frequency of his use of fricative + nasal clusters. In final position, the frequency of nasal + obstruent (stop or fricative) and final stop + [s/z] combinations can be increased. At this time, it would be appropriate to address regular plurals (or possessive or third-person singular) with Bryan; gains can be made in both phonology and morphology through work on nasal or stop clusters with final [s/z] morphological markers. Other nasal + obstruent (e.g., -*mp* or -*mz*) clusters also would be promising. In addition, the emergence of final fricative + stop clusters (thus far, in the form of one instance of -*sk*) can be encouraged. Of course, though eventually they will have to be addressed, initial and final clusters with liquids would be a major challenge at this point, as Bryan does not produce any such clusters. In fact, target liquids consistently are either omitted or substituted with [w].

Summary

Do-it-yourself independent analysis forms are an option for identifying the consonants, vowels, and consonant clusters that can be produced by the child. Word forms elicited by using articulation or process test pictures can

Initial Consonant Clusters

Name: Age:
Date: Examiner:
Source of sample: Size of sample:

Indicate with check mark, a specific number or specific percentage those clusters that occur in the child's speech. (Note: If the child produces an "illegal" cluster that does not normally occur in English, list it as "other.")

Two-element clusters

Obstruent + liquid

pr-___	pl-___	pj-___		br-___	bl-___	bj-___	
tr-___		tj-___	tw-___	dr-___		dj-___	dw-___
kr-___	kl-___	kj-___	kw-___	gr-___	gl-___	gj-___	gw-___
						mj-___	
						nj-___	

fr-___	fl-___	fj-___	
θr-___		θj-___	θw-___
	sl-___	sj-___	sw-___
ʃr-___			

hj-___
vj-___
lj-___

[s] + obstruent

sp-___   st-___   sk-___   sm-___   sn-___

Other:

Note: The glide [j] occurs far more often in initial clusters in British than in American English.

Three-element clusters

spr-___	spl-___	spj-___	
str-___		stj-___	
skr-___	skl-___	skj-___	skw-___

Other:

Final Consonant Clusters

Name: Age:
Date: Examiner:
Source of sample: Size of sample:

Indicate with check mark, a specific number or specific percentage those clusters that occur in the child's speech. (Note: If the child produces an "illegal" cluster that does not normally occur in English, list it as "other.")

Two-element clusters

Nasals

-mp___   -mt___   -md___ -mf___   -mθ___   -mz___
          -nt___   -nd___   -nθ___   -ns___   -ntʃ___   -ndʒ___ -nz ___
                    -ŋk___   -ŋd___   -ŋz ___

Stops

          -pt___   -bd___   -pθ___   -ps___   -bz___
                                               -tθ___   -ts ___   -dz___
          -kt___   -gd___   -ks___   -gz___

Fricatives

          -ft___   -vd___   -fθ___   -fs___   -vz___
          -θt___   -ðd___   -θs___   -ðz___
-sp___   -st___   -sk___   -zd___   -zm___
          -ʃt___   -ʒd___
          -tʃt___   -dʒd___

Liquids

-lp___   -lt ___   -lk___   -ld___   -lm___   -ln___
                              -lv___   -lf___   -lθ___   -ls___   -ltʃ___   -ldʒ___ -lz___

Other:

Three-element clusters

-mps___
          -nts___   -nst___   -ntʃt___   -ndʒd___
                    -ŋks___   -ŋst___
-lps___   -lts___   -lks___   -lst___   -ltʃt___   -ldʒd___

Other:

FORM 3-4.
Final consonant clusters.

Initial Consonant Clusters

Name: *Bryan*

Date: *5/17/93*

Source of sample: *APP-R*

Age: *3;11*

Examiner: *SLV*

Size of sample: *75 words (32 with clusters in them)*

Indicate with check mark, a specific number or specific percentage those clusters that occur in the child's speech. (Note: If the child produces an "illegal" cluster that does not normally occur in English, list it as "other.")

Two-element clusters

Obstruent + liquid

pr-___	pl-___	pj-___		br-___	bl-___	bj- ___	
tr-___		tj-___	tw- ___	dr-___		dj- ___	dw-___
kr-___	kl-___	kj- *1*	kw-___	gr-___	gl-___	gj- ___	gw-___
						mj-___	
						nj- ___	

fr-___	fl-___	fj-___
θr-___		θj-___	θw-___
	sl-___	sj- *1*	sw- *8*
ʃr-___		

hj-___
vj-___
lj- ___

[s] + obstruent

sp- *2*   st- *1*   sk-___   sm- *1*   sn- *1*

Other: *fw-: 3; ʃw-: 1*

Note: The glide [j] occurs far more often in initial clusters in British than in American English.

Three-element clusters

spr-___	spl-___	spj-___
str-___		stj-___
skr-___	skl-___	skj-___	skw-___

Other: *stw-: 1*

EXAMPLE 3-3.
Initial consonant clusters.

Final Consonant Clusters

Name: *Bryan*   Age: *3;11*

Date: *5/17/93*   Examiner: *SLV*

Source of sample: *APP-R*   Size of sample: *75 words (32 with clusters in them)*

Indicate with check mark, a specific number or specific percentage those clusters that occur in the child's speech. (Note: If the child produces an "illegal" cluster that does not normally occur in English, list it as "other.")

Two-element clusters

Nasals

-mp___   -mt _1_   -md___ -mf___ -mθ___   -mz_1_

          -nt _6_   -nd _1_   -nθ___ -ns___   -ntʃ _1_ -ndʒ _1_ -nz _2_

                   -ŋk___   -ŋd ___   -ŋz___

Stops

          -pt___   -bd___   -pθ___ -ps___   -bz___

                                             -tθ___ -ts _1_   -dz_1_

          -kt___   -gd___   -ks___   -gz___

Fricatives

          -ft___   -vd___   -fθ___ -fs___   -vz___

          -θt___   -ðd___   -θs___   -ðz___

-sp___   -st___   -sk _1_   -zd___ -zm___

          -ʃt___   -ʒd___

          -tʃt___   -dʒd___

Liquids

-lp___   -lt___   -lk___   -ld___ -lm___ -ln___

                             -lv___ -lf___ -lθ___   -ls___   -ltʃ___ -ldʒ___ -lz___

Other: *-bs: 1*

Three-element clusters

-mps___

          -nts___   -nst___   -ntʃt___ -ndʒd___

                   -ŋks___   -ŋst___

-lps___   -lts___   -lks___   -lst___   -ltʃt___ -ldʒd___

Other: *None.*

EXAMPLE 3-4.
Final consonant clusters.

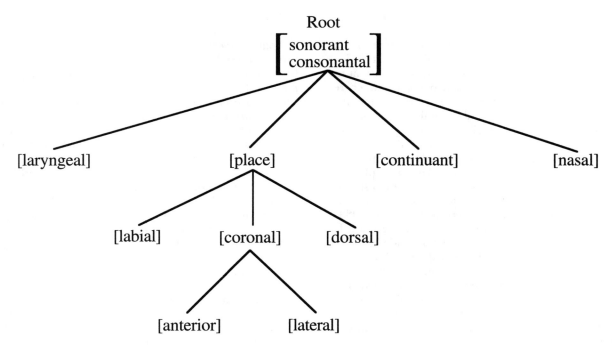

FIGURE 3-1.
Feature geometry tree for English. (Adapted from JJ McCarthy. Feature geometry and dependency: A review. *Phonetica* 1988;43:84–108.)

provide data for these analyses to supplement samples of spontaneous speech as needed.

FEATURE GEOMETRY

Feature geometry is the aspect of nonlinear phonology that deals with the features of speech sounds and how they behave. Just as segments, syllables, and words are, the features are seen as one level of the phonological hierarchy. Within that level, they are further hierarchically arranged as *major* and *minor features* within categories of features that tend to operate together or in similar ways.

Two major goals of feature geometry emerge. One is minimizing the number of features used to describe the phonology of each language in a maximally efficient manner. The other is discovering the hierarchical relationships among the features so as to make predictions about the manner in which the presence or behavior of one feature in the language might affect the presence or behavior of another.

Dinnsen's prediction (1992) that children will not acquire any liquids until they first have acquired some fricatives or affricates is an example of the latter goal. Efficiency in feature representation, the first goal, is gained from taking advantage of universal and language-specific defaults. Because the contrasts within a language are important for this process, this aspect of feature geometry is discussed in Chapter 4.

Both goals of feature geometry motivate the current feature terminology. One example is the fact that the terms [alveolar] and [palatal] are subsumed under the

feature [coronal] (tongue-tip). Alveolar sounds are considered to be [+ coronal + anterior] and palatals are considered to be [+ coronal − anterior]. This distinction simplifies describing phonological patterns that affect both alveolars and palatals. Such patterns are common, so one should be able to describe them efficiently. The fact that a certain sound is coronal seems to have more impact on the phonological patterns in which it is involved than whether it is an anterior coronal (i.e., an alveolar) or not (i.e., a palatal). Because coronality has more impact on the behavior of phonological elements than does anteriority, [coronal] occupies a spot higher in the feature geometry hierarchy than does [anterior]. These principles are represented graphically in feature trees.

Feature Geometrees

Linguists draw treelike structures to represent the hierarchical nature of the relationships among features. The top of the tree is called the **root node**; the feature categories hang down below (as usual, in a configuration opposite from that of a real tree). Two types of trees are drawn: those that represent all the feature options available for a particular language and those that represent the features of a particular sound. Myriad technical arguments have been expressed for preferring certain feature geometry configurations over others, and the issues are far from resolved. However, one possible representation of the feature geometry of English (based on McCarthy, 1988) is shown in Figure 3-1.

Each location on the tree is referred to as a **node** (e.g., the root node, the laryngeal node), and the items that hang below each node are called the **daughters** of that **mother node**. Not surprisingly, place of articulation is a very important node. Two branches within the feature tree are specified for place of articulation and correspond to the distinction between supralaryngeal features (correlating to aspects of articulation above the glottis) and those that are laryngeal. The laryngeal branch includes voicing, glottal consonants ([ʔ, h]), and some other laryngeal features that are primarily relevant to languages other than English. The supralaryngeal place of articulation branch is divided tentatively for English into labial, coronal (tongue-tip and blade), and dorsal (back of the tongue, which is velar in English; McCarthy, 1988). The [coronal] node is subdivided further for English by the features [anterior] (tongue-tip versus blade, as in [s] versus [ʃ]) and [lateral] (to distinguish [l], which is lateral, from [r], which is not). The very minor status of [lateral], hanging well below the feature [continuant], corresponds to children's relatively late acquisition of liquids. The feature [continuant] is much higher up in the tree, in keeping with children's tendency to acquire at least some fricatives before they have developed a contrast between [l] and [r].

Relationships among the nodes are determined by evidence from the way in which features pattern together in the languages of the world and in specific languages. Various types of evidence are used to determine whether features are at the same levels in the hierarchy or depend on one another. The arguments associated with some of these types of evidence are extremely technical, involving detailed analyses of languages other than English. The simplest type of evidence comes from the way in which various features behave when assimilation occurs. The basic principle provides that, if some feature high in the tree is assimilated, all lower features must be assimilated as well. A higher feature (e.g., sonorant) never will assimilate without lower features (e.g., labial) assimilating too. However, lower features may assimilate without higher features doing so. In total assimilation, all features are assimilated; the two sounds become identical. In partial assimilation, only some (lower) features become the same. For instance, the nonsonorant labial [f] could assimilate to the palatal sonorant glide [j] in two ways:

1. By becoming sonorant, in which case the lower place and continuant nodes also would "come along for the ride." In this scenario, [f] would change both its manner and its place of articulation, and both consonants would emerge as [j], as in [jɔɪjɚ] for *foyer*. This change reflects total assimilation.
2. By becoming palatal (i.e., becoming [ʃ] under the influence of [j]) without becoming sonorant as well, yielding, for example, [ʃɔɪjɚ] for *foyer*. The lower, place, nodes would change without the higher, sonorant, node's changing. This change reflects partial assimilation, as the place but not the manner of articulation has changed.

For ease of exposition, the assimilation arguments are the focus here as the justification for the feature geometry of English is sketched. The basic premise provides that features that tend to change together must occupy the same level in the tree and be dominated by the same mother node. A feature that sometimes can change alone is presumed to occupy a level lower than a feature that always changes in conjunction with other features. Thus, for example, because place can change independently of manner (continuant and nasal nodes) and vice versa, neither dominates the other. They must occupy the same level.

The place of articulation groupings were based in part on the fact that, when assimilation occurs, all the place features typically change together. For instance, if some other consonant assimilates to [w], which is both [+labial] and [+dorsal], that consonant will become both [+labial] and [+dorsal] as well. Because [labial], [coronal], and [dorsal] often act together and in the same ways, the assumption is that they must be daughters of the same node. Similarly, [anterior] and [lateral] occur together. For example, a consonant that assimilates to [l] in one place feature will assimilate also on the other place feature, never on only one of these. Therefore, these two elements must hang together. If assimilation changes a sound from or to coronal, the victim of the assimilation will take on the anteriority and the laterality of the causative sound also. Therefore, these two must hang from the coronal node.

In contrast, we know that place and manner of articulation do not always operate together. A child may assimilate a stop to a fricative by producing both as stops (i.e., the same manner of articulation) without changing the place of articulation of either one (e.g., *coffee* produced as [kɔpi]). On the other hand, the child also could produce both at the same place of articulation without changing the manner of either one (e.g., *coffee* produced as [pɔfi]). Thus, place and manner do not necessarily work together (although they may). Because they appear to be independent of each other, neither one can be the daughter of the other; they must be separate and occupy the same level in the tree.

Two distinctions are made within manner of articulation: continuant (fricatives, liquids, and glides versus stops) and nasal. They do not operate as one category, either. Assimilation can change the continuance of a segment without changing its nasality. In some dialects of English, for example, the continuant [z] becomes the noncontinuant (stop) [d] before the noncontinuant (nasal stop) [n], but it retains its oral (non-nasal) production. The standard example of this continuant assimilation without nasal assimilation is the pronunciation of *business* as [bɪdnɪs] (McCarthy, 1988). Therefore, although a certain place node groups all the place-of-articulation features together, no manner node exists to group all manners of articulation together. Nasal and continuant are separate nodes at the same level in the hierarchy.

Two feature distinctions always operate together and change only if the entire segment changes: [sonorant] (differentiating vowels, liquids, glides, and nasals from the less tonal stop, fricative, and affricate obstruents) and [consonantal] (differentiating consonants from vowels). These features change only in total assimilation, when all

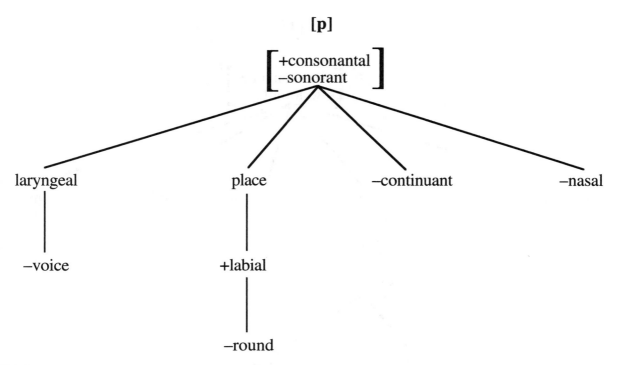

FIGURE 3-2.
Feature specification for /p/.

features of one sound become identical to all features of the other. Therefore, these features are considered to be inseparable from the segment itself or, in tree analogy, inseparable from the root of the tree. These two features are termed the *major sound class features* because they occupy the highest level in the hierarchy.

The feature tree for a particular sound is similar to that for the language as a whole, except that it is far simpler. Only those features that are needed within the language to distinguish between that particular sound and all other sounds of the language are specified. Thus, the feature specification for /p/ might be something like the tree shown in Figure 3-2. Such a diagram illustrates the hierarchical relationships among the features far better than does the old Chomsky and Halle (1968) feature specification for [p]:

$$\left\{\begin{bmatrix} -\text{syllabic} \\ +\text{consonantal} \\ -\text{sonorant} \\ -\text{nasal} \\ -\text{continuant} \\ +\text{anterior} \\ -\text{coronal} \\ -\text{back} \\ -\text{high} \\ -\text{low} \\ -\text{voice} \end{bmatrix}\right\}$$

Additionally, this system allows more straightforward descriptions of some articulatory differences between sounds. For instance, in previous phonological theories, the affricates [tʃ] and [dʒ] were differentiated from [ʃ] and [ʒ] via the feature [anterior], which was given a plus value for the affricates (because the stop portions of the affricates are alveolar) and a minus value for the fricatives (which are wholly palatal). This distinction implied that affricates are wholly anterior, although they are not. The fricative portions of these affricates are not anterior; they are palatal when they occur within an affricate just as they are when they occur alone. Thus, the anteriority of the affricate actually changes over the course of its production. Because the feature hierarchy is now an entity separate from the phonotactic structure of the word, it no longer is necessary to specify only one value of each feature per consonant or vowel slot in the word. Therefore, phonetic changes can be indicated as they occur—in midsegment. The features for [tʃ] now can be diagrammed as illustrated in Figure 3-3, with two values of anterior and two values of continuant, representing the fact that these values change in the course of producing the segment.

Implications of Feature Geometry for Intervention

Feature geometry has some direct implications for phonological intervention, many of which have yet to be tested thoroughly through research. Clinical phonologists (e.g., Bernhardt, 1992b; Stoel-Gammon & Stemberger, 1994) hypothesized that children will learn the features from the top (the root) down. They will master the distinction

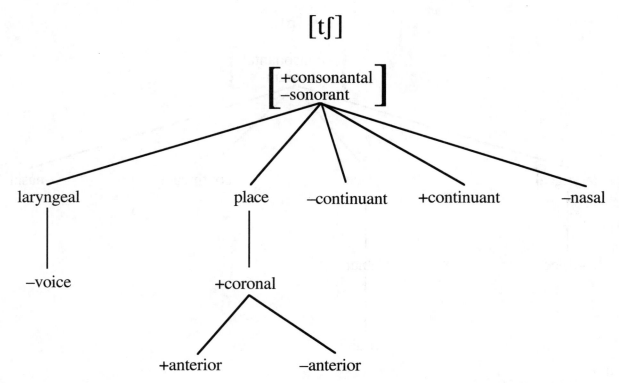

FIGURE 3-3.
Feature specification for /tʃ/.

between consonants and vowels and between sonorants and nonsonorants very early on. New nodes will be added one by one, from top to bottom (Beers, 1996; Rice & Avery, 1995). This very basic prediction is known to be true, in fact: Only the most severely affected children lack at least one consonant-versus-vowel contrast in their repertoire, even if the consonant is only a glottal stop. The distinction between glottal and nonglottal consonants also is acquired promptly and easily by most children. Similarly, the contrast between obstruents (e.g., stops) and sonorants (e.g., nasals) already is well established as one that is acquired very early. A reasonable hypothesis holds that slightly farther down the tree, the contrast between glottal and supraglottal consonants (e.g., [ʔ] versus [p]) will be mastered long before the child learns the distinction between coronal consonants that are or are not anterior (e.g., [s] versus [ʃ]).

The feature tree is, in fact, one of the bases for Dinnsen's proposal (1992) about levels of acquisition of sound classes. His levels correspond roughly to levels within the feature hierarchy (see Figure 3-1), although some minor differences exist. (Dinnsen's levels are repeated here for the reader's convenience.)

- Level A: vowels, glides, voiced stops, nasals, glottals
- Level B: level A sounds + voicing contrast for stops
- Level C: level B sounds + some fricatives or affricates
- Level D: level C sounds + one liquid consonant (lateral [l] or nonlateral [r])

- Level E: level D sounds + more liquids *or* more obstruents (e.g., fricatives or affricates)

Level A requires mastery of the features consonantal (vowels versus consonants), sonorant (stops versus nasals and glides), and laryngeal (oral versus glottal consonants). Typically, the child at this point is also mastering at least one distinction at the upper level of the place node (e.g., labial versus coronal), although Dinnsen does not address this issue. At level B, some laryngeal node features appear (voicing). At level C, a continuant node distinction occurs as fricatives (which are [+continuant]) emerge. Similarly, at level D, a distinction appears at the lowest level within the place category, as granddaughter node [lateral] emerges. Presumably, the higher place node categories—labial versus coronal versus dorsal—have developed during this time as well, but Dinnsen states that these properties are not as predictable as are manner features.

Thus, for those with good visual-spatial skills, seeing the levels of phonetic development hierarchically organized on a tree clarifies the gradual addition of feature distinctions within the child's phonological system. Visualizing the hierarchical relationships facilitates the prediction of features that may represent the next step for a child.

The terminology of feature geometry also can facilitate the description of a child's phonological status. For example, a child who produces only glottals (e.g., [h, ʔ]) could be said to be "lacking a place node" (i.e., having no supralaryngeal places of articulation). A therapy goal then would be to establish the child's place node. In choosing among possible therapy goals, the clinician could target more major place contrasts higher in the tree (e.g., coronal versus dorsal) before trying to teach the child the lower contrasts, such as those *within* the coronal node (anterior, lateral).

With respect to generalization, intervention on features within one node is hypothesized to be more likely to trigger generalization to other feature specifications within that node. For instance, therapy that focuses on one aspect of the place node could generalize to other aspects of place. In contrast, no manner node exists, so this type of generalization of learning would not be expected from therapy that addresses some aspect of manner. In other words, facilitating a coronal versus labial contrast might lead to spontaneous progress in the development of the coronal-versus-dorsal contrast (i.e., mastering velars), but facilitating a nasality contrast should have no effect on the continuant versus noncontinuant contrast. Similarly, given that the laryngeal node is separate from the other nodes relating to place of articulation, progress on contrasts within that node (e.g., differentiation of voiced versus voiceless sounds, or differentiation of [h] from [ʔ] in a very severe case) might not be expected to have an impact on any other contrasts. However, Gierut (1996a,b) made the specific claim that children acquire the features of their languages in cycles, alternating the acquisition of laryngeal contrasts (e.g., glottal versus supraglottal or voiced versus voiceless) with the acquisition of supralaryngeal contrasts. In her studies, children who are ready for a laryngeal cycle according to her criteria, for example, can be rushed through that cycle and into the next, a supralaryngeal cycle, if a supralaryngeal target is addressed in therapy. Thus, choosing an out-of-phase therapy target can speed the child's phonological learning process, according to Gierut (1996a,b).

Yavas (1997) claimed that children who are developing phonology normally always substitute more primary features (sonorant, continuant, coronal) for more secondary features. Primary features, especially sonorant, are not replaced by others. Only children with phonological disorders, he stated, sometimes do the reverse, gliding fricatives, stopping liquids and glides, backing coronals, and fricating stops. Substitutions of lower features for higher features are deviant, as they are not found in children who are developing normally. Thus, if Yavas is correct, the direction of substitutions as modeled on the feature geometry tree can provide an indication of the degree of deviance of a child's phonological system.

Summary

Feature geometry involves categorizing speech sound features according to the phonological patterns in which they co-occur. Linguists then draw trees to represent the hierarchical relationships among the categories. The major sound class features [sonorant] and [consonantal] are the most basic. Other nodes include a laryngeal category (for voicing, [h], glottal stops, etc.), a place of articulation category, and two manner features (continuant and nasal) that are not categorized together because they occur independently.

ARTICULATORY PROGRAMMING

In 1955, Hockett (p. 210) made an apt analogy to explain the relationship between the abstract unit we call a **phoneme** and the actual speech sounds that emerge from our mouths:

> Imagine a row of Easter eggs carried along a moving belt; the eggs are of various sizes, and variously colored, but not boiled. At a certain point, the belt carries the row of eggs between the two rollers of a wringer, which quite effectively smash them and rub them more or less into each other. The flow of eggs before the wringer represents the series of impulses from the phoneme source. The mess that emerges from the wringer represents the output of the speech transmitter.

In other words, speaking does not involve producing one distinct phoneme after another; articulatory commands for speech sounds are integrated highly with one another for maximum efficiency. Similarly, the acoustic information that listeners use to comprehend others' messages are not divisible into neat little phoneme-sized packages. Therefore, the type of model of speech sound features presented to this point is far from the reality of on-line speech programming.

Gestural Phonology

Gestural phonology, as described by Browman and Goldstein (1986, 1992) and Kent (1997), is a response to this problem. It is a more grounded (articulatory) approach to phonological features. Rather than focusing on characteristics of individual consonants and vowels, this theory is based on the movement patterns required to make the transition from one segment into another. The emphasis is on **gestural scores**: phonological plans for producing such integrated phonological units as syllables and words. Gestural scores highlight **phase relations** among various articulators. This is the time dimension.[11] Separate tiers are used to model the articulators: velum, tongue body, tongue-tip, lips, and glottis. This is the space dimension. A gestural score for the word *pad*, adapted from Kent (1997), is given in Figure 3-4.

This figure shows that, during the entire production of the word *pad*, the tongue body is positioned with a widened pharyngeal cavity appropriate to the production of the vowel. This pharyngeal posture overlaps in time with the lip closure at the beginning of the word, and the alveolar tongue-tip closure at the end of the word. For the production of the [p], the lips close first, then the glottis

---

[11] I am grateful to Kristine Strand, an Einstein fan, for calling this space-time analogy to my attention.

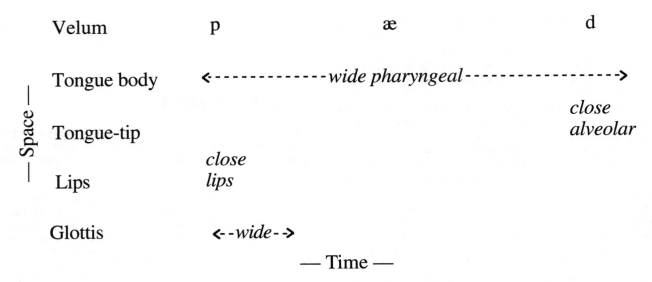

FIGURE 3-4.

Gestural score for *pad*. (Adapted from RD Kent. Gestural phonology: Basic concepts and applications in speech-language pathology. In Ball MJ, Kent RD [eds]. ***The New Phonologies: Developments in Clinical Linguistics.*** **San Diego: Singular, 1997, 247–265.)**

opens wide for the voiceless consonant. The open glottis overlaps with the vowel posture, increasing the voice onset time (as appropriate).

Implications of Gestural Phonology for Intervention

Gestural phonology suggests possible underlying patterns in children's speech that are not easily detectable from phonetic transcription alone. Alice, described earlier, demonstrated a consistent word recipe involving palatal consonants and vowels, especially in medial and final position. The exact consonants or vowels that occurred varied quite a bit, but typically they sounded as if they were produced with the blade of the tongue raised to the palate. Thus, her word pattern, based on an earlier babble vocal motor scheme, was described far more easily as an articulatory gestural score with a high (palatal) tongue body than in terms of specific consonants and vowels. A similar claim was made for Emma, with her alternating labial-alveolar pattern in both babble and early words, by Goodell and Studdert-Kennedy (1991) and by Studdert-Kennedy and Goodell (1992). Emma, too, was inconsistent in the exact consonants that she produced, but their places of articulation were predictable. Queller (1994, 1995) proposed similar gestural bases for child production patterns, although he did not advocate gestural phonology per se. For example, he illustrated that the inconsistent degree of palatalization present in the word productions of 16-month-old Timmy (also discussed earlier and by Vihman et al., 1994) can be described more accurately as a gradual narrowing of the vocal tract than as the production of particular consonants or vowels.

These examples demonstrate the utility of a gestural perspective on child phonology. Regularities often become more easily identifiable in children's word recipes when they are seen as gestural scores rather than as series of independent segments.

CHAPTER FOUR

Contrast

THE IMPORTANCE OF CONTRAST

The most critical function of a phonological system is that of differentiating messages. If all words sound the same or the differences between them are random, we cannot communicate. If the number of contrasts in a language is reduced, the effectiveness of that language will be compromised.

The importance of contrast can be seen at an even more basic level if animal languages are compared to those of humans. Animals' simple communication systems include very limited numbers of contrasts. Many animal species use particular signals to identify themselves as one of a group, to attract members of the opposite sex, or to indicate danger. Italian honeybees, for instance, have a comparatively complex language for communicating about food. They perform three contrasting dances that indicate the distance of the food from the hive (less than 20 feet, 20–60 feet, and more than 60 feet). The rates and angles at which they dance provide further information about the distance to the food and the direction in which it is located. The enthusiasm with which they dance is an indicator of the quality of the food (Fromkin & Rodman, 1978). They are, however, unable to express the exact type of food, the dangers that might be encountered along the way, their means of travel (e.g., walking versus flying), or any information about vertical direction (e.g., "It's straight up!" Yule, 1996). Thus, within the bee communication system, a few contrastive features of dance *form* are available for indicating distance, direction, and food quality. In comparing this system to the number of contrastive features typically available within the phonology alone of a human language (including many phonotactic and phonetic contrasts), however, it is evident that the bee system is extremely limited. When other sources of contrast within human languages—such as the ordering of sounds into words and words into sentences—are considered, the contrastive potential of our communication system appears vast.

Languages of the World

Contrast is a major player in the constant struggle between ease of production and ease of perception. Less extreme speech sounds are easier to pronounce, yet more difficult to differentiate perceptually. Sounds that are very similar to each other may be difficult to distinguish in articulation and perception. Singletons are easier to produce than are clusters, but singletons alone may not yield sufficient contrast. Simple vowel (V) and consonant-vowel (CV) syllables are easier to produce than are syllables with diphthongs and complex clusters. Yet, as indicated in Chapter 2, restricting itself to such simple syllable shapes leaves Hawaiian with only 162 possible syllables in contrast to Thai's 23,638 possible syllables (Crystal, 1987). Hawaiian has to compensate for its limited syllable variety with extremely long words.

In addition to inventory limitations of this sort, phonological patterns may reduce **phonotactic** contrast (e.g., by reducing clusters to singletons). Phonological patterns may also reduce contrast between sounds or sound classes, a contrast that is termed **phonemic**. For example, when fricatives are stopped (e.g., /f/ is pronounced as [p]), the contrast between fricatives and stops is lost. When a phonological pattern eliminates the contrast between two word shapes, phonemes, or sound classes, this contrast is said to be **neutralized**. Reducing the number of contrasts available in a language reduces the communicative potential of the speakers. A balance must always be maintained if contrast is to be preserved.

The need to preserve contrast is clearly evident in the histories of languages. Phonological change often appears to operate without regard for its potentially major impact on the lexicon of the language (Bynon, 1977). However, if phonological changes occur and reduce the potential for contrast, one can expect further changes—either phonological or not—to restore the potential for contrast in some other way. In many cases, the same number of contrastive segments will be available both before and after the change but with a somewhat different distribution. These cases are termed **sound shifts**. Two of the most famous cases in the development of the language that eventually came to be known as English are the First Consonant Shift (also known as *Grimm's law*) and the Great Vowel Shift.

The First Consonant Shift occurred as the ancient precursor to the Germanic languages split off from the rest of the Indo-European languages. Before the shift, the consonant system included voiceless, voiced, and aspirated voiced stop consonants (Table 4-1).

Every one of these consonant sound classes shifted, with voiceless stops becoming pronounced as voiceless fricatives, voiced stops becoming pronounced as voiceless stops, and voiced aspirated stops becoming pronounced as voiced stops. Thus, the resulting consonant system still included voiceless and voiced stops (although now in different words) but now also included voiceless fricatives[1] (Bynon, 1977; Fromkin & Rodman, 1978), as shown in Table 4-2.

The results of this change are still evident today. Certain English words that contain fricatives correspond to Romance language words that contain voiceless stops (e.g., *father*: *père* in French, *padre* in Spanish; *three*: *trois* in French, *tres* in Spanish). Furthermore, certain English words containing voiceless stops correspond to Romance language words that contain voiced stops (e.g., *two*: *deux* in French, *dos* in Spanish; Fromkin & Rodman, 1978). Although many changes had occurred in this sound shift, the same potential for phonological contrast remained available.

Similarly, in the Great Vowel Shift, all the long vowels in fifteenth-century English shifted upward in the vowel triangle (with the highest vowels falling off into diphthongs), but the same number of vowel contrasts as before were available afterward. The specific changes that occurred are shown in Table 4-3 (adapted from Bynon, 1977, and Fromkin & Rodman, 1978).

---

[1]/x/ is a voiceless fricative.

TABLE 4-1.
Pre-Shift Consonant System

p	t	k
b	d	g
bʰ	dʰ	gʰ

Note: Superscript "h" indicates aspiration.
Source: Adapted from T Bynon. *Historical Linguistics*. Cambridge: Cambridge University Press, 1977; and V Fromkin, R Rodman. *An Introduction to Language* (2nd ed). New York: Holt, Rinehart and Winston, 1978.

TABLE 4-2.
Post-Shift Consonant System

f	θ	x
p	t	k
b	d	g

Source: Adapted from T Bynon. *Historical Linguistics*. Cambridge: Cambridge University Press, 1977; and V Fromkin, R Rodman. *An Introduction to Language* (2nd ed). New York: Holt, Rinehart and Winston, 1978.

TABLE 4-3.
Great Vowel Shift

Middle English	Modern English	Example
[iː]	[aɪ]	[miːs] → [maɪs] (mice)
[uː]	[aʊ]	[muːs] → [maʊs] (mouse)
[eː]	[i]	[geːs] → [giːs] (geese)
[oː]	[uː]	[goːs] → [guːs] (goose)
[ɛː]	[eː]	[brɛken] → [breːk] (break)
[ɔː]	[oː]	[brɔːken] → [broːk] (broke)
[aː]	[eː]	[naːmə] → [neːm] (name)*

*Other changes also have affected the pronunciation of this word.
Note: The colon represents increased segment duration.
Source: Adapted from T Bynon. *Historical Linguistics*. Cambridge: Cambridge University Press, 1977; and V Fromkin, R Rodman. *An Introduction to Language* (2nd ed). New York: Holt, Rinehart and Winston, 1978.

The pre-shift vowel qualities are still represented in English spelling four centuries later, which is why some related words in writing look more similar than they actually sound. Tense and lax vowel pairs (i–ɪ, e–ɛ, u–ʊ, o–ɔ) formerly occurred in alternation, depending on the morphological structure of a word, as in such word pairs as [dəvín] ("duhveen") and [dəvíniti]. Thus, at that time, it was sensible to write both vowels with the same letter (in this case, *divine* and *divinity*, with the letter *i* representing both [i] and [ɪ]). These word pairs were affected by the shifting of the tense vowels, so the alternations now often occur between vowels that differ in their articulatory positions as well as in their degree of tenseness. The spellings remain the same as before the shift, but the phonetic relationships now are less clear. Examples include *divine–divinity*, *sign–signal*, and *crime–criminal* (previously [i–ɪ], now [aɪ–ɪ]); *serene–serenity*, *please–pleasant*, and *clean–cleanliness* (previously [e–ɛ], now [i–ɛ]); and *sane–sanity* and *humane–humanity* (previously [a–æ], now [eɪ–æ]; Fromkin & Rodman, 1978).

Sometimes, phonological changes can lead to homonymy, which is a lexical loss of contrast (i.e., a loss of contrast in the vocabulary of the language). This loss is not a problem unless the two words that have become homonymous are used in similar contexts. As Susan Niditch (personal communication, 1996), a professor of religion at Amherst College, once remarked, "[I]f you're at a tea party, you'll understand that someone is saying, 'Please pass the cookie' and not, 'Please pass the gorilla.'"

California vowels can serve as a real-life example. In this state, the distinction between [ɑ] and [ɔ] has been neutralized (lost). *La* and *law*, *caught* and *cot*, *naught* and *not*, and others now are homonym pairs in that dialect. As far as is known, Californians do not compensate in any way for this loss of contrast, probably because few pairs of homonyms actually cause confusion. Similarly, in parts of the Northeast, the [æ] sound is raised to the extent that, in some dialects of Boston, the names *Anne* and *Ian* sound identical. Again, however, the neutralization of this high-low vowel contrast does not yet appear to have triggered any compensatory mechanisms.

When a conflict of this sort, called a **homonymic clash**, does result from loss of contrast, usually it is resolved lexically. Put simply, people change their word use to make their meanings clear. In Texas English, for instance, where [ɛ] is raised before nasals, *pen* and *pin* are pronounced in the same way: [pɪn]. To reduce the resulting confusion,

Texans talk about "ink pins" ([ɪŋk pɪnz]) when they refer to such writing implements.

Another example of homonymic clash relates to another vowel sound shift. In Old English, the verb /læːtɑn/ had a meaning similar to our current verb *let*: to allow to remain. The Old English verb /lɛttan/ had an almost opposite meaning: to hinder, prevent, or obstruct. Then the vowel /æː/ shifted to [ɛ], owing to a general vowel reorganization in the language. The result was two verbs both pronounced in a fashion similar to that of our current verb *let*. Thus, if someone were to say, "Pray you let us not see our mother" (Simpson & Weiner, 1989), this could mean either "Please don't allow us to see our mother" or "Please don't prevent us from seeing our mother." Imagine the confusion if someone were to yell, "Let him go!" after an escaping thief. Eventually, one of the two meanings had to disappear from use to reduce such ambiguity. Today, *let* has only one meaning.

An example of a homonymic clash resulting from a series of sound changes comes from the Gascony region of France. In some parts of this region, the most common word for rooster was *gallus*, borrowed from Latin. The word for cat was *gattus*, from the Latin word *cattus*. However, a morphophonological change occurred that shortened words of this type, eliminating the *-us* ending, yielding *gall* (rooster) and *gatt* (cat). When another following phonological change replaced the *ll* with [t] in final position, a conflict arose: Was [gat] to refer to cats or to roosters? The cats won, and the word *coq* (which was already in existence but used less frequently) became the label most commonly used for roosters in place of [gat].

TABLE 4-4.
Joan's Homonyms

bought, buckle, button, pocket, spot, bad, bark, bent, bite, black, pat, block	[bɑt]
bowl, boy, pea, pear, ball, bare, bear, beer, blow, blue	[bu]
bread, break, brick, pig, put, bead, bed, bird, board, boat, boot	[bʊt]

Source: Adapted from D Ingram. *Procedures for the Phonological Analysis of Children's Language.* Baltimore: University Park Press, 1981.

This led to a popular saying in France, "In Gascony, the cat killed the cock" (Bynon, 1977).

A further example of this sort from the history of English is provided by the word *ass*. Originally, this word was used only to refer to donkeys. However, a similar word, *arse*, was used to refer to the buttocks. As the language changed and many dialects became "*r*-less" (e.g., the infamous Boston "Pahk ya kah in Hahvad yahd and play cahds"), the contrast between [ɑɚ] and [æ] was neutralized, and these two words came more and more to resemble each other. Through guilt by association, *ass* lost its popular use, and the far safer word *donkey* largely replaced it (Funk, 1978). Some etymologists believe that the *rooster* meaning and the obscene slang meaning of the word *cock* may have clashed in a similar fashion. The former derived from Indo-European *ku-*, meaning "rounded hollow thing" or "egg" and the latter from the Indo-European *kak*, meaning "male genitalia." This reputed clash is disputed by others (Ciardi, 1980).

Sometimes, the solution to a homonymic clash is phonological rather than lexical. In modern-day American English, medial alveolar stops are flapped, with the tongue just briefly touching the alveolar ridge. This process creates a sound ([ɾ]) that actually is quite close to the Spanish singleton *r* sound (as in *para*). As a result, the contrast between such words as *latter* and *ladder* could be lost because the medial /d/s and /t/s both are flapped. No difference exists any longer between the consonants in the two words; phonologists say /t/ and /d/ are *neutralized* in medial position. However, the contrast is maintained by the duration of the [æ] sound. The vowel is prolonged (as indicated in the International Phonetic Alphabet [IPA] by a colon) before the voiced /d/ and is shortened before the voiceless /t/: [læ:ɾɚ] (a device to climb on) versus [læɾɚ] (the last one mentioned). Usually, vowel duration is not *phonemic* (contrastive) in English, but it serves a contrastive function in this case to compensate for the neutralization of the original contrast.

In summary, a brief excursion into the mysteries of historical linguistics and language change illustrates the importance of phonological contrast in languages. If different words come to be pronounced too similarly, often confusion will result. Under these conditions, some other aspect of the language (word use, other aspects of phonology, etc.) must change to re-establish communicative efficiency.

Child Phonology

Children have smaller numbers of phones and word shapes to use in forming words, with a resulting decrease in the number of contrasts available to them. However, they also have smaller vocabularies, so less contrast is needed. Do children avoid homonymy, and do they change their word use to limit its occurrence? In other words, do they give priority to ease of production or to ease of perception? These questions have arisen in the child phonology literature.

Ingram (1975) hypothesized that some "apparently unnatural or at least unmotivated" phonological patterns in children's early word attempts may be attributable to children's attempts to avoid homonymy. Vihman (1981), on the other hand, argued that homonymy is viewed by the child as a small price to pay for using the smallest number of word forms possible. Indeed, she claimed that some children actually seek homonymy as a means of maximizing their vocabularies in the face of limited phonological capacities. A young child who re-uses the same word form for several word meanings can have a larger vocabulary without greater articulatory effort.

Ingram (1985) proposed a broader perspective encompassing both these points of view. His proposal was based on the give-and-take among three factors in early phonology: vocabulary size, phonetic inventory size, and amount of homonymy. If the vocabulary grows beyond the phonetic capacity, he argued, homonymy will increase. This change will be tolerated to a certain point. However, eventually the increase in homonymy will exert pressure on the system, encouraging the child to explore new phonetic options. In this view, alternating periods of increasing and decreasing homonymy would be expected in early phonology.

Ingram (1981) provided an analysis of a child with a high degree of homonymy. This child, Joan (initially described by Velten, 1943), produced a large number of homonyms at 1 year, 10 months. This behavior may have been due, in part, to the fact that she already had a vocabulary of 175 words. She also produced a relatively wide variety of speech sounds for a child her age. However, she had a strong preference for monosyllables, which restricted the number of different word shapes she could produce. Some of her most overused homonymic forms and the words that they were intended to represent[2] are listed in Table 4-4. Even with contextual cues, such a high level of homonymy surely must have caused confusion for Joan's listeners.

Lleó (1990) took the issue beyond the very earliest periods of phonological development, demonstrating that the tolerance of homonymy is a strategy available to the child later in phonology as well. Lleó provided examples to show that limitations on the phonetic and phonotactic repertoires may motivate the child to be more tolerant of higher levels of homonymy so as to expand her vocabulary. The

---

[2]As Denise Segal (personal communication, 1996) reminded me, some of these homonyms may also have semantic sources, of course. For example, *button* and *buckle* could be grouped easily into one semantic category by a child of this age.

child (Laura) whom she studied, for instance, actually demonstrated increased homonymy during a period in which her phonetic repertoire was increasing. This increase was unexpected; a larger phonetic repertoire should have improved the potential for contrast. Lleó's explanation was that the child was also attempting far more multisyllabic words at this time but was able to produce only monosyllabic and disyllabic word shapes. She could not produce all of the syllables in the words she wanted to say. Therefore, longer words were reduced to homonymous disyllabic forms. For example, the long words *escombraries* (garbage), *sabatilles* (slippers), and *Tobias* (a name) were merged into a two-syllable form, [píes], for a time. The lack of available phonotactic contrast (no more than two syllables per word) was a more overwhelming factor than was the increased availability of phonetic contrast (more sounds). When the child's phonotactic repertoire eventually grew to include trisyllabic forms, the amount of homonymy in her lexicon decreased.

In short, the multiple factors that operate on a developing phonology—including vocabulary size, phonetic inventory, and phonotactic inventory—will influence the amount of contrast available within the system. If the number of possible contrasts is too small for the child's lexicon, homonymy may increase. This state of affairs may be relatively acceptable for the child whose motivation during that period is lexical rather than phonological. If the child is able to communicate despite many homonymous forms, he or she will be less motivated to vary phonetic and phonotactic repertoires. This state of affairs is quite common in early phonology, when children's attempts at communication are fairly context-bound and adults are usually able to guess at their meanings despite ambiguous phonological information. As the child's vocabulary and semantic intent continue to grow, however, lack of contrast begins to have a noticeable impact on his or her communicative effectiveness. At this time, homonymy will be less tolerable, and the system will have to grow in some respect to accommodate an unmanageable vocabulary size.

In summary, children do not avoid homonymy consistently. In fact, during certain periods of phonological development, they may be very tolerant of homonymous forms because of the phonetic or phonotactic limitations within their systems that reduce the potential for contrast. However, a trade-off occurs between the simplicity of homonymy and the efficiency of unambiguous communication. When successful communication is significantly affected by too many homonyms, the phonological system is likely to change. If it cannot change (owing to phonological disorder), the child may begin to supplement oral communication with gestures or pantomime or become very frustrated.

TYPES OF CONTRAST

Languages make use of many different types of phonological contrast. Several possible sources of contrast are addressed in previous chapters, including contrasts by number of syllables (e.g., *Toto* versus *toe*), syllable shapes (*hope* versus *hoe*; *sip* versus *slip*), distributions of the same segments in different word positions within the same syllable or word shape (e.g., *top* versus *pot*), and stress patterns (cóntrasts contrást; presént the présents). Languages other than English may use types of contrast that English does not use (e.g., the use of word pitch in tone languages).

Suprasegmental Contrast

Languages of the World

Contrast is not achieved only by variations on sound segments themselves. For instance, the amount of overlap between two contiguous sounds may differentiate a word from a phrase. As discussed in Chapter 2, the difference between the word *nitrate* and the phrase *night rate*, for instance, lies in the perceived degree of overlap that occurs between the [t] and the [r]. In *nitrate*, the [ɑɪ] is prolonged, and the [tʰ] is articulated fully; in *night rate*, the [ɑɪ] is cut short with a glottal stop instead of a fully articulated [tʰ], which serves the psychological function of separating the /t/ from the following /r/.

Stress patterns can be useful also for achieving contrast. In most dialects of American English, for example, such verbs as *presént*, *convért*, *contrást*, and *subjéct* receive stress on the final syllable of the word, whereas such nouns (and adjectives) as *présent*, *cónvert*, *cóntrast*, and *súbject* receive initial stress (Hyman, 1975). Stress patterns may also represent the grammatical chunks into which a phrase should be divided. When an adjective + noun phrase achieves the status of a nominal (noun) compound, its stress pattern changes. A big difference is seen, for instance, between a *hót dóg* (overheated canine; approximately equal stress) and a *hót dòg* (barbecue food; less stress on *dog*). Other pairs of phrases that differ only by stress include *a gréen hóuse* versus *a gréen hòuse* (for plants) and *a bíg wíg* (large hairpiece) versus *a bíg wìg* (important person). In my husband's family, chocolate cake is such a favorite that its label has achieved compound status as *chócolatecàke* (as opposed to *chòcolate cáke*).

Stress patterns also achieve contrast at the sentence level in English; the stressed word can change the implied meaning of an entire sentence. Sentence-level stress focuses the listener on ideas that the speaker intends to highlight or contrast in the sentence:

I didn't know he stole the jewels. (but you knew)

I *didn't* know he stole the jewels. (You said I did.)

I didn't *know* he stole the jewels. (I suspected.)

I didn't know *he* stole the jewels. (I thought she did.)

I didn't know he *stole* the jewels. (I thought he borrowed them.)

I didn't know he stole *the* jewels. (the important ones)

I didn't know he stole the *jewels*. (I thought he stole something else.)

In English, pitch serves to signal pragmatic or syntactic contrasts only. For example, a question typically is understood when the speaker uses rising intonation, even if the utterance is in sentence form (e.g., "You're going to the Bahamas?"). Some dialects in New York demonstrate a (stereo)typical use of a rise-fall pitch pattern on the middle and then at the end of the sentence to indicate sarcasm or a surprised question. Used on the foregoing question, for instance, it would indicate that going to the Bahamas is a very stupid idea or at least totally unexpected. The contrast value of this intonation pattern is demonstrated by the following humorous story:

> A man sees the following poem on the window of a dry-cleaning establishment:
> > My name is Fink
> > And what do you think
> > I press pants for nothing
> Deciding to take advantage of this good deal, he brings in several pairs of suit pants. When he picks them up, however, Mr. Fink asks him for $5 per pair. When the man questions the charge, the dry cleaner says, "My name is Fink and what do you think—I press pants for *nothing?*"

As we saw in Chapter 2, in some other languages, pitch patterns—tones—may differentiate one word from another. The most famous example of this is the four Chinese words all pronounced segmentally as [ma], each with its own tone (Crystal, 1987). Speakers of nontonal languages may have difficulty in mastering such a different system or even in attending to these contrasts. For several months, this author tutored a Chinese-Vietnamese woman whose children's names differed only in tone (e.g., *Phung* with high tone for her daughter and *Phung* with low tone for her son) and was unable to learn to differentiate the boy's name from the girl's.

Child Phonology
Suprasegmental effects such as tone are not as critical to English phonology as to the phonologies of other languages. Furthermore, many of the stress effects that do have an impact on English phonology affect only multisyllabic words and are therefore learned later by many children. However, stress patterns are highly relevant to children's speech production. They are more likely to preserve syllables that occur within trochees (strong syllable + weak syllable, as in *cámel*) than those that occur within iambs (weak syllable + strong syllable, as in *giráffe*; Gerken, 1994a,b). This preference for trochees is seen at the sentence level as well (Gerken, 1991; Gerken & McIntosh, 1993). However, most children do not learn to contrast trochaic versus iambic stress patterns (e.g., *cóntrast* versus *contrást*) until the majority of their phonological learning is complete.

It is important to note, however, that some English-learning children may use suprasegmentals contrastively in ways that are not directly borrowed from the adult language. Jaeger (1997) described an English-speaking child who was developing normally and who temporarily used word pitch as if English were a tone language. This author also worked with a child who used fundamental frequencies ranging from 70 to 700 Hz to differentiate words that

he could not differentiate segmentally. For example, a very high, sharply falling pitch pattern was used with [ʌbʌ] to request *open*; a flat contour with the same sequence of segments ([ʌbʌ]) meant *elephant*. He undoubtedly borrowed the basic idea from English, as Americans do tend to use a falling pitch pattern when cueing a child to say "open" as a request; labels are modeled somewhat more monotonically.

Another of this author's clients, this one with developmental verbal dyspraxia (DVD), used intonation (pitch, duration, and loudness) to modify his idiosyncratic words for *big* and *little*. Both were pronounced [mɑmə], but if this form meant *big*, the syllables were prolonged and resonant, with a lilting pitch pattern. It sounded like (but of course was not) a non-Italian's attempt to say *mama mia* with an Italian accent. *Little* was produced in a quiet monotone. Both productions were supplemented by appropriate hand gestures to enhance the contrast. "Holly," another child who had DVD, used [bijə, bɛə, bɪʊ] to express a variety of [b]-initial words; she disambiguated *baby* by whispering and *pig* with a gesture (SL Velleman, 1994).

For most English-speaking children and adults, pitch patterns express syntactic, pragmatic, social, or emotional contrasts rather than phonological ones. However, stress patterns are important even to early word learning. Furthermore, suprasegmental effects are one possible source of contrast that children may seek to apply unconventionally if they are unable to add contrast to their systems in a more conventional manner.

Summary
Any aspect of speech production that can be controlled under conditions of rapidly changing articulatory configurations can be used contrastively. Children in need of additional phonological contrast within their systems may exploit available production differences, including prosodic differences, in ways that are not exhibited by mature speakers of the same language.

Segmental Contrast

Languages of the World
The many different types of phones that may occur in languages and child phonologies are addressed in Chapter 3, but their contrastive role has not been discussed. Yet some pairs of phones that are acoustically and articulatorily different do contrast; they serve to differentiate word meanings in the language (e.g., *top* versus *cop* versus *cot*). The functions of other pairs of phones may overlap partially or even completely.

All languages do have some sounds that differ randomly in association with one another, with no linguistic rule reliably predicting when each will occur. In American English, for example, speakers may neglect to pronounce word-final /t/ as such. Often, it is substituted by [ʔ] (e.g., "I've [gɑʔ] a [koʔ]" rather than "I've [gɑtʰ] a [kotʰ]"). The point at which this occurs typically depends on sociolinguistic factors, such as the formality of the situation and the status and dialect of the speaker. The glottal stop [ʔ]

also routinely substitutes for /t/ in the medial position of certain words, such as *curtain* ([kəˀən]) and *button* ([bʌˀən]), except in very formal speech or **citation contexts** (e.g., reading a word list). Native speakers of American English are typically not consciously aware of these alternations in pronunciation. They might classify a person who always used [tʰ] in such words as *curtain* or *coat* as very formal or putting on airs but probably would not be able to explain why they formed this opinion of that person. However, they would be very confused by a person who randomly alternated [d] and [g]; that person would be unintelligible.

PHONEMES. The phones of a language that perform the critical function of differentiating words are called *phonemes*. Phonemes can be identified through the use of *minimal pairs*. These pairs are words with different meanings that differ by only one sound. Rhyming words, in which the initial phonemes contrast, are one type of minimal pair that comes easily to mind: *goat–coat, seat–sheet, man–pan, national–rational*, and so on. However, the phoneme contrast within a minimal pair can occur also in other positions of the word: *goat–got, seat–sit, mat–map, batter–battle, better–beggar, ridicule–reticule, formication–fornication*, and so on. The presence versus absence of one sound can be critical also to a minimal contrast: *preference–reference, blouse–louse, bolster–boaster, ten–tent, pea–peat, peat–eat*, and so on. Word pairs that are spelled similarly but do not sound almost the same, of course, do not count as phonological minimal pairs (e.g., *bead–dead, breath–break, cone–gone*).

What minimal pairs tell us is that the sounds that differ from one member of the pair to the other change the meanings of the words, and that they are therefore *contrastive* sounds, or *phonemes* within the language. A sound that changes the meaning of a word when it is substituted for another sound (e.g., /t/ and /r/ in *tent–rent*) is a phoneme in that language. Phonemes are indicated in IPA through the use of slashes (e.g., /b/).

Each language has its own set of phonemes, chosen from the larger set of all speech sounds used in the language. The same types of principles apply to the sets of *phonemes* selected by different languages as to the (larger) sets of sounds: Ideally, the pronunciation of phonemes in a language should be easy, as should differentiating them from one another. Phones that are acoustically too similar (e.g., the voiceless labiodental fricative [f] and the voiceless bilabial fricative [ɸ]) are not used contrastively within a language (Maddieson, 1984). One can most efficiently determine the phonemes of a language (or of a child's phonological system) by obtaining a (large) sample of words and looking for minimal pairs. The examples of minimal pairs (including rhyming words) given earlier help to identify some of the phonemes of English: /p, t, k, g, m, n, s, ʃ, l, r, o, ɔ, i, ɪ/. Multiple minimal pairs within a set, such as *mat, hat, pat, tat, cat, rat, sat, that, bat, fat, gnat*, and *vat*, yield the highest level of confidence that the appropriate phonemes have indeed been identified. Typically, the phonemes correspond for the most part to those sounds of the language that are represented by an alphabetic writing system (if the language has one) and to those sounds of

TABLE 4-5.
Burmese Nasal Minimal Pairs

Word	English Gloss
ma	healthy
m̥a	order
na	pain
n̥a	nostril
ŋa	fish
ŋ̥a	rent

Note: The circles under the letters indicate voicelessness.
Source: Adapted from LH Hyman. *Phonology: Theory and Analysis*. New York: Holt, Rinehart and Winston, 1975.

which the speakers are consciously aware. (Can you think of some exceptions from the English alphabet?)

The phonemes of some other languages represent contrasts rarely heard even in noncontrastive contexts in English. Voiced versus voiceless nasals, for instance, are contrastive phonemes in Burmese, as the minimal pairs given in Table 4-5 illustrate (Hyman, 1975).

If English speakers used such voiceless nasals throughout their speech, speech-language pathologists might question their velopharyngeal status and send them to an ear, nose, and throat specialist. Despite such speakers' apparent vocal deviance, however, listeners would most likely have no trouble understanding what they were saying. Voiceless nasals do not contrast with voiced nasals in English, although voiceless nasals do occur in clusters with [s] in casual speech. The /m/ in *smoke*, for example, usually is pronounced as [m̥] ([sm̥ok]). Although [smok] and [sm̥ok] are acoustically different, they have exactly the same meaning in English, so no lexical confusion could result.

ALLOPHONES. The *allophones* of a phoneme are variant pronunciations of that phoneme that may differ from one word production to another within the same language, either consistently or inconsistently, without changing word meanings. In the previous example, the use of [m̥] versus [m] in the word *smoke* is determined by the speaker's speech style and formality; no semantic difference is intended or inferred. Therefore, [m̥] and [m] are allophones of the same phoneme, /m/. In the examples given earlier, the use of [t] versus [ˀ] (e.g., [kotʰ] versus [koˀ] for *coat*) in final position in English changes the sounds of the words but does not change their meanings. Because of the type of alternation that they exhibit, these two sounds ([t] and [ˀ]) are said to be allophones in **free variation** in final position.[3] Either one may occur in final position of a word without changing the meaning of that word: [mætʰ] and [mæˀ] may sound slightly different, but they both have exactly the same meaning (*mat*). Therefore, [t] and [ˀ] are both allophones of the English phoneme /t/. Furthermore, the speaker's decision whether to use a fully released [tʰ] versus [ˀ] at the end of the word *mat* is a social, not a

---

[3]These two allophones are not in completely free variation, of course, as [ˀ] does not occur in initial position or in most consonant clusters.

phonological, choice. If the conversation is informal and the listener has no hearing or comprehension problems, glottal stop likely will be chosen. If the situation is formal or ease of perception is a paramount concern, a fully released [tʰ] will be used. In the intermediate situation, the speaker may opt for an unreleased but supraglottal [t˺].

Another example of free variation is the use of glottal stop in medial position in American English. In most dialects, this allophone shows up after a stressed vowel in such words as *button*, *Latin*, and *curtain* ([bʌʔɪn, læʔɪn, kɚʔɪn]). Many New Yorkers use glottal stop medially in *little*, *gentle*, *shuttle*, and the like as well. However, in careful speech, most Americans pronounce the [tʰ] allophone, as it sounds more formal and correct and perceiving it is also easier. The choice is dictated completely by social circumstances, not by any aspect of the phonology of English per se. Using either allophone in the wrong situation might raise questions about the person's social status or attitude but would not cause confusion.

Other pairs or groups of allophones may be in **complementary distribution**. In these cases, the two phonetic variants substitute for each other in highly predictable ways. In other words, although the use of one allophone or the other does not change the meaning, people are consistent in their choices of the allophone to use in a given phonetic context. The choice is not a social one; it is dictated by ease of production. For example, as indicated earlier, [m̥] and [m] are both allophones of the English phoneme /m/. However, the point at which each will occur is predictable: The voiceless allophone comes after [s]. This devoicing of /m/ occurs because it is easier to produce a voiceless nasal immediately after the voiceless [s]; formality and intelligibility do not play a major role. No one would be confused by a speaker who used the wrong nasal allophone in a particular word position, but some extra effort would be required from the speaker to do so, and some people might think that that person had an accent (or possibly velopharyngeal insufficiency).

Another example of complementary distribution from English relates to the so-called *dark l* allophone. In English, the articulatory gesture for /l/ consists of both retracting and lowering the tongue dorsum and raising the tip of the tongue toward the alveolar ridge. In final position and before velars, the lowering and retracting is earlier and more extreme, yielding a velarized, or dark, [l]. This lowered, retracted [l] is more vocalic, and the light [l] is more consonantal (Sproat & Fujimura, 1993). The contrast is evident in producing such pairs as *milk–lick*; the [l] in *milk* both feels and sounds less consonantlike. Dark [l] is made with less tongue contact because the tongue is retracted and lowered in the mouth. For these reasons, dark [l] is actually more vowellike than are other [l] allophones. However, most speakers are totally unaware of the difference. They produce dark [l] in final position and before velars, but they think that they are producing light [l] all the time. If someone actually did produce a light [l] in these dark [l] contexts, it would have very little impact on listeners' perceptions, although it might sound as though the person were speaking somewhat carefully. This tendency for

listeners to fail to notice a light [l] substituted for a dark [l] is due to the fact that light and dark [l] are allophones of the same phoneme and therefore are irrelevant to English speech perception processing.

The predictable patterning of light and dark [l] may account for the frequent tendency of children to vowelize [l] in just those positions in which it is dark: in final position and before velars (e.g., [mɪʊk] for *milk*). Children may be hearing dark [l]s, recognizing their vowellike nature, and assuming that a vowel goes there (e.g., they may assume that the word actually is /mɪʊk/). Unlike the substitution of a light [l] for a dark [l]—substitution of one allophone for another—vowelized [l]s usually are noticed, because vowelized [l] is almost identical to [ʊ] and /l/ and /ʊ/ are different, contrastive phonemes. Listeners are very sensitive to phonemic contrasts, even if the two sounds (e.g., /l/ and /ʊ/) are more similar in acoustic or articulatory properties than are some allophone pairs (e.g., dark and light /l/). Thus, listeners tune in to vowelization errors (substitution of a vowel in place of a liquid). They tell the child to say /l/ instead of /ʊ/, and they show the child how to put the tongue-tip on the alveolar ridge, although this position actually is not correct for dark [l].

For this reason, speech-language pathologists must be careful in modeling such allophones as dark [l] to children. The allophone that actually occurs in the word should be modeled, not the allophone that we consciously associate with the letter. It is hardly surprising that children are resistant or slow to learn when speech-language pathologists model light [l] for them (with the tongue-tip on the alveolar ridge) and insist that this sound is correct in *pull* and *milk*; it is not. What the child hears the clinician say within these words actually is dark [l], and it is acoustically much closer to the [ʊ] sound that the children do produce. If we model dark [l] for our clients, they will be more likely to believe us and also more likely to hear the contrast that we wish them to learn (in this case, dark [l] versus [ʊ]).

Another English-language allophonic pattern that may cause clinicians to judge children overly harshly is that of voicing alternations. As discussed in previous chapters, English voiceless stop phonemes (/p,t,k/) actually have some allophones that overlap with those of the voiced stop phonemes /b,d,g/. English voiced and voiceless stops actually differ more in aspiration (the voiceless having it and the voiced not) than in voicing per se. The stops that American phonologists term *voiced* (/b,d,g/) actually are voiceless unaspirated, whereas the *voiceless* are also voiceless but usually are aspirated. However, in consonant clusters with [s], English speakers produce voiceless unaspirated stops for the sounds that we spell as *p*, *t*, *k*. Thus, the consonant sounds in [s] + stop clusters actually are acoustically the same as the English so-called voiced stops. For instance, an accurate IPA transcription of a careful pronunciation of the word *dot* really would be [tɑtʰ]: The initial *d* is voiceless unaspirated, just as is the *t* in *stop* ([stɑp]). This factor may be a contributor to Caleb's confusion (noted in Chapter 2; DePaolis, personal communication, 1997), created when, in response to his mother's reference to the next door neighbor, he protested, "It's not a store!"

TABLE 4-6.
German Voice Contrast: Initial Position

Word	English Gloss
Buste	bust
Puste	breath
dann	then, moreover, thereon
Tann	pine forest
Gabel	fork
Kabel	cable

Note: In German, nouns are capitalized. Glosses are taken from PH Glucksman. *World-Wide German Dictionary.* Greenwich, CT: Fawcett, 1961. Letters in bold represent voice contrast.

TABLE 4-7.
German Voice Contrast: Medial Position

Word	English Gloss
Qua**bb**e	jellyfish
Qua**pp**e	tadpole
lei**d**er	unfortunately; alas!
Lei**t**er	leader, manager
Man**d**el	almond, tonsil
Man**t**el	mantle, cloak
Klin**g**en	to clink, tinkle
Klin**k**en	to operate (e.g., a latch)

Note: Glosses are taken from PH Glucksman. *World-Wide German Dictionary.* Greenwich, CT: Fawcett, 1961. Letters in bold represent voice contrast.

TABLE 4-8.
German Voice Contrast: Final Position

Word	Pronunciation	English Gloss
Ra**d**	[rɑːt]	wheel
Ra**t**	[rɑːt]	counsel
Bun**d**	[bunt]	alliance, league
bun**t**	[bunt]	multicolored
schlu**g**	[ʃluk]	struck, beat (past tense)
Schlu**ck**	[ʃluk]	gulp, sip

Note: The colon represents increased segment duration. Glosses are taken from PH Glucksman. *World-Wide German Dictionary.* Greenwich, CT: Fawcett, 1961. Letters in bold represent neutralized voice contrast.

Both the /d/ phoneme in *door* and the /t/ phoneme in *store* actually are voiceless unaspirated.

The *t* in *top* is even more voiceless; it is voiceless aspirated ([tʰɑp]). Thus, when children produce such words as *stop* without the initial [s] and we perceive *dop*, telling them that they have voiced the initial /t/ is incorrect. In fact, they merely have maintained the appropriate voicing for that allophone of /t/, as it would be pronounced if the [s] also had been produced. A child who pronounces *stop* as [tɑp] (to our ears, *dop*) and *top* as [tʰɑp] actually is maintaining appropriately the contrast between the two words. The child who produces *both* words as [tʰɑp] has not maintained the English voicing contrast. If we train children to say [tʰɑp] for *stop*, they *then* may incorrectly produce [stʰɑp] once they master [s] clusters, which obviously would be inappropriate.

Sometimes a pair of sounds or sound classes may be in contrast (phonemic) in some word positions but allophonic in others. One example of this comes from German. German does have a voicing contrast, such that, for instance, voiced stops can be found in some of the same positions as voiceless stops but in different words. In these cases, just as in English, the occurrence of voice (or lack of voice) signals a meaning difference. Some examples of contrast in initial position are given in Table 4-6.

In contrast to the English t/d voicing contrast that is neutralized in medial position (*latter–ladder*; see previous discussion), voice is contrastive in medial position for all places of articulation in German, as shown in Table 4-7.

However, all stops typically become voiceless in final position. Therefore, as Table 4-8 illustrates, words ending in final voiced stops become homonymic with words ending in final voiceless stops.

The distinction between voiced and voiceless stops is lost in final position, resulting in *partial neutralization* of the contrast. Fortunately, the number of word pairs affected by this partial neutralization is small, and usually context helps to differentiate them.

SURFACE AND UNDERLYING REPRESENTATIONS. When a word actually is pronounced, each phone may be affected in some way by the other phones within the word. A nearby nasal may cause slight nasalization, a velar may cause backing, a rounded vowel may cause rounding, and so on. The production of each phone may be affected also by its position in the word, without any meaning change. As mentioned previously, for example, /t/ often is produced as [ʔ] in word-final position in English.

In this sense, a speaker cannot produce a phoneme in its pure, unadulterated state within a word. The phoneme itself is an abstract mental concept, representing the speech sound which the speaker intends to produce. The sound actually produced is some allophone (whether in free variation or in complementary distribution) of that phoneme.

Because phonemes are viewed as abstract units that cannot actually be produced, the phonemes in a word sometimes are termed the **underlying representation** of the word: the word in its conceptual state before the vagaries of motor planning and motor control become involved. The word as it actually is pronounced—using allophones of the intended phonemes—is termed the **surface representation**. In traditional generative phonology, linguists sketched out word derivations, showing in a step-by-step process the way in which the surface form of a word was derived from the underlying form as phonological rules or processes applied (see Chapter 5) and as sounds were affected by each other and by the overall shape of the word.

FUNCTIONAL LOAD. The notion of phoneme as a functional (i.e., contrastive) phonological unit has been illustrated. However, not every phoneme is as useful as every other to the language. Some phonemes, such as stops in English, are included in many words and involved in many contrasts; they have a high **functional load**. Others, such as [ʒ], play a very minor role in the language as they differentiate only a small set of words; they have a low functional load.

Functional load is, of course, related to ease of perception and ease of production. Those phonemes that are articulated easily and are perceptually salient tend to have higher functional loads for the same reasons they are more commonly found in the languages of the world, in babbling, and in early child vocabulary. If two phonemes within a language are perceptually very similar, at least one of them will likely have a low functional load. In English, for instance, both /f/ and /θ/ are phonemes despite the fact that perceptually they are easily confused (Velleman, 1988). The language has protected itself by including few minimal pair words. Those pairs that do exist typically include at least one word that is either uncommon, archaic, or slang (e.g., *fie–thigh, fink–think*), or they include words from different parts of speech (e.g., *thin–fin*). These pairings do not eliminate all possible confusions,[4] but they do minimize them.

It is important to note that, although functional load is related to the frequency of occurrence of a phoneme, the two may be very different. For example, [ð] is an extremely frequent phoneme in English, but it is used almost exclusively in articles and other fairly redundant function words (*the, that, there,* etc.). Thus, its frequency of use is quite high, but its functional load is quite low. Although it may be noticeable, it is rarely confusing when a nonnative speaker substitutes, for example, [z] or [v] for [ð]: "Zee cat is on zee roof."

SUMMARY.   Segmental contrast is achieved via phones that signal meaning contrasts within a language. Not every phone is contrastive; sets of phones that alternate with each other without changing meanings are individually called *allophones*. Collectively, the allophones from each set represent the outward manifestation of one *phoneme*. Allophones may occur in free variation or in complementary distribution with one another. Phoneme contrasts may be neutralized in certain contexts. The frequency of occurrence of a phoneme is less important than its contrastive value within the language, which is known as its *functional load*.

Child Phonology

FROM SYLLABLE TO SEGMENT.   Children, regardless of their linguistic environments, do not acquire phonology by learning one phoneme at a time and then sticking them together. They first master syllable and word shapes through an extensive period of prelinguistic speech practice (babbling) and then use their best-learned shapes as the basis for words. As the child's lexicon increases and the amount of homonymy becomes unworkable, reorganizations occur and may trigger the emergence of seg-

mental contrast. Once segmental contrast enters the picture, the child's variability in production of segments that contrast with others may decrease (Rice, 1996). In other words, children may produce contrastive phonemes more consistently than other sounds.

"Timmy," whose phonology was analyzed by Vihman et al. (1994), is a case in point. His words and babble were so similar that distinguishing them was difficult for a period of almost 6 months. At 10–11 months, he produced one monosyllabic word shape, [bɑ]. He used this syllable in the presence of balls, blocks, and boxes and to imitate other [b] words, such as *basket, bell, boat, book,* and *button* and, by 15 months, *bird, brush, bunny, baa*. From 11 months on, he used another favorite word shape [kɑkɑ], usually in disyllabic form, to refer to *kitty, quack-quack, car, duck, key,* and *Teddy*. Because of the phonotactic and phonetic contrast between the two word forms, they do not form a true minimal pair. Thus, it cannot be said that Timmy really had two consonant phonemes, although admittedly he did appear to be categorizing words as either labial or not. Rather, he had two production patterns. His overuse of these two simple patterns greatly limited the amount of contrast that was possible within his lexicon. As a result, he had an extremely high level of homonymy.

At 14–15 months, a change occurred as Timmy began to be creative with his [C + ɑ] syllable pattern. He appeared to select consonantal features from target words and attach them to his favorite vowel [ɑ] in a productive manner. For instance, *eye* (phonetically very similar to [ɑj] in adult English) became [jɑ], and [βɑ] was used for words containing consonants with labials, frication, or both (*Ruth, fire, flies, flowers, plum*). Such forms as [nɑ] for *nose* and [mɑ] for *moo* and *moon* followed. At this point, then, Timmy could be said to have a clear set of minimal pairs. However, we certainly cannot say that he had vowel phonemes: No vowel contrast whatsoever was evident in his vowel system, as one single element ([ɑ]) cannot contrast with itself.

A similar lack of contrast can be seen when we consider the nouns in the lexicon of Holly (from SL Velleman, 1994), the 28-month-old who had DVD. Holly's classes of homonymous words at 2 years, 4 months, were the following:

[b] nouns (*bunny, bear, bird, baby* [whispered], *bell, pig* [with gesture], *Bert*)	[bijə, bɛə, bɪʊ]
Other nouns (*tree, kitty, coffee,* and others with nonlabial initial consonants; often unglossable)	[tʰ, tˢ, dɪ], coronal (alveopalatal) click

As with Timmy's words, Holly's nouns appeared to be based on two favorite, overused word shapes. Each word shape had a few variants, but the variants were interchanged in an unsystematic manner; they were not contrastive. It cannot be said that Holly had the phonemes /b/ and /t/ at that point, as these consonants were inseparable from their word shapes. Some words (especially within the [b] noun class) were disambiguated slightly by using vocal or gestural cues: *Baby* was whispered, and *pig*

---

[4]This author once discussed deaf counseling with her sister for 15–20 minutes in a noisy subway car before finally making a comment about sign language, thereby discovering that her sister had been talking about *death* counseling!

TABLE 4-9.
"Alice"'s Initial Minimal Pairs

blanket	[bɑji]
bottle	[pɑji]
mommy	[mɑji]
dolly	[dɑji]
daddy	[tɑji]
(good)night	[nɑji]

Source: Adapted from MM Vihman. Early syllables and the construction of phonology. In Ferguson CA, Menn L, Stoel-Gammon C (eds). *Phonological Development: Models, Research, Implications.* Parkton, MD: York Press, 1992, 393–422; and MM Vihman, SL Velleman, L McCune. How abstract is child phonology? Towards an integration of linguistic and psychological approaches. In Yavas M (ed). *First and Second Language Phonology.* San Diego: Singular, 1994, 9–44.

TABLE 4-10.
"Molly"'s Endings for *Bang* at 1;1.8

[bæː]
[bæʔ]
[bæ̆k]
[bæːŋ]
[bæːɪn]
[bæːini]
[bæŋⁿi]

Note: The colon represents increased segment duration.
Source: Adapted from MM Vihman, SL Velleman. Phonological reorganization: A case study. *Language and Speech* 1989;32:149–170.

TABLE 4-11.
"Molly"'s Final Nasal Pattern at 1;3.24

button	[pɑnə]
round	[hɑnʌ]
around	[wɑnə]
Ernie	[hʌnə]
Brian	[pɑnə]
down	[tænə]
Granma	[næmʌ]
hand	[hɑnɛ]
bang	[pɑnə]
green	[kʏni]
in	[ɪni]
name	[nɛmi]
Nicky	[ɪnni]

Source: Adapted from MM Vihman, SL Velleman. Phonological reorganization: A case study. *Language and Speech* 1989;32:149–170.

was accompanied by a gesture. Therefore, Holly appeared to have intended contrast. Despite this, her intelligibility was severely affected by her limited phonetic and phonotactic repertoires.

As a child's phonological system emerges, segmental contrast may be available to a limited extent, with word shapes continuing to play a role. Such is the case of "Alice" (studied by Vihman, 1992, and Vihman et al., 1994). At 15 months, she produced a convincing set of minimal pairs, but the contrast lay in the initial consonants only, as shown in Table 4-9.

Although she did produce a variety of other word shapes, this palatalized form was clearly a favorite; its ease of production for her may have facilitated her development of initial phonemic contrasts in words of this and similar shapes. By holding the rest of the word form constant, she may have been more able to experiment with and master the initial phoneme contrasts.

Both Timmy and Alice appeared to develop segmental contrasts in initial position first, but this is not necessarily always the case for other children. "Molly," whose phonology was studied by Vihman and Velleman (1989), appeared to focus more on final position. She demonstrated word-final production patterns for both nasals and voiceless obstruents. The chronology of the emergence of word-final nasal segments in her speech was as follows.

At 1 year, 26 days, Molly first attempted words that had a nasal in final position in the adult form: *bang, balloon, button.* However, although *bang* was produced with a final nasal, the others were not. In fact, no consistent production pattern was discernible:

bang	[bɑɪŋ]
balloon	[bʏɛʰ][5]
button	[bʌʔ]

(Note: Transcriptions throughout examples from Vihman & Velleman, 1989, are somewhat simplified for clarity.)

At 1 year, 1 month, 8 days, by using a final velar nasal in keeping with her production pattern for *bang,* Molly imitated *down* as [tæŋ], as though she were trying out an established pattern on a new word. She also experimented with a wide variety of different endings for *bang* (Table 4-10).

After this experimental period, Molly appeared to settle on the (C)VN:V (e.g., [bæŋːi]) pattern as her preferred way of producing nasal-final words. This pattern appeared to have the advantage of making the final nasals more salient by placing them in medial position (before a vowel). By 1 month later, Molly was even restructuring other word types in accordance with her newly established word recipe. Some words with medial nasals in the adult form, and eventually even one word with a target *initial* nasal (*Nicky*), were pronounced in this way. Some examples are given in Table 4-11.

Molly's focus on a pattern for producing final nasals in medial position actually reduced the contrast within her system in one respect. Molly's mother noticed that *button, balloon, banana,* and *bunny* had become indistinguishable, as now all were produced as [pʌn:ə] or [pɑn:ə]. This change may have seemed to her mother like regression. However, the use of this production pattern increased the contrast within Molly's system by providing an easy frame for producing final consonants, so the contrast between, for example, [n] and [m] could be maintained. Furthermore, at the same time as her final nasal production pattern became evident, a final obstruent pattern also was emerg-

---

[5]*Baby gamma* [ʏ] is an upper mid-back unrounded vowel (Pullum & Ladusaw, 1986).

TABLE 4-12.
"Molly"'s Final Obstruent Pattern

glasses	[kɑkʰi]
red	[watʰ]
book	[pʰʊkʰ]
house	[haʊtʰ]
that	[tɑtʰ]
Ruth	[hʌtʰ]
oink	[hokʰ]
peek	[pikʰ]
pig	[pʰɪkʰ]
stuck	[kʰɑkʰ]
walk	[wakʰə]
work	[hʌkʰ]
tock	[tʰakʰi]
block	[pʰakʰ]
click	[kʰɪkʰ]
clock	[kʰɑkʰ]

Note: Superscript "h" indicates aspiration.
Source: Adapted from MM Vihman, SL Velleman. Phonological reorganization: A case study. *Language and Speech* 1989;32:149–170.

TABLE 4-13.
"C"'s Use of Clicks

some	[ləm]
this	[ðɪǀ]
upside-down	[əlaɪdaʊn]
shark	[lɑɚk]
touch	[təǀ]
bridge	[bwɪdǀ]
stove	[lov]
snake	[lneɪk]
school bus	[kulbəǀ]
treasures	[twɛləǀ]
jelly	[lɛwi]

Source: Adapted from LM Bedore, LB Leonard, J Gandour. The substitution of a click for sibilants: A case study. *Clinical Linguistics & Phonetics* 1994;8:283–293.

ing. This pattern (Table 4-12) also appeared to be based on making final consonants as salient as possible, in this case by appending a final vowel (as she had done for nasals) or a very strong aspirate release, or both.

As a result of these two patterns, Molly's segmental contrasts in final position were quite clear. However, note that still not all her contrasts were parallel to the contrasts of the adult system. For instance, *tock* and *clock* were not minimal pairs in her speech at that time, although *click* and *clock* and *block* and *clock* were.

Thus, children with similar phonetic repertoires may use the phones available to them in very different ways, such as achieving contrast in initial position (as Alice did) versus final position (as Molly did). See Ingram (1996) for further discussion.

ACCURACY VERSUS CONTRAST. It is important to note that the development of contrast does not necessarily depend on the accurate production of each phoneme or allophone relevant to that contrast. Neither Timmy nor Alice, for example, produced their words in an adultlike manner. Yet both had sets of minimal pairs by 14–15 months and therefore did achieve a kind of segmental contrast within the contexts of their own phonological systems.

Bedore et al. (1994) provided an example of a child who maintained sound class contrast in a very unusual way. This child ("C"), a 4-year-old monolingual English speaker, produced dental clicks ([ǀ]) in place of all sibilants ([s, z, ʃ, ʒ, tʃ, dʒ]). These clicks, which are produced by flattening the anterior portion of the tongue behind the teeth to create suction, sometimes were combined with stops by this child to represent the stop + fricative combinations called *affricates*. Furthermore, C used clicks to mark morphologically important fricatives: third-person singular, possessives, and noun plurals were indicated with a click. Some examples are given in Table 4-13.

This child was stimulable for sibilants and began to produce them all in an adultlike manner after a very brief period of intervention (four sessions) focused only on /s/. The authors noted that *click* had been C's favorite sound since her earliest word productions and that dental clicks are acoustically similar to sibilant sounds (similar noise spectra). They also speculated that using a click rather than stops to substitute for sibilants avoided the problem of increasing the functional loads of [t] and [d]. However, using one phone (click) to substitute for an entire sound class must have been less and less effective for a child whose vocabulary was likely to have been growing quickly. This may account, in part, for her extremely rapid learning once her attention was focused through therapy on the appropriate production patterns.

Another striking case of contrast without articulatory accuracy was reported by Howard (1993). She described a child with cleft palate, "Rachel," whose phonetic repertoire included very few standard English phones. Phones that could be produced in an adultlike manner were restricted to [m, b, f, θ, w, j, ʔ]. The other phones Rachel used are considered "deviant" by English speakers. They included non-English places of articulation (e.g., uvular and pharyngeal), manners of articulation (e.g., ingressive air flow), and combinations of features (e.g., voiced velar glide, labiodental nasal).

Despite these deviant phonetic characteristics, Rachel enjoyed a "high level of intelligibility," and she was "exceptionally resistant to therapy" (Howard, 1993, p. 300). On investigation, it was determined that this child's phonotactic repertoire was adultlike. She was able to produce even three-element consonant clusters. Furthermore, she was using her unusual set of phones to signal most contrasts within English phonology. She was particularly successful at maintaining the nasal-oral contrast and the continuant contrasts (stops versus fricatives versus affricates). For example, she contrasted nasal versus oral stops by using a uvular nasal for the former and a glottal plosive (combined with place of articulation cues, such as lip closure) for the latter. She contrasted stops versus fricatives by achieving complete closure somewhere in the vocal tract for stops and by achieving friction somewhere for fricatives. Place and voicing contrasts were maintained less successfully, but evidence indicated that Rachel was attempting to make these distinctions. For instance, she distinguished stops from affricates by using a sequence of closures for the affricate, in keeping with English phonology. However, neither the stops nor the affricates were produced in a form that closely resembled adult articulation of such contrasts, as illustrated here:

tap   [ʔæʔʰ]

yes   [jɛʔ]

jam   [ʔjæm]

In Rachel's speech, [ʔ], [j], and [ʔj] were contrastive elements representing stops, glides, and affricates, respectively. Furthermore, affricates were produced as conjunctions of two consonantal elements, as in typical English. Similarly, the alveolar-palatal contrast from the English fricative series (e.g., s/ʃ) was signaled by using labialization to mark palatals. This tendency mirrors the lip-rounding that typically does accompany production of palatal fricatives:

Sue [ʐu]   shoe [ʐʷu]

sock [ʐɒʔʰ]   shop [ʐʷjɒp̄ʰ]

(Note: [ʐ] represents a voiceless palatal fricative—[ç]—with audible nasal escape; [ʐʷ] is the labialized version of the same. See Duckworth et al., 1990, for details.)

Thus, Rachel maintained contrasts between appropriate English phonological categories while using few of the appropriate articulatory characteristics of the phonemes or sound classes in question. Howard speculated that Rachel's resistance to therapy resulted from her reluctance to dismantle a complex system of contrasts that, after all, was working for her. Intervention in such cases must be designed in such a way as to do as little damage as possible to the functioning aspects of the system while gradually replacing the deviant elements with more appropriate ones. Unfortunately, Howard did not indicate how (or, indeed, whether) this end was achieved in Rachel's case. In any case, Rachel is a perfect example of a child who managed to maintain most of the contrasts within the language without being able to produce a number of the phones with which they usually are maintained.

Heselwood (1997) provided a similar example of an adult who was severely dysfluent. This patient used a voiced nasal click to represent sonorants and a non-nasal click to represent obstruents. With these substitutions, he was able to maintain all the contrasts expected in adult English.

In summary, early and delayed or disordered children's phonologies may exhibit a certain amount of tension between reliance on well-practiced word patterns or favorite sounds and the need for contrast. Some children manage to communicate with very little contrast (and therefore a high degree of homonymy) for certain periods. However, as their vocabularies grow, new solutions must be sought to increase the potential for contrast, or they will be unintelligible. Some children's—and adults'—unusual solutions may increase contrast in a manner that largely parallels, but does not match, the normal adult phonology.

PHONEMES AND ALLOPHONES: SURFACE AND UNDERLYING REPRESENTATIONS IN CHILD PHONOLOGY.   The issue of children's underlying representations has generated much intellectual heat in the past (beginning with such authors as Braine 1974, 1976; Macken, 1979; Moskowitz, 1975; Smith, 1973; and Stampe, 1969), and undoubtedly it will continue to do so for some time to come. We focus here on those aspects of the debate that bear most directly on actual clinical practice.

The fundamental question to be posed is, "What do children know and when do they know it?" Other questions follow. Do children store the full phonetic form of each word that they learn? Are children aware of the full adult form of each word they attempt to produce, or are children's production targets sometimes an incomplete or incorrect version of the adult word? If children do store the full adult phonetic forms in their recognition (perception) memory, do they store them less accurately in their production memory bank, or is the word accurately stored in one location only, with "output rules" that turn an accurate perceptually based memory into an inaccurately produced word?

Children's Perceptions of Contrasts.   A few studies of children's discrimination (speech sound perception) have shown a relationship between nonadult perception and nonadult production of specific, acoustically difficult contrasts. Children who do not do well at producing certain contrasts also perform poorly at discriminating those same contrasts (e.g., /f/ versus /θ/; Velleman, 1988). However, children can discriminate many other pairs of error phonemes despite their substitutions of those same phonemes. Clearly, misperception does not account for the majority of children's phonological simplifications. (For further discussion see, for example, Barton, 1980; Eilers & Oller, 1976; Hoffman et al., 1983; Kornfeld, 1971; Locke, 1980; Maxwell & Weismer, 1982; and Velleman, 1988.)

Despite what appears to be mostly accurate perception, young and disordered children often do distort the adult forms of words in a significant manner, including cases of migration or metathesis across intervening elements (e.g., [uz] for *zoo*; Leonard & McGregor, 1991; and [gɑbi] for *buggy*; Berman, 1977). Such cases are quite rare in adult phonology. Fee (1991), Fikkert (1991), Lleó (1992), Macken (1993), McDonough and Myers (1991), Menn and Matthei (1992), Ohala (1991), Velleman (1992), Vihman et al. (1994), and others have proposed that young or disordered children, regardless of what they may be capable of perceiving, may have simplified phonological output representations of words. In other words, their production plans may be simpler than their perceptual abilities would suggest. For example, children who have a preferred production template at a given time may seem to ignore a reasonable amount of perceived word-specific information. Such children may use the phonetic or phonotactic patterns that they have established as production templates rather than using the actual adult form of the word, even if they know at some level how the word should sound.

In fact, in some cases one can be reasonably sure that a child is choosing (subconsciously, of course) not to use the proper adult form of the word, as the child's earlier fairly

TABLE 4-14.
"Nathan"'s Use of [d] and [n] (Hypothetical)

doggie	[dɔdi]
cookie	[dʊdi]
go	[do]
mom	[nɑn]
more	[nod]
no	[no]
butter	[dʌdʌd]
bye	[dɑɪ]
pig	[dɪd]
shoe	[du]
feather	[dɛdʊd]
sing	[dɪn]
string	[dɪn]
blue	[du]
basket	[dædæd]
monster	[nʌnʌd]
first	[dɪd]

accurate word forms appear to "regress" as the words come to conform more closely to one another. One example of this sort was described for "J" (Macken, 1978) in Chapter 2. J temporarily sacrificed the segmental accuracy of the initial sibilant fricative /s/ in *silla* (Spanish for *chair*) to increase the number of syllables to two. He was capable of producing a sibilant at the beginning of the word, and his first form of *silla* did include an initial [ʃ] ([ʃːɑ]). However, when he increased the length of the word to include both syllables, he gave up producing a fricative in initial position at all ([kɪjɑ], [tɪːjɑ]). Clearly, he had perceived the initial fricative; his stopping of this fricative was a phonological choice, not an articulatory necessity.

This case and Molly's apparent regression illustrate that children may choose not to use information that they have in planning their productions of words. However, whether the apparently unused information about the word is still available somewhere in their brains to assist in discriminating that word from others, or whether it is filtered completely out of the incoming auditory signal, is not certain. *Children's Awareness of Contrasts.* One group of researchers has carefully considered children's **phonological knowledge** (i.e., the information about the underlying representation of the word that is available to the child's speech production–planning mechanism). In works such as Barlow (1996), Dinnsen and Elbert (1984), Elbert et al. (1984), Elbert and Gierut (1986), and Gierut (1985), the authors have conducted clinical research to demonstrate that this factor may predict learning curves and improvement resulting from phonological intervention. Specifically, they claim that those children who appear to have stored more complete information about the adult form of the word are more likely to gain and generalize from remediation than are those who have stored little such information.

Unfortunately, it is impossible to assess a child's phonological knowledge directly. This information must be inferred either from the child's phonemic perception (a process fraught with difficulties) or from the child's production patterns. Elbert and Gierut (1986) and their col-

leagues opt for the second of these routes. They use a variety of different means for identifying the child's use of phonemic contrasts and for inferring the child's awareness (knowledge) of these contrasts. First, they determine the child's phonetic repertoire, including the distribution requirements that operate on this repertoire. For instance, consider a child who uses fricatives and voiceless stops only in final position, voiced stops only in initial and medial positions, and no liquids in any words. Given this information, they are able to determine those sounds that are used contrastively by the child. If the child uses fricatives only in final position, a fricative-stop *phoneme contrast* is not possible in initial or medial position but may be possible in final position. Thus, the child has some limited "knowledge" of fricatives as contrastive elements. If voiced stops are used in initial and medial positions only, and voiceless stops in final position only, no voiced-voiceless stop contrast is possible. Voiced and voiceless stops are in *complementary* distribution (i.e., predictably occurring in distinct word positions). They are *allophones* rather than phonemes with respect to each other, because they do not contrast with each other. If no contrast occurs ever, it is less likely that the child has any phonological knowledge of that contrast. In this hypothetical case, liquids may be neither phonemes nor allophones because they simply do not occur in the child's speech.

Sometimes one discovers a contrast that is not immediately evident. For example, a child who produces both *pig* and *pick* as [pɪ] may appear to have no knowledge of final voicing contrasts—or even of final consonants at all. Yet, if the same child pronounces *piggie* as [pɪgi] and *picky* as [pɪki], one infers that the child must know that *pig* contains a final consonant and that it is voiced, even though the child cannot pronounce it as such. Therefore, Elbert and Gierut (1986) advocated the second step of searching for minimal pairs in a variety of phonological and morphological contexts (*piggie* as well as *pig*, *digging* as well as *dig*, etc.). In one study (Barlow, 1996), children with more phonological knowledge produced less variable forms of target sounds. However, in other studies, such as Velleman (1988), children's variability initially increased when they became aware of a phonemic contrast (specifically /f/ versus /θ/).

Dinnsen and Elbert (1984), Elbert et al. (1984), and Gierut (1985) demonstrated that children make the most progress on aspects of adult phonologies about which they have the most knowledge. For instance, children who appeared to omit final consonants yet showed some evidence of knowledge that they exist (such as the hypothetical, previously described child who says [pɪ] for *pig* but [pɪgi] for *piggie*) made more progress and generalized better in remediation than did children who showed no such awareness of the existence of final consonants in adult speech (Dinnsen & Elbert, 1984).

Some examples should help to clarify the issues of phonemes and allophones in children's phonological systems. First, consider the data in Table 4-14 from a hypothetical child called "Nathan." Looking at Nathan's use of [d] and [n], one can see that he uses them contrastively. Both phones occur in all word positions and before the same vowels. Furthermore, there are minimal pairs in all word positions:

TABLE 4-15.
"Jacob"'s Harmony

| [dædum, gɑkɑ, dædæ, dɑitɑ, gigʌ, didi, dejdɑ] | thank you |
| [geikʌ, dedɑ] | Jacob |

Source: Adapted from L Menn. *Pattern, Control, and Contrast in Beginning Speech: A Case Study in the Development of Word Form and Word Function.* Bloomington, IN: Indiana University Linguistics Club, 1978a.

[do]—[no]   (*go* versus *no* and *more*)

[dʌdʌd]—[nʌnʌd]   (*butter* versus *monster*)

[dɪd]—[dɪn]   (*pig* versus *sing*)

The phones [n] and [d] differentiate words in Nathan's system. If one is substituted for another, it will make a different word. Therefore, *n* and *d* are said to be separate phonemes for Nathan, and slashes are used to indicate this: /n/, /d/. Similarly, Nathan uses a variety of vowel phones, and many of these are contrastive:

[dɔdi]—[dʊdi]   (*doggie* versus *cookie*)

[dʌdʌd]—[dædæd]   (*butter* versus *basket*)

These vowels are separate phonemes for Nathan because they function to add contrast to his system, and slash notation is used to indicate this: /ɔ/, /ʊ/, /ʌ/, /æ/.

Sometimes, a child is able to produce only inconsistently both members of a phonotactic or phonetic contrast pair, with no predictable phonological pattern. The phones involved in this type of variability typically are termed *allophones* in free variation, as discussed earlier with respect to adult phonologies. For example, Menn's "Jacob" (Menn, 1978a) produced variant forms of each word with different (usually harmonized) consonants in different productions, shown in Table 4-15.

For Jacob, [d] and [g] clearly are not distinct phonemes. They vary randomly with each other. Although the two consonants in one word typically will agree in place of articulation (although not always, according to Menn), it is unpredictable whether that place of articulation will be alveolar or velar in a given production of the word. Therefore, [d] and [g] are allophones in free variation for Jacob at this stage.

Other children's patterns may appear similar at first glance but differ in important ways. Consider the data from Bleile (1991) in Table 4-16. Initially, one may expect d/g minimal pairs within this set, but only vowel minimal pairs are found (e.g., *di–du, go–gæ*). When one looks more closely, it is evident that [d] and [g] are allophones in complementary distribution. Specifically, [d] occurs before high vowels (as it requires the tongue-tip to be up), and [g] before lower vowels (as the tongue-tip typically is lower for [g]). This pattern resembles the CV babble patterns identified by Davis and MacNeilage (1990). As Bleile (1991) pointed out, the vowels actually are providing the only contrast.

Acoustic Studies of Contrast. A strong note of caution is necessary here. Studies of acoustics such as those of Kornfeld

TABLE 4-16.
Consonant Allophones

tea	[di]
toe	[go]
go	[go]
goose	[du]
key	[di]
train	[gæŋ]
dress	[gə]
dog	[gæ]
clue	[du]
cloud	[gæ]

Source: Adapted from KM Bleile. *Child Phonology: A Book of Exercises for Students.* San Diego: Singular, 1991.

(1971), Macken and Barton (1979), Weismer et al. (1981), and Velleman (1988) have demonstrated that some children who appear to demonstrate either a lack of contrast or a pattern of allophones in fact may be maintaining a phonemic contrast, although not well enough. Such children may be differentiating words articulatorily by producing two sounds or sound classes contrastively within words. However, due to motor limitations, these children may produce the sounds or sound classes in such a way that the difference is not perceived by adult English speakers (except, in some cases, by parents or speech-language pathologists who are accustomed to the children's speech).

In the three examples described by Weismer et al. (1981), final stops were omitted from all words. If no final stops are present, of course the voicing contrast cannot be preserved in final position—or can it? Two of the three children actually lengthened the vowels in words that should have had final *voiced* stops only. They produced such words as *cab* with prolonged vowels ([kæ:]) and such words as *cap* with shorter ones ([kæ]). Although in American English, most speakers actually do tend to produce longer vowels before voiced than before voiceless stops, listeners expect to hear the final consonant as well, so these children previously had not been given credit for maintaining this contrast. Yet, these subjects were actually contrasting voiced versus voiceless final consonants in a sense, by way of the preceding vowels. This strategy parallels that used by English speakers to maintain the contrast between such word pairs as *ladder* and *latter*.

Kornfeld (1971) reported a similar finding for children who were labeled as *gliders*. They appeared to be producing [w] for adult /r/ and /l/. Kornfeld found acoustic differences between their attempted glides (/w/) and their attempted liquids (/l/, /r/), even though all three sounded the same to the adult ear. Thus, these children presumably were attempting to differentiate [w] from the liquids but were unable to do so in a manner that listeners could detect.

From the most functional point of view, the children in these studies still were neutralizing the contrasts in question because the articulatory distinctions that they were making could not be perceived and therefore did not make the children any more intelligible. However, prognosis for improve-

TABLE 4-17.
Child Partial Neutralization (Hypothetical)

go	[doʊ]
dough	[doʊ]
coat	[tot]
duck	[dʌk]
tuck	[tʌk]
egg	[ɛk]
dad	[dæt]
hat	[hæt]
quack	[twæk]
dog	[dɔk]
good	[dʊt]
bad	[bæt]
bat	[bæt]
pat	[pæt]

ment is considered to be far better for children who are producing a contrast at any level (perceptible or not) than for children who apparently are unaware of the distinction to be made. Articulatory attempts at phonological contrast provide one more piece of evidence about the child's phonological knowledge, which is predictive of outcome (Dinnsen & Elbert, 1984; Elbert et al., 1984; and Gierut, 1985).

As in adult phonologies, child phonologies may include pairs of sounds (or sound classes) that are in contrast in some contexts but neutralized in others. Often, voicing is the contrast that is *partially neutralized* in child speech, just as it is in German. Consider the sample in Table 4-17.

Considering initial position, one can see that voiced and voiceless stops do contrast there, as they do in adult English. Minimal pair contrasts, such as *duck* versus *tuck*, are maintained. However, in final position, all consonants are devoiced. No contrast exists in the child's productions of *bad* versus *bat*. Therefore, the voicing contrast is neutralized in final position only in this child's phonology, just as it is in German.

Summary. Phonemes are minimal speech-sound units that convey a lexical meaning difference between two words. They help speakers to distinguish one word from another. Pairs of sounds that are not in contrast with one another may be allophones in free variation (random occurrence of one or the other) or allophones in complementary distribution (predictable occurrence of one or the other). The contrastive use of two different phones is an important indicator of phonological knowledge and may predict progress in therapy.

IMPACT OF PHONOTACTICS ON CONTRAST. Although phonemes typically have "gotten all the press," phonotactic contrasts can have a major impact on the child's communicative effectiveness as well. Timmy, the child who produced very limited forms for several months, is a case in point. His two initial word forms, [ba] and [kaka], both included only CV syllable shapes. Furthermore, they did not contrast consistently by number of syllables, as the *kaka* words sometimes were produced as [ka] only. Even as his repertoire began

to expand at 14–15 months, the words he added were still in CV(CV) form: [ja], [βa], [na], [ma]. Homonymy continued to be pervasive. For instance, [ja] was used for *ear*, *eye*, and *hair*, and [ma] was used for *moo*, *moon*, *mushrooms*. At 16 months, he added vowel contrast to his system with [bi], [bu], [ki], [ku], and the like. Limited phonotactic contrast also finally was added, as minimal pairs that differed in number of syllables (e.g., [ba] for *block/peg*, [baba] for *baby*, *bracelet*) began to occur. This new phonotactic differentiation added significantly to his potential for contrast. However, syllables continued to be limited to CV form (no clusters or final consonants), and therefore words remained restricted to CV and CVCV options.

Grunwell (1981) provided another example of a child who had limited contrast within his system, owing to phonotactic limitations. This child produced neither clusters nor final consonants. As a result, homonymy was frequent in his speech. Examples included the use of the syllable [ti] to express *tea*, *tree*, *cheese*, *key*, *string*, and *queen*.

Velten's child (as described by Ingram, 1981) is another case in point. She was able to produce a variety of phonemes in CV and CVC word shapes. However, her restriction to monosyllables led to very widespread homonymy, with up to 12 meanings for one word shape. Similarly, Lleó's subject (1990) reverted to homonymy at a later time. Although her phonetic repertoire was growing, she was stuck with one- and two-syllable word shapes at a time when she was attempting many trisyllabic words. As a result, many multisyllabic words were reduced to shorter, homonymic forms.

Thus, a limited phonotactic repertoire has just as much potential for restricting communicative contrast within a child's phonological system as does a limited phonetic repertoire.

FUNCTIONAL LOAD. Functional load is vital to the assessment of contrast in children's systems and to the selection of intervention targets. Children may be quite tolerant of homonymy as the cost of an increased vocabulary size until their systems become nonfunctional as a result. The overuse of a particular phoneme or word or syllable shape is one of the factors that may decrease the level of contrast in children's systems, rendering the children unintelligible. Holly, the child with DVD, and Timmy, the younger, normally developing child, have been described earlier as examples of children who overused their favorite word shapes. Other children may overuse particular phones. "Mike," a 4-year-old described by Pollock (1983), was a case in point (Table 4-18).

Mike had two consonant phonemes in his phonological system. Clearly, /d/ and /n/ *were* separate phonemes because they contrasted. For instance, [da] (*balls*, *got*, *stand*, and *sun*) and [na] (*right*) were minimal pairs. However, note that these two phonemes were doing all the consonantal work in Mike's communication system. Their very high functional loads resulted in a great deal of homonymy—for example, [da] expressed four different meanings. As a result, Mike was very unintelligible. Nathan, described earlier in the chapter, was very similar in that /d/ and /n/ had very high functional loads as the only consonants within his system.

TABLE 4-18.
"Mike"'s High Functional Load for Alveolar

balls	[dɑ]
dish	[dɪ]
fast	[dæ]
got	[dɑ]
hat	[næ]
mask	[næ]
right	[nɑ]
stand	[dɑ]
sun	[dɑ], [dɑn]
tent	[dɛ]

Source: Adapted from KE Pollock. Individual preferences: Case study of a phonologically delayed child. *Topics in Language Disorders* 1983;3:10–23.

Grunwell (1982) provided another example. As we saw in Chapter 2, 6-year-old "Martin" coalesced all fricative + liquid/glide consonant clusters and some stop + liquid/glide consonant clusters into [f]. This same phone also served to represent several other fricatives and affricates, as seen in Table 4-19.[6]

Although /f/ certainly was not the only consonant phoneme in Martin's speech, clearly it was overworked in initial position. In comparison to adult English /f/, Martin's /f/ was doing quadruple duty. From a relational analysis standpoint, this one sound represented adult singleton /f/, /f/ clusters, singleton fricatives and affricates, and clusters with fricatives and affricates. Its use had been overgeneralized even to some clusters with stops. Specifically, those stop + liquid clusters that adults tend to affricate in casual speech (e.g., *drinking*) were produced as [f] by Martin. In fact, a further examination of Martin's word forms provides even deeper insight. The words given in Table 4-20 illustrate that [v]—[f]'s voiced counterpoint—also had a high functional load, but in medial and final position. Thus, labiodental appears to have been a favored place of articulation for Martin, with voicing dependent on word position. It is clear that the frequency of occurrence and the functional loads of [f] and [v] in this child's speech were far too high.

In summary, children with limited phonotactic repertoires, especially those who are unable to get beyond particular phonotactic templates, may have reduced potential for contrast. This situation may hold temporarily even for children with age-appropriate phonetic and phonemic repertoires. Children who rely too heavily on particular phonemes, resulting in inappropriate functional loads, may also evidence poor intelligibility owing to lack of contrast.

IMPLICATIONS FOR REMEDIATION

A child whose phonology does not allow for sufficient contrast will not be able to communicate effectively. Specifying the amount of contrast needed is difficult, as such needs depend in large part on the child's communicative

[6]The [a]/[ɑ] distinction made by Grunwell is a contrast of British English not found in most dialects of American English.

TABLE 4-19.
"Martin"'s High Functional Load for [f]

cheese	[fi]
chimney	[fɪmni]
drinking	[fɪnʔɪn]
farm	[fɑm]
feather	[fɛvə]
flag	[fav]
flower	[fɑʊə]
juice	[fuʔ]
sandwiches	[famwɪʔɪ]
scissors	[fɪvə]
ship	[fɪp]
sleeping	[fiʔm]
strawberries	[fɔbɛɹi]
string	[fɪn, fɪm]
sugar	[fʊvə]
swimming	[fɪmɪn]
thread	[fev]
thumb	[fʌm]
train	[feɪm]
tree	[fi]

Source: Adapted from P Grunwell. *Clinical Phonology.* Rockville, MD: Aspen, 1982.

TABLE 4-20.
"Martin"'s High Functional Load for [v]

feather	[fɛvə]
flag	[fav]
thread	[fev]
scissors	[fɪvə]
sugar	[fʊvə]
bridge	[bɪv]
pig	[bɪv]
cage	[geɪv]
color	[kʊvə]
finger	[fɪnvə]
red	[ʊev]

Source: Adapted from P Grunwell. *Clinical Phonology.* Rockville, MD: Aspen, 1982.

situation. Vocabulary size, mental age, familiarity of listeners, and motivation are just a few of the factors that determine the necessary amount of contrast. Intelligibility (especially as reported by very familiar listeners, such as parents) and frustration level are key indicators of insufficient contrast.

It is important not to forget that a child with limited phonological resources may attempt to maintain contrasts in an unexpected manner. Rachel, the child with cleft palate who used unusual phones to parallel English contrasts, and the children with nonfunctional phonologies who used prosody in unusual ways to introduce more contrast into their systems are examples of this behavior.

Independent Versus Relational Assessment

As with all other aspects of child phonology, analyzing and assessing a phonological system can be accomplished in two ways: independently and relationally. To assess contrast *independently*, sources of contrast within the child's own forms must be identified without consideration for the target forms. For example, if [b] and [β] function to differentiate words within the phonological system, they will be considered to be contrastive phonemes within that system, regardless of the fact that they are not distinct phonemes in adult English. Specifically, if *bear* and *bare* are produced distinctly by a child as [bɛ] and [βɛ], they will not be considered to be homonyms within that child's phonology. Regardless of their status in the ambient language, they are contrastive for the child.

To assess contrast *relationally*, the contrasts produced by children are compared directly to those of the adult language. The children's speech is analyzed to determine whether they have neutralized any contrasts that are present in the adult phonology (e.g., by substituting one for the other). The phonology of each child's lexicon is investigated to identify homonymy in the child's system that does not parallel adult homonymy.

Thus far, independent analysis of the child's system itself has been the main focus in this book. Relational analysis is one major focus of Chapter 5. In the following section, independent analysis will continue to be emphasized (i.e., assessing the child's system as a system rather than comparing it to other, adult systems). However, some relational analysis procedures also are presented.

Many types of contrast can be assessed by extending the analysis of the data organized via procedures previously discussed. These are reviewed here, listed according to considerations that arise from a contrast perspective.

Child Production of Contrastive Word Shapes

As indicated in Chapter 2, various aspects of word shape can be assessed using do-it-yourself forms. First, identification of the child's phonotactic repertoire (using Forms 2-1 through 2-3) can be used to determine the occurrence of initial consonants, final consonants, and consonant clusters in the child's speech. These elements alone can yield a variety of contrasts within the developing phonological system:

- Initial consonant versus initial vowel
- Final consonant versus final vowel (open versus closed syllable)
- Clusters versus singleton consonants

Additionally, the occurrence of multisyllabic words, reduplicated syllables, or harmonized forms is a very strong indicator of the amount of syllable or word contrast available. The following questions are relevant here:

- *Word length*: Are words with different numbers of syllables available to the child in speech production? In other words, is word length (in syllables) contrastive (*p* versus *peepee*)?
- *Reduplication*: If word length in syllables is contrastive, is the content of those syllables also contrastive? For example, can the child contrast *potato* versus *tomato* or only *toe*

versus *Toto*? Children who frequently reduplicate may not be able to contrast syllables within a word.

- *Harmony/assimilation*: Is the child able to produce words with two (or more) different consonants (or vowels) within a word? If all consonants (or vowels) within a word harmonize with one another, many possible contrasts are eliminated (e.g., *top* versus *pop*; *pot* versus *tot*; *baby* versus *beebee*).
- *Consonant-vowel combinations*: Can consonants and vowels freely combine, or are specific consonants restricted to co-occurrence with certain vowels or vice versa? If both *baa* and *bee* cannot occur, for instance, featural variety within syllables is limited.

Forms 3-1 through 3-4 (Consonant Repertoire, Vowel Repertoire, and Cluster Repertoires), which facilitate the identification of the child's phonetic repertoires, are useful for answering questions such as the following:

- Do all consonants occur in all positions, or are some restricted to initial, medial, or final positions, limiting possible contrast? (Recall Leonard and McGregor's subject [1991], who always produced fricatives in final position, even if they occurred in initial position in the adult word and even if the result was a final consonant cluster. For this child, *oops* and *soup* would be homonyms: [ups].)
- Is it possible for two different consonants to occur consecutively? Restrictions on adjacent consonants reduce the contrast made available by the production of clusters versus singleton consonants. (Recall Martin's use of a singleton [f] to represent most consonant clusters as well as some singleton fricatives.)
- Do strong distribution requirements exist in the form of a word recipe and require certain features to occur in a certain order? (Recall Berman's "Shelli" [1977], who always produced velar first [before labial or alveolar] in the word. Although she was not reported actually to have produced these words, presumably such pairs as *gum* and *mug* would have been homonyms for her: [gʌm].)

In addition, the clinician can search for phonotactic minimal pairs and simply list them to aid in identifying the contrasts the child appears to be making. For instance, Joan, the highly homonymic child described by Ingram (1981; based on Velten, 1943) was restricted to monosyllabic words; word length was not contrastive within her system. However, she did show some evidence of phonotactic contrast. Her three favorite homonymic word shapes were [bɑt], [bu], and [bʊt]. These word shapes differed in their vowel qualities but also in the presence versus absence of a final consonant. On the basis of this evidence, then, one is able to hypothesize that Joan could use CVC versus CV word shapes as a source of contrast within her otherwise somewhat limited phonotactic system, even though she could not use CV or CVC versus CVCV.

In short, the more varied the syllable and word shapes that children can control productively, the more contrast will be available to them.

Child Production of Contrastive Sound Classes

The sounds that children can produce can be combined in a wide variety of ways to increase the number of contrasts within their systems. A first look for contrastive sound classes may be made using Forms 3-1 through 3-4. Sound classes that are missing from the phonetic inventory clearly are not available for such purposes. For example, if children lack fricatives in all positions, fricatives clearly are not available to contrast with other consonant phonemes. The same holds for individual phonemes—for instance, if [s] is never used, it cannot participate in phonemic contrasts.

Another important aspect of contrast that can be gleaned from these phonetic inventory forms is the occurrence of contrast across positions. It is common for children to have self-imposed nonadult restrictions on the sound classes that they use in certain word positions. Some questions that often are useful in this respect include the following:

- *Voicing*: Is the child able to contrast voiced elements with voiceless elements at the same position in the word? For example, do both voiced and voiceless stops occur in initial position, or in final position? If, for instance, all voiced stops occur in initial position whereas voiceless stops occur in final position only, they cannot possibly contrast.
- *Frication*: Do fricatives and stops occur in the same word positions? Often, fricatives will occur in final position only, with stops occurring in all but final position. Again, no contrast is possible if the two sound types do not show up in the same places.
- *Velar consonants*: Do all places of articulation occur in all word positions? It is not unusual for a child to produce velars in final position only. Other places of articulation may occur in all positions (in which case, contrast is possible but only in final position) or may occur in all except final position (in which case, contrast with velar is not possible, as the place of articulation features are in complementary distribution).

Any sound classes that have restricted distributions of these types will participate in a limited number of contrasts.

Another simple do-it-yourself strategy is to search for phonetically similar words within the speech sample collected from the child. In a small sample (e.g., 200 words or less), one would not expect to find very many minimal pairs, but pairs or even triplets that differ by only two segments rather than one segment (*near-minimal pairs*) can often be found. Examples of such near-minimal pairs could include *strike-swipe*, *Parker-Harper*, and *pray-clay* as evidence that [k] and [p] are in contrast. Phones that occur in several such contrastive sets are highly likely to be separate phonemes in the child's system.

Consider again the data from Molly at 14–15 months of age. Molly tended to focus on final position, and many of her words had very similar endings. Despite this, several minimal pairs or near-minimal pairs occurred within her speech sample, as illustrated in Table 4-21.

The occurrence of these pairs clearly indicates that Molly used several different consonants (e.g., [p] versus

TABLE 4-21.
"Molly"'s Minimal Pairs

Minimal Pairs/Triples	Near-Minimal Pairs
[panə], [wanə]	[hanʌ], [hʌnə]
[hanʌ], [hanɛ]	[næmʌ], [nɛmi]
[pʰakʰ], [kʰakʰ]	[pikʰ], [pʰɪkʰ]
[kʰakʰ], [kʰɪkʰ]	[tatʰ], [tʰakʰi]
[pʰukʰ], [pʰɪkʰ], [pʰakʰ]	[kakʰi], [kʰakʰ]
[tatʰ], [watʰ]	
[kʰɪkʰ], [pʰɪkʰ]	
[hautʰ], [hʌtʰ]	

Source: Adapted from MM Vihman, SL Velleman. Phonological reorganization: A case study. *Language and Speech* 1989;32:149–170.

[w] and versus [k]; [t] versus [w]) and vowels (e.g., [a] versus [ɪ] versus [ʊ]; [aʊ] versus [ʌ]; [æ] versus [ɛ]) contrastively. Therefore, each of these phones probably functioned as a distinct phoneme within her system. Note that aspirated versus unaspirated stops (e.g., [kʰ] versus [k]) may also have been contrastive; further data would confirm or disconfirm this possibility.

If locating minimal pair (or near-minimal pair) words is difficult, minimal pair syllables can be also sought in a child who (unlike Molly) does produce varied bisyllabic words. For example, if the child says [badʊ] for *bottle* and [dadi] for *daddy*, the two initial syllables of these words provide some evidence for a b/d contrast: [ba] versus [da]. The two final syllables—[dʊ] versus [di]—support a ʊ/i contrast. Form 4-1 provides a framework for listing such contrasts systematically, such that minimal pairs, near-minimal pairs, and syllable-minimal pairs that provide evidence for the same contrast can be listed in one row.

Sample data are provided in Example 4-1 from 5½-year-old "Christine." The sample was small; therefore, few minimal pairs were identified. She had extremely few words of more than one syllable, so minimal syllable pairs within longer words were rare. She had several vowel contrasts, however, and a limited stop versus fricative versus nasal contrast (/s/ versus /p/) in final position. In initial position, she contrasted /w/ versus /m/ and /j/ versus /m/ (both glide versus nasal) and /n/ versus /m/ (alveolar versus labial). It is interesting to note that all these contrasts—in both initial and final positions—include a labial as one member of the pair. Clearly, labial was a well-established place of articulation for Christine, one that she was able to use as a basis for phonemic contrast.

In many cases, one of the diagnostic questions that must be addressed concerns the child's substitutions: What phones does the child produce for various target adult phonemes? This question is most familiar to most clinicians. To answer this question, relational analysis must compare adult forms to child forms.

Forms just like do-it-yourself Forms 3-1 and 3-2, renumbered and relabeled as Forms 4-2 and 4-3, can be used also as tools for relational phonetic-phonemic analysis. This analysis is accomplished by using the phones listed on the forms to represent the phonemes of adult English. Above

Word and Syllable Contrasts

Name: Age:
Date: Examiner:
Source of sample: Size of sample:

Contrast	Minimal pair words	Minimal pair syllables	Near-minimal pairs
Example: b - k	<u>b</u>i - <u>k</u>i *bee - key*	be<u>b</u>i - mʌŋ<u>k</u>i *baby - monkey*	<u>b</u>æt - <u>k</u>æp *bat - cap*

FORM 4-1.
Word and syllable contrasts.

Word and Syllable Contrasts

Name: *Christine*
Date: *10/20/90*
Source of sample: *spontaneous conversation*

Age: *5;4*
Examiner: *SLV*
Size of sample: *55 words*

Contrast	Minimal pair words	Minimal pair syllables	Near-minimal pairs
i - ɑɪ	mi - mɑɪ *me - mommy*		
i - ʌ - æ - u	di - dʌ - dæ - du *see - stuff - that - too*		
s - p - m	ʌs - ʌp - ʌm *us - up - home*		
w - m	wɑɪ - mɑɪ *why - mommy*		
j - m ɛ - æ			jɛs - mæs *yes - mask*
n - m		n̲æ̲s̲di - mæs n̲a̲s̲ty - mask	

EXAMPLE 4-1.
Word and syllable contrasts.

Consonant Phoneme Substitutions (Relational Analysis)

Name: Age:
Date: Examiner:
Source of sample: Size of sample:

Indicate substitutions beside (presumed) target phonemes (e.g., f^b). Mark phonemes that are not attempted with an X, and those that are omitted with Ø.

	Labial	Interdental	Alveolar	Palatal	Velar	Glottal	Other/notes:
Initial							
Stops	b		d		g		
	p		t		k		
Nasals	m		n				
Glides	w			j			
Fricatives	v	ð	z	ʒ			
	f	θ	s	ʃ		h	
Affricates				tʃ, dʒ			
Liquids			l	r			
Medial							
Stops	b		d		g		
	p		t		k	ʔ	
Nasals	m		n		ŋ		
Glides	w			j			
Fricatives	v	ð	z	ʒ			
	f	θ	s	ʃ		h	
Affricates				tʃ, dʒ			
Liquids			l	r			
Final							
Stops	b		d		g		
	p		t		k	ʔ	
Nasals	m		n		ŋ		
Fricatives	v	ð	z	ʒ			
	f	θ	s	ʃ			
Affricates				tʃ, dʒ			
Liquids			l				

Note: [r] not listed in final position as [ɚ] is a rhotic **vowel**. Medially, [r] should be counted only where it is consonantal (*around*), not vocalic (*bird*).

FORM 4-2.
Consonant phoneme substitutions (relational analysis).

Vowel Phoneme Substitutions (Relational Analysis)

Name: Age:
Date: Examiner:
Source of sample: Size of sample:

Indicate substitutions beside (presumed) target phonemes (e.g., ʊ˞). Mark with an X any phonemes not attempted.

	Front	Central	Back
Simple vowels			
High			
Tense	i		u
Lax	ɪ		ʊ
Mid			
Tense	e		o
Lax	ɛ		ɔ
Low		ʌ,ə	
	æ		ɑ
Diphthongs			
			ɔɪ
			ɑɪ
			ɑʊ
Rhotic vowels			
High			
	iɚ		uɚ
Mid			
	ɛɚ		ɔɚ
Low		ɚ	
		ɑɚ	

FORM 4-3.
Vowel phoneme substitutions (relational analysis).

TABLE 4-22.
"Holly"'s Homonyms

Child Homonymic Forms	Meanings
[bijə, beə, bɪʊ]	bunny, bear, bird, baby (*whispered*), bell, pig (*with gesture*), Bert
[tʰ, tˢ, dɪ], coronal click	tree, kitty, coffee

Source: Adapted from SL Velleman. The interaction of phonetics and phonology in developmental verbal dyspraxia: Two case studies. *Clinics in Communication Disorders* 1994;4:67–78.

or beside the phoneme listed for each consonant and vowel sound in the language, the clinician should write the actual phone produced. Multiple substitutions should be listed in order of frequency of occurrence, with most frequent substitutions listed first.

Correct productions may be listed or not, as appropriate to the situation. In cases in which the child sometimes produces the correct form but sometimes substitutes, listing the occurrences of the correct form is helpful: On looking at the form later, the clinician will know that the correct phone was produced and will know the relative frequency of its use. For example, $v^{b,v,w}$ would indicate that the child most often substituted [b] for /v/, next most often produced it correctly, and least often substituted [w].

In Example 4-2, the substituted phones of a hypothetical child ("Johnny Stopper") are listed in italics. As in analyzing the child's phonetic repertoire, these forms are then scrutinized for gaps in sound classes. Such gaps may occur either with respect to those sounds produced correctly (e.g., velars never produced correctly) or with respect to those sounds that are attempted (e.g., velars never attempted). Phones that occur often as substitutes for adult phonemes are also appropriate candidates for functional load analysis, as described in the next section.

It is evident from the data on the Example 4-2 and 4-3 forms that this child lacked the following sound class contrasts: fricative-stop, liquid-glide, velar-alveolar, rhotic-nonrhotic vowel, and simple vowel-diphthong.[7] However, the fact that /k/ sometimes was produced as [k] in medial and final position (indicated by the fact that both [t] and [k] are listed there) indicates that the velar-alveolar contrast may be emerging. Therefore, this contrast would be an appropriate goal for remediation.

Note that the variants of each assumed target phoneme are listed; presumably they are the allophones of that phoneme. For instance, Johnny's phoneme /k/ had the allophone [t] in all positions and the additional allophone [k] in medial and final positions. As one cannot predict (as far as can be determined from the form) the one that will occur in medial and final positions, these allophones

---

[7]In fact, Johnny may not even have been aware of some of these contrasts. One of the drawbacks of relational analysis is that it assumes that the child is fully aware of adult word forms and that his speech production target is the adult form. In reality, we cannot be sure of the child's underlying representation without more in-depth analysis of his phonology, preferably including discrimination probing and acoustic analysis of the contrasts in question.

are considered to be in partially free variation. His /l/ phoneme had the allophones [j] and [w] in initial and medial position, also in free variation with each other. In final position, [ʊ] always occurred. Because the **environment** (position of occurrence) of the [ʊ] allophone is predictable (final position), [ʊ] is considered to be in complementary distribution with the other two allophones of /l/ ([j] and [w]).

Another important question that can be addressed using this type of relational analysis is whether the child was avoiding any adult phonemes. If velars, for instance, are never attempted, this has important implications for remediation. To avoid velars (but not other places of articulation), the child must be able to discriminate velars from other places of articulation. Furthermore, avoidance indicates awareness that this sound class is difficult. Although the avoidance of a sound class (or a phoneme) may have an important impact on the child's communication (as words that contain those sounds will not even be attempted), the clinician should recognize that resistance will undoubtedly occur when the child is pressed to produce avoided sounds.

In the case of Johnny Stopper, rhotic diphthongs were never attempted. Johnny clearly avoided words that include such vowels, although he did attempt words with [ɚ]. The speech-language pathologist who worked with Johnny should have been aware of this in choosing target words for other sounds (e.g., *lair* would not have been a good target word for the production of [l], as Johnny would have been reluctant to attempt such a word). His willingness to at least attempt [ɚ] might have offered a window into this sound class if the production of rhotic vowels had been targeted in therapy. Johnny's lack of attempts at [ɜ] in initial and final position were not of concern, as this phoneme is quite rare in the language and therefore few opportunities are available for its production in a speech sample.

In short, segmental contrast can be determined by identifying potentially contrastive sound classes within the child's speech, by identifying minimal and near-minimal pairs in the child's speech, and by considering the child's substitutions for assumed target phonemes.

Evidence Regarding Contrast within the Child's System

Grunwell (1985) and Ingram (1981) suggested looking for homonyms in children's productive vocabularies. An appropriate worksheet can be created easily for those children for whom it appears appropriate, simply by listing word shapes and meanings under two headings. This type of worksheet is illustrated in Table 4-4 for Joan (Ingram, 1981) and in Table 4-22 for Holly, the child with DVD. Note that this is not a relational analysis, as the target (adult) forms are not compared to the child forms; only the target *meanings* are relevant.

The important information to be gleaned from this exercise is that Holly (in this case) had at least two sets of homonymic forms, each of which represented a wide variety of up to seven target words. Furthermore, in each case,

Consonant Phoneme Substitutions (Relational Analysis)

Name: *Johnny Stopper* Age: *4;10*

Date: *8/8/98* Examiner: *SLV*

Source of sample: *free play* Size of sample: *150 words*

Indicate substitutions beside (presumed) target phonemes (e.g., f^b). Phonemes marked with an X were not attempted in this sample. Ø indicates that the sound was omitted.

	Labial	Interdental	Alveolar	Palatal	Velar	Glottal	Other/notes:
Initial							
Stops	b		d		g^d		
	p		t		k^t		
Nasals	m		n				
Glides	w			j			
Fricatives	v^b	$ð^d$	z^d	**X**			
	f^p	$θ^t$	s^t	$ʃ^t$		h	
Affricates				$tʃ^t$, $dʒ^d$			
Liquids			$l^{w,j}$	r^w			
Medial							
Stops	b		d		g^d		
	p		t		$k^{t,\,k}$	**X**	
Nasals	m		n		$ŋ^n$		
Glides	w			j			
Fricatives	v^b	$ð^d$	z^d	$ʒ^d$			
	f^p	$θ^t$	s^t	$ʃ^t$		h	
Affricates				$tʃ^t$, $dʒ^d$			
Liquids			$l^{w,j}$	**X**			
Final							
Stops	b		d		g^d		
	p		t		$k^{t,\,k}$	**X**	
Nasals	m		n		$ŋ^n$		
Fricatives	v^b	$ð^d$	z^d	**X**			
	f^p	$θ^t$	s^t	$ʃ^t$			
Affricates				$tʃ^t$, $dʒ^d$			
Liquids			$l^ʊ$				

Note: [r] is not listed in final position as [ɚ] is considered to be a rhotic **vowel**. Medially, [r] should be counted only where it is consonantal (*around*), not vocalic (*bird*).

EXAMPLE 4-2.
Consonant phoneme substitutions (relational analysis).

Vowel Phoneme Substitutions (Relational Analysis)

Name: *Johnny Stopper*   Age: *4;10*
Date: *8/8/98*   Examiner: *SLV*
Source of sample: *free play*   Size of sample: *150 words*

Indicate substitutions beside (presumed) target phonemes (e.g., $\upsilon^{\eth}$). Mark with an X any phonemes not attempted.

	Front	Central	Back
Simple vowels			
High			
Tense	i		u
Lax	ɪ		ʊ
Mid			
Tense	e		o
Lax	ɛ		ɔ
Low		ʌ,ə	
	æ		ɑ

Diphthongs

ɔɪ^{ɔ,ɪ}

aɪ^{a,ɪ}
aʊ^{a,ʊ}

Rhotic vowels

	Front	Central	Back
High	X		X
Mid	X		X
Low		ɚ^{ə}	X

EXAMPLE 4-3.
Vowel phoneme substitutions (relational analysis).

TABLE 4-23.
"Ellen"'s Unintelligible Utterances

bɔdə
bidə
bububu
bʌdə bʌ bʌdə
ʌbububibu
ɔdɔtʰ
bʊdɪvʊ
ʌdʌbabaɪ
aʔl
bʊdæ
bʌdʊ
bʌnəmaʊ
bʌdʌmbʌ
bʌdʌ

Note: Superscript "h" indicates aspiration.

TABLE 4-24.
"Martin"'s Substitutions

Child Phone	Assumed Target Phonemes	Restrictions/Environments
[f]	/f/	Initial position
	/f/ clusters	Initial position
	Other fricatives, affricates	Initial position
	Clusters with fricatives	Initial position
	Clusters with affricates	Initial position
	Stop + /r/ clusters	Initial position; infrequent
[v]	Nonlabial stops	Medial, final positions
	Voiced fricatives	Medial position
	Voiced affricate /dʒ/	Final position
	/l/	Medial position

Source: Adapted from P Grunwell. *Clinical Phonology.* Rockville, MD: Aspen, 1982.

the homonymic form included two or more variants, or **allomorphs** (e.g., *bunny* could be [bijə], [bɛə] or [bɪʊ]). Clearly, this reduced her intelligibility significantly. The fact that she was using paralinguistic cues (whisper, gesture) to help to distinguish her homonyms indicated that she was aware of the inefficiency of her speech for communication purposes.

Another possible independent analysis that does not refer even to target meanings is the analysis of unintelligible forms. Often, it is quite revealing to look for commonalities among the phonetic forms for words that were unintelligible. Identification of such commonalities can assist the speech-language pathologist in determining factors contributing to unintelligibility. For example, if all unintelligible forms are multisyllabic, clearly multisyllabic words should be a target for intervention. "Ellen" produced the unintelligible utterances shown in Table 4-23 at 2 years, 3 months.

These words share a heavy reliance on [b], on a pattern of labial-alveolar consonant alternation (e.g., [bɔdə, bidə, bʌdə bʌ bʌdə]), and on reduplication (e.g., [bububu, ʌbububibu]). Ellen's intelligible utterances were re-examined with these apparent preferences in mind, and the intelligible utterances were found to exhibit the same patterns. Reduplication and a heavy functional load for labials had already been identified, but Ellen's labial-alveolar consonant alternation had not been noticed until these unintelligible forms were examined. It is likely that this combination of preferences significantly reduced the contrasts available within Ellen's production vocabulary and that it was responsible for much of her unintelligibility.

For relational analysis of child phones that have high functional loads, as suggested by Grunwell (1985), a self-created worksheet also is appropriate. Such a worksheet is created easily by taking the information from Forms 4-2 and 4-3 and simply listing each of the child's phones in one column and the adult phones to which each appears to correspond in another. A third column could be used for the specific environments (positions) in which the substitution occurs. As an example, Martin's [f] and [v] (Grunwell, 1982) are listed in Table 4-24, along with all the adult

phonemes that they appear to represent: most fricatives and affricates, clusters with fricatives and affricates, some stops, some liquids, and some stop + liquid clusters. This simple chart clearly confirms the clinician's suspicions that Martin was using labiodental fricatives for far too wide a variety of functions.

In sum, the additional contrast information that can be determined from a speech sample includes functional loads, homonymy, and preferred patterns.

THE NONLINEAR PHONOLOGY APPROACH TO CONTRAST

Trees

In Chapter 2, treelike models are used to demonstrate the relationships among various elements of phonotactic structure (segments, syllables, words, etc.). In Chapter 3, other tree structures are used to model the relationships among phonological features. The impact of information about the contrastive functions of these elements in particular languages (or in particular children's phonologies) does not complicate matters. Rather, it enables speech-language pathologists to determine simplification strategies for "pruning" those branches of the trees that are not functional in a particular phonology.

It has often been proposed that children's earliest underlying representations are word-based: Young children are more aware of the overall shape of the word than of its individual elements (e.g., segments). This awareness is exemplified by the high level of variability that children may show in the production of early words: The gestalt is constant, but the details are inconsistent. Other evidence includes the patterns of assimilation, metathesis, reduplication, and syllable reduction that affect the entire word. These whole-word patterns are quite frequent in early phonologies.

The most parsimonious account of any phonology includes only those elements that *must* be specified. For instance the feature [uvular] is relevant to French (because

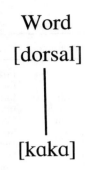

Word

[dorsal]

|

[kɑkɑ]

car, kitty, quack, Teddy

FIGURE 4-1.
"Timmy"'s [kɑkɑ] tree.

of the French uvular *r* sound), but including this feature in descriptions of English is unnecessary; it is not contrastive or even phonetic in our language. It is useless to mention something that has no function in the phonology. Similarly, if children's phonologies clearly operate at the word level, it is unnecessary to propose syllable or segment levels in their underlying representations. In other words, only relevant levels of the word should be addressed in any hypothesis about a particular child's phonological system. (For further discussion of this point, see Bernhardt & Stoel-Gammon, 1997; Dinnsen, 1996a,b, 1997; Stemberger & Stoel-Gammon, 1991; Stoel-Gammon & Stemberger, 1994.)

As indicated in Chapter 2, trees are used to model phonologies. The branches of a tree indicate the options available within a phonology. For example, if the phonology of language X includes words of more than two syllables (as all adult phonologies do), the model will have to include a level for syllables and a level for feet, representing pairs of syllables. In contrast, if a child's phonology only permits monosyllables (like that of Joan Velten), including a foot level is senseless. Each word will be exactly one syllable, and essentially no difference will exist between the word level and the syllable level in that child's phonology. In the absence of a difference between a word and a syllable, including both levels is not necessary; a word level alone will be sufficient. Another way of saying this is that the word is *nonbranching*: No branches appear below it, because it is the child's most fundamental level at that time. Several phonologists have supported the idea of representing child phonologies with minimal underlying structures of this sort (Iverson & Wheeler, 1987; McDonough & Myers, 1991; Menn & Matthei, 1992).

The simplest possible phonology predicted by current theory would be one that included only CV syllables (Demuth, 1996; Demuth & Fee, 1995; Fee, 1996; Fikkert, 1994), with minimal feature contrasts from one word to the other. Timmy, the child studied by Vihman et al. (1994), is a case in point. His first word productions were

restricted to <bɑ> and <kɑ(kɑ)>. These word shapes were used for many different lexical items. No vowel other than [ɑ] was produced; in other words, no vowel contrast was demonstrated. The number of syllables in the <kɑ(kɑ)> words was inconsistent and therefore noncontrastive. Two-syllable exemplars of <kɑ(kɑ)> did not have consistently different meanings from one syllable, [kɑ], tokens. Any <kɑ(kɑ)> word could be produced either way. Thus, the distinction between the syllable level and the word level was irrelevant for contrast purposes. In fact, voicing also was inconsistent; sometimes, the <kɑ(kɑ)> words were produced with [g] and the <bɑ> words with [p]. The only consistent phonetic difference between semantically different lexical items was the use of the place features typically associated with [b] versus those associated with [k]. Therefore, place of articulation (labial versus dorsal or velar) was the only distinctive feature Timmy had. Furthermore, he never produced labial and dorsal within the same word; [bɑkɑ] or [kɑbɑ] were not possible.

As no evidence could substantiate that Timmy differentiated syllables from words or segments within syllables, and no vowel contrast was available, the consonant place of articulation appeared to be a feature of the entire word. As discussed in Chapter 2, this application of one feature to whole words is called *autosegmentalization*. Recall that this term infers that the feature applies at a level above the segment. The feature [dorsal] can be assumed to have been autosegmentalized in Timmy's early speech because no evidence indicated that segments or even syllables were relevant units for him. Therefore, Timmy's tree structure for a word such as *car* would be as given in Figure 4-1.

The other features of the word—including the occurrence of the vowel [ɑ]—were completely predictable (i.e., noncontrastive). They are considered to be *defaults*; they are characteristics that would occur in any word that was not specified otherwise. In fact, if some words were specified as dorsal, any words not so specified obviously would be labial; other choices are not possible. Because it was the first phonetic characteristic that Timmy ever used in words, [labial] was considered to be Timmy's default consonant feature specification. Thus, in a word such as *ball*, no features needed to be specified; [bɑ] was his most likely word shape. When no other specifications were included, he would produce this syllable. Another way of saying this is that the syllable [bɑ] was Timmy's default: "When in doubt, say [bɑ]." Any words in this category would have even simpler underlying representations. No specifications would be required because *everything* was predictable. This simple underlying representation is illustrated in Timmy's <bɑ(bɑ)> tree (Figure 4-2).

Underspecification

Representations that are simplified due to defaults are said to be **underspecified**. Underspecification theory states that nothing should be put in the underlying representation that does not have to be there. What does belong are unpredictable things. If something is predictable (phonetically or phonologically), no reason mandates wasting (mental) storage space on it. The point has been made

Word

|

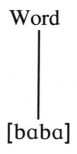

[bɑbɑ]

ball,   block,   box

FIGURE 4-2.
"Timmy"'s [bɑ] tree.

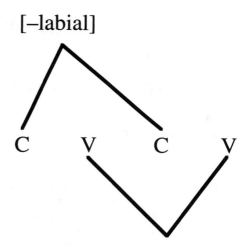

[dædæ], [gɑkɑ], etc.: *thank you*

FIGURE 4-3.
Minimal specification for "Jacob"'s *thank you*. (C = consonant; V = vowel.)

before: Linguists do not bother to put in underlying representations for English words the fact that all English consonants are [–uvular]. The uvular place of articulation is never used in English, so mentioning it is superfluous. Furthermore, liquids, nasals, and glides in English are not marked as [+voice] because they do not occur contrastively in voiceless versions, even though some other English consonant types do include voiceless versions. Voicing is a distinctive feature for English, but is not distinctive within the subclasses of liquids, nasals, and glides.

Similarly, if a child never used any consonants other than [g] and [k], mentioning [+velar] at all would be redundant in that child's underlying representations.[8] Independent analysis of this phonological system would be very simple with respect to consonant place of articulation. For such a child, consonant feature choices would not exist. All consonants would be automatically velar. Of course, this underspecification of place of articulation would also be a very important fact to note in the *contrastive* phonological analysis. Addition of places of articulation likely would be an early therapy goal, just as learning uvulars would be an important goal for any American who wanted to speak French with an authentic French accent.

Jacob (Menn, 1978a) provided another example of very simple structure. Because velar and alveolar consonants appeared to be allophones in free variation in his speech from 14 months up to 18 months (in such word productions as [dædum, gɑkɑ, dædæ, dɑitɑ, gigʌ, didi, dejdɑ] and, rarely, [gædə, gɑjdʌ] for *thank you*), a feature that can refer to both must be included in the underlying representation. The vowel within the word appears to be quite random, with some tendency to vowel harmony and a contradictory tendency to a front vowel-back vowel pattern. Which feature should be used to encompass the possibility of either [g] or [d]? The most obvious choice is to indicate that the word was never produced with [b] (or [p]) by specifying

the feature as [–labial]. Given these facts, Jacob's underlying representation for *thank you* might appear as it does in Figure 4-3. This representation shows that the two consonants agree in features and are nonlabial. The vowels, also, are shown to agree in this figure.

Because neither the phonetic details nor the predictable phonological patterns determining the production of each consonant and vowel segment are spelled out in the underlying representation, the underlying segments (e.g., Timmy's representations) are said to be *underspecified*. Underspecification allows speech-language pathologists to identify and clear away the predictable aspects of a phonology and therefore is valuable in studying a disordered phonology. Using an underspecification approach, the clinician can determine the levels (word, syllable, segment) and elements (i.e., the units at each level) that are functional (contrastive) and those that are not. Underlying representations in which almost everything is underspecified, such as Timmy's and Jacob's, provide very little basis for contrast and, therefore, very little basis for effective communication.

The Behavior of Defaults

In fact, underspecification can explain many phenomena in child phonology that otherwise seem quite mysterious. For instance, coronals often assimilate to (take on the place of articulation of) velars and labials. For example, a /g/ or /b/ consonant in a word will *spread* its place feature to a /d/ in the word, changing the /d/ to [g] or [b] (e.g., *doggie* becomes [gɔgi] or *bottle* becomes [bɑbɑ]). However, in the event of a place error not due to assimilation (e.g., in a one-consonant word), often an alveolar substitutes for

---

[8]Note that for dealing formally with underspecification of features, various systems are available (other than the +/– system described here). They are reviewed in Steriade (1995).

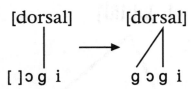

FIGURE 4-4.
Velar assimilation in *doggie*.

the presumed target consonant (especially a velar, as when *go* becomes [do]). Similarly, stops assimilate to nasals or fricatives in such productions as [min] for *bean* or [fʌf] for *puff*. However, stops also substitute for nasals and especially for fricatives in nonassimilatory errors, such as [du] for *zoo* (Stoel-Gammon & Stemberger, 1994). Why do certain types of errors result in the production of more alveolars or more stops, whereas others reduce the frequency of these types of consonants?

The most basic universal, unmarked features are the defaults of the phonological system. The most common consonant manner feature, [stop], is one such default. Therefore, when no other consonant manner feature is specified, a stop will be produced. ("When in doubt, produce a stop.") Similarly, [coronal] (alveopalatal) is the most universal, least marked consonant place feature. Therefore, it does not need to be specified. If no consonant place feature is indicated, a coronal will be produced. Thus, if any consonant is unspecified in the underlying representation (for whatever reason) and no neighboring specified feature can spread to fill in the features, [coronal] or [stop] automatically will fill in at the surface. That is, as the output is planned, any unspecified portions of the mental representation of the word automatically will be produced with these default characteristics. The default status of these features explains why they are most likely to substitute for other features (e.g., stops are substituted for fricatives in stopping, coronals are substituted for velars in fronting).

Why are these same features more likely to be lost through assimilation? The lack of specification makes [stop] and [coronal] more vulnerable to spreading by other features. At the underlying level, segments that should be pronounced with stops or coronals are not specified: Those features automatically will be provided at the output level if the slots are still unfilled. However, the result of this underspecification is that unfilled feature specifications occur at the underlying level. If one consonant in the word is specified to be [+dorsal], for instance, and another is unspecified, the [dorsal] feature can spread easily into the empty place specification to fill the gap. No other specification has to be deleted for the entire word to become velar, as would be necessary if the victim consonant were specified, for example as [labial]. The default now will not have the opportunity to appear, as the feature specification for that slot has already been filled. This concept is illustrated in Figure 4-4.

Another example of this concept was provided by Goad (1996) using Amahl's data from Smith (1973). She pointed out that this child treated /l/ in a manner similar to that of /r/ and /j/. Thus, she proposed that he had a general "semivowel" phoneme with no associated place feature, which encompassed all three of these adult targets. Because this semivowel phoneme had no place feature, these target phonemes were especially susceptible to place harmony (e.g., resulting in [giŋ] for *ring*, [gɔk] for *lock*, and [dewiːbuːn] for *telephone*).

Bernhardt (1992a) and Stoel-Gammon and Stemberger (1994) proposed further that those segments that are the least specified (e.g., coronals and stops) are generally learned first in the process of phonological development. In one sense, this argument is circular. Recall that those features designated unmarked and therefore considered to be underspecified in underlying representations are so chosen in part owing to their ease of acquisition and in part to their frequency of occurrence in the phonetic repertoires of the languages of the world. In other words, features and phones that are easily learned are used by many languages and therefore are considered to be unmarked. To then make the claim that the most unmarked sounds (e.g., stops and coronals) are easily learned really does not shed a great deal of light on the matter. However, such assimilation and substitution data as those presented by Stoel-Gammon and Stemberger (1994) and discussed earlier do provide additional evidence for these choices for remediation.

Dinnsen (1996a,b) added to the discussion by pointing out that underspecification in children may be context-specific. For example, a child may have a particular stop as the default consonant in initial position but have a certain fricative as a final position default. Then, different features could be underspecified in different word positions.

Summary

The nonlinear theories of defaults, autosegmentalization, and underspecification highlight those aspects of a phonology that are, in a sense, the most automatic. Identifying the most immutable aspects of a phonology accomplishes two ends. First, it leads to the identification of those aspects of the child's phonology that are the most habitual and the most systematic. Overcoming these patterns (e.g., the use of a default consonant or a default phonotactic pattern) through intervention may be very difficult, yet very important. Second, in this way, the nonautomatic aspects of the child's phonology are segregated from the automatic aspects. These nonautomatic underlying structures and elements are the source of contrast in the system and therefore provide the basis for effective communication. They represent the choices available to the child for the production of distinct word shapes. Thus, the speech-language pathologist's role is to break down the child's reliance on inappropriate defaults and to build on the contrastive elements.

CHAPTER FIVE

Phonological Patterns

Three major perspectives are possible regarding phonological patterns: *rules*, *processes*, and *constraints*. In this chapter, these terms are defined and compared and contrasted, and examples highlight the historical order in which these three theories were developed. All reflect the goal of identifying broader patterns within the child's speech. Classes of sounds as well as specific segments, and classes of word positions (e.g., syllable-final, word-initial) as well as specific environments (e.g., following [f]) are examined. These strategies facilitate the clinician's descriptions of the child's production (and misproduction) of the language. Although theoretical differences exist among the approaches, from a very practical standpoint all serve this same purpose. Each has advantages and disadvantages in assessing a child's phonology. The best solution may be to understand all three and to use each as appropriate to a specific situation.

In this chapter, the theoretical background, guiding principles, and clinical implications of each approach are reviewed. Then relationships among these pattern types are described using specific clinical examples.

PHONOLOGICAL PATTERN TYPES

Generative Phonology: Rules

Overview
Generative rules are statements about relationships among phonological elements at different phonological levels. The assumption is that the stored, underlying form of a word undergoes certain predictable changes on its way to the surface, pronounced form of the word. Some of these alterations—those that are closest to the surface levels—are assumed to be totally phonetically based. In other words, they are seen as articulatory (physiological) rather than phonological (cognitive). Other rules are viewed as more abstract linguistic patterns that each language may or may not choose to implement. Some of these patterns reflect interactions between the phonology and the grammar (especially morphology) of the language. Others are more purely phonological. Rules that are phonetically natural (i.e., make sense from a physiological point of view) and those that are in keeping with known phonological universals are valued more highly by linguists working within this model. However, no specific, strict criteria for naturalness have been set within the theory.

The most crucial principles of generative phonology, most of which have been incorporated into later models as well (e.g., Ingram, 1997) are the following (based on Dinnsen, 1984; Vihman, 1996):

- Phonological patterns can be described by formulating statements using precise and explicit notation.
- Segments are decomposable into feature complexes (i.e., sets of distinctive features).
- Both an underlying, abstract level of phonological representation and a surface phonetic level exist.

- Phonological rules describe regular relationships between the underlying levels and the surface levels of phonologies.
- Phonological rules are not totally independent of one another. The existence of one may affect the nature or the impact of another.

Each of these ideas is discussed in depth in the immediately following sections.

Precise and Specific Notation
The information included in any phonological rule must include the **element** that will change, the **change** that it will undergo, and the **environment** in which this change will occur. In traditional generative phonology, the element typically would be a phoneme or a class of phonemes (e.g., stops). The change would consist of alterations in feature specifications, such as [+voice] becoming [–voice]. Sometimes, the change would involve deletion or insertion (epenthesis) of an element. Typically, the environment would include the syllable or word position of the element in question (e.g., initial position) or the neighboring segments (e.g., between vowels, before [p]). Thus, a typical rule might state that stops (the elements) become unaspirated (the change) after a word-initial [s] (the environment).

Feature Complexes
These pieces of information are typically expressed using features and phonological symbols whenever possible in order to capture phonological generalizations. Decomposing segments into features allows one to be both more specific and more general: more specific in the sense that only those features critical to the operation of the rule are specified, and more general in the sense that any segment with that feature (or those features) can be expected to be subject to that rule in the correct environment. For example, in this author's dialect, [s] often is pronounced as [ʃ] before [r]. Thus, *groceries* is pronounced [groʃriz], *nursery* as [nɚʃri], and so on. The sibilant undergoes palatal assimilation: The /s/ is palatalized before [r]. This change occurs because [r] is produced with the tongue raised toward the palate (as it is for [ʃ]) rather than toward the alveolar ridge (as it would be for [s]). For ease of production, the sibilant is produced at the same place as the following liquid. Specifying the places of articulation rather than using the letter symbols reveals the motivation for the rule.

Regularity of Phonological Rules
The speech pattern just described could be stated in the following terms: Alveolar sibilants become palatalized in the environment before palatal liquids. Using → to indicate *become* and / to indicate *in the environment*, the following could be written:

alveolar sibilants → palatalized / before palatal liquids

Adding _____ to indicate the location of the occurrence, we get:

alveolar sibilants → palatalized /_____ palatal liquids.

The blank line indicates that the location of the alveolar sibilant that will change is, in this case, just before [r].

In current linguistic theory, [alveolar] actually is not the preferred feature used to describe such consonants as /s/. The broader term, [coronal] (alveopalatal) is used. This term implies the use of the tongue-tip in the formation of the sound. Alveolars are specified as [+anterior] (farther forward in the mouth), and palatals are [−anterior] ("minus anterior," or nonanterior). The use of this feature terminology would change the rule to the following:

anterior coronal sibilants →
    nonanterior /_____ nonanterior liquids.

Although this change adds one more feature to the left of the rule, it makes clearer exactly what is changing articulatorily. The sibilant is being produced farther back in the mouth, in the palatal area, in anticipation of a palatal consonant.

Using feature notation, with features in square brackets ([ ]), + to indicate a feature, and − to indicate the opposite of that feature, this rule becomes:

$$\begin{bmatrix} +\text{anterior} \\ +\text{coronal} \\ +\text{sibilant} \end{bmatrix} \rightarrow [-\text{anterior}] \; / \underline{\quad} \begin{bmatrix} -\text{anterior} \\ +\text{liquid} \end{bmatrix}$$

This rule may be too specific, however. On both the input side and the environment side of the rule, both the manner and the place of articulation have been specified. Does the alveolar (anterior coronal) have to be a sibilant to undergo this change? Does the palatal (nonanterior coronal) have to be a liquid to trigger the change?

The answer to the first question is no. This specific rule, in fact, is one example of a more general rule in which palatals affect preceding alveolars. For instance, the /t/ in *mattress* and the /t/ in *train* are pronounced as [tʃ] in this author's dialect as well ([mætʃrıs], [tʃreın]): They are palatalized in assimilation with the following [r]s. In other words, all anterior coronals lose their anteriority (i.e., are pronounced farther back) in anticipation of the palatal liquid [r]. Thus, the [+sibilant] specification on the input side of the rule can be dropped:

$$\begin{bmatrix} +\text{anterior} \\ +\text{coronal} \end{bmatrix} \rightarrow [-\text{anterior}] \; / \underline{\quad} \begin{bmatrix} -\text{anterior} \\ +\text{liquid} \end{bmatrix}$$

In this dialect, however, the change in place of articulation does not show up before other palatals,[1] so [+liquid] must remain. A related pattern applies in certain dialects of

TABLE 5-1.
Fe?fe?-Bamileke Consonant-Vowel Assimilation

Output Form	Gloss
[vɑp]	to whip
[tʃɑk]	to seek
[fat]	to eat

Source: Adapted from LH Hyman. *Phonology: Theory and Analysis.* New York: Holt, Rinehart and Winston, 1975.

British English, in which /s/ is palatalized before the palatal glide [j] in such words as *assume*: [əʃjum]. In other words, the anterior coronal /s/ is produced in a less anterior position prior to the nonanterior coronal glide [j]. In these dialects, the manner features on the environment side of the rule (the portion after the →/ that specifies where the change will occur) would refer to glides rather than to liquids. Note that both these rules are phonetically natural; producing two consecutive segments at the same place of articulation is easier than changing the tongue position from alveolar to palatal between segments.[2]

Hyman's (1975) example of consonant-vowel assimilation from Fe?fe?-Bamileke, in which the vowels [ɑ] and [a] are affected by the consonant following, illustrates the usefulness of features. As the reader may recall, the vowel [ɑ] occurs before [k] and [p], and the vowel [a] occurs before [t] (Table 5-1).

In some ways, this pattern is confusing: [a] is a more front vowel than [ɑ], which accounts for its co-occurrence with [t]. However, why does the more front vowel not co-occur with [p], which surely is one of the most front consonants possible? Why should [p] and [k] behave similarly when they are articulated so differently? Is this a phonetically unnatural rule?

The answer lies in a more careful consideration of the articulatory facts, which are represented in the phonological model. In fact, [t] is produced with the tongue-tip raised; neither [k] nor [p] involves the tongue tip. The vowel [ɑ] is low and back. For accurate production of [ɑ], the tongue must be lowered mostly via lowering the mandible itself. The vowel [a], being less back and also less low, requires less lowering. Therefore, the tongue tip has less far to travel from [a] to [t] than from [ɑ] to [t]. These facts are captured in the jargon of phonology by grouping the consonants that require tongue-tip raising into the category [coronal]. This feature is far more useful in this case than would be a feature that simply refers to the frontness of the consonant. The rule can now be written as follows:

$$\begin{bmatrix} +\text{vocalic} \\ +\text{low} \end{bmatrix} \rightarrow [-\text{back}] \; / \underline{\quad} \begin{bmatrix} +\text{consonantal} \\ +\text{coronal} \end{bmatrix}$$

---

[1]Acoustic analysis might well reveal some degree of palatalization before any type of palatal. However, the palatalization is not sufficient in other cases to be detectable to the untrained listener. It has been claimed that an underlying /t/ in such words as *donation* and *creation* (from *donate* and *create*) and an underlying /d/ in such words as *explosion* and *erosion* (from *explode* and *erode*) became palatal fricatives historically under the influence of the high front vowel following. The phonetic basis for this change is that [i] is produced using an articulatory configuration similar to that used in the production of palatal consonants. Thus, the alveolars become palatal in preparation for the palatal vowel. (As no palatal stops exist in English, they also become fricatives.)

[2]Of course, the tongue movement really would not occur *between* the segments because, in running speech, segments overlap: No *between* exists. The tongue would begin to move during the [s] and complete its transition by mid-[r].

TABLE 5-2.
Feeding Rule Order

Rule	piece of string
Underlying form	/mpundo/
Voicing assimilation	[mbundo]
Cluster simplification	[mundo]

Source: Adapted from M Kenstowicz, C Kisseberth. *Topics in Phonological Theory.* New York: Academic Press, 1977.

TABLE 5-3.
Rule Order Blocks Application

Rule	piece of string
Underlying form	/mpundo/
Cluster simplification	Does not apply
Voicing assimilation	*[mbundo]

Note: The asterisk indicates a form that does not occur in the language.
Source: Adapted from M Kenstowicz, C Kisseberth. *Topics in Phonological Theory.* New York: Academic Press, 1977.

It states that a low vowel is articulated farther front in the mouth before a coronal (tongue-tip) consonant.

One assumption behind the proposed underlying representation versus surface structure dichotomy was that only the critical (unpredictable) information about any word should be stored in the mental lexicon. Predictable patterns or rules also would be stored, but less neurological space would be taken up (it was hypothesized) by a set of simple forms plus a set of rules than by several sets of related forms for each root word. For example, if 250 words were subject to the same morphophonological rule (e.g., plural), storing 250 words plus one rule would be more efficient than storing 500 words (the unchanged forms plus the changed forms). Thus, *create* and *creation*, which differ not only in the addition of the *-ion* ending but also in the surface pronunciation of the underlying /t/, would not each need a separate slot in the mental lexicon. *Create* and *-ion* would each be stored once, with a predictable rule indicating the changes that the /t/ must undergo when the *-ion* is added (see footnote 1). Similarly, a set of rules would take care of the vowel alternations in such word pairs as *clean-cleanliness, nation-national,* and *harmony-harmonious,* so that each version of each word would not have to be stored separately.

Impact of Rules on One Another

Neighboring segments within a word are not the only phonological elements that interact. Generative rules themselves may have an impact on one another. For example, the application of one rule may make it possible for another rule to apply later. In Mwera, a Bantu language, for instance, a cluster simplification rule is found (Kenstowicz & Kisseberth, 1977). Voiced stops are deleted after a nasal. For example, the cluster /mb/ would be pronounced as [m]. This rule normally would not apply to such clusters as *mp-*, in words such as *mpundo* (*piece of string*), because voiceless stops usually are not affected. However, another rule causes voiceless stops to become voiced after nasals. This change is a form of voicing assimilation: The voiceless stop becomes voiced under the influence of the preceding voiced nasal. The voicing assimilation rule results in *mp-* becoming *mb-*. The [b] can then be deleted by the cluster simplification rule. The first rule *feeds* the second, making it possible for the second rule to apply. Thus, as shown in Table 5-2, the two rules interact to create the final result.

If the rules were to apply in the reverse order, the /p/ would not be deleted by the first rule, as it would become voiced only after the deletion rule already had failed to apply, as shown in Table 5-3.

The fact that [mbundo] is not a possible output form—no native speaker of Mwera pronounces this word in this way—indicates that the rules must apply in the previous, feeding order. In some other language or dialect, they could apply in the other, *bleeding* (blocking) order.

Generative phonologists have demonstrated also that, in many languages, phonology and morphology interact. Although English is a fairly morphology-poor language (i.e., there are relatively few bound morphemes), morphology-phonology interactions can be identified even in the English language. For example, recall that English speakers routinely assimilate the voicing of certain morphological endings, such as plural ([kæts] versus [kɪdz]), third-person singular ([kɪks] versus [dʒɔgz]), possessive ([pɑps] versus [bɑbz]), and past tense ([kɪst] versus [bʌzd]), although the assimilation is not reflected in English spelling. Similarly, the various forms of the prefix *in-* (meaning, roughly, *not*) are *phonologically conditioned.* The morpheme changes to match the surrounding phones. The nasal assimilates to match the place of articulation (and sometimes even the manner of articulation) of the consonant following, and English speakers spell the words as they say them to the extent that the alphabet allows. This assimilation yields such words as *inept, impossible, indelible, illegal,* and *irreverent.*

These cases pose an additional difficulty for rule writing, however. The pronunciation of the plural, for example, will depend on the sound that immediately precedes it; one general rule cannot be written. The affix *-in* poses even more of a problem: It may change both place and manner of articulation. How can one rule be written to describe every possible change? Additionally, if individual rules have to be written for each case, wherein lies the benefit? To do so would be quite inefficient.

To deal with cases of this sort, phonologists adopted the use of the symbol α (Greek *alpha*). It was used in rules such as:

$$[\text{+nasal}] \rightarrow [\alpha \text{ place}]/\_\_\_+ \begin{bmatrix} \text{+consonantal} \\ \alpha \text{ place} \end{bmatrix}$$

This rule states that nasals[3] will agree in place of articulation with following consonants. The positioning of the alphas indicates that the two places of articulation would

---

[3]The morphophonological rule applies specifically to the prefix *in-*, but this pattern of "homorganic nasals," which agree in place of articulation with a following obstruent, is, in fact, fairly general in casually spoken English.

TABLE 5-4.
Yawelmani Vowel Harmony

Output Form	Gloss
[hɔyɔhin]	named
[gɔphin]	took care of an infant
[hudhun]	recognized
[cuyɔhun]	urinated

Source: Adapted from CW Kisseberth. On the abstractness of phonology: The evidence from Yawelmani. *Papers in Linguistics* 1969;1:291–306. Cited by LH Hyman. *Phonology: Theory and Analysis.* New York: Holt, Rinehart and Winston, 1975.

be the same. In other words, if the following consonant were labial, the nasal would become labial; if it were coronal, coronal; if it were dorsal, dorsal. The alpha symbol is like a little marker within the rule: Everything that has this marker will agree with anything else within the rule bearing this same marker. In this case, the place of articulation of the nasal will become the same as the place of articulation of the consonant following.[4]

The + after the blank line in the rule indicates a morpheme boundary. In other words, the nasal is the last phoneme within a prefix, and it is being influenced by the initial consonant in the stem of the word (or by the initial consonant of another prefix, as in *ir + re + duc + ible*). This morpheme boundary symbol indicates that the rule does not apply to such monomorphemic words (words with only one morpheme) as *infant* (i.e., English speakers are less likely to say [ɪmfənt] than [ɪmpɑsɪbəl], except perhaps in very fast speech).

Alpha notation can be used also for cases of harmony at a distance, as in Kisseberth's example (1969) of vowel harmony from Yawelmani. Recall that, in this language, the vowel /i/ in the past tense suffix *-hin* (roughly equivalent to *-ed* in English) is pronounced as [u] if there is a previous [u] anywhere in the word (Table 5-4).

In this case, however, the environment is more complicated. Consonants or even entire syllables may intervene between the vowel that undergoes the change and the vowel that triggers (or causes) the change. One option in such cases is to use X to represent some amount of irrelevant phonological material in the environment. The rule could be written, then, approximately in this fashion:

$$/i/ \rightarrow [+back]/ \begin{bmatrix} +vocalic \\ +back \end{bmatrix} X + h\_\_n$$

This rule states that /i/ will become [+back] in agreement with any vowel that comes before it in the word. Other vowel features will not be changed. Thus, the suffix vowel will be pronounced as [u] whenever a back vowel precedes it. Any elements in between will be ignored.

Again, + indicates a morpheme boundary. In this case, the past-tense morpheme occurs at the end of the verb, so + is used between the stem of the verb and the past-tense ending. This symbol helps express the idea that the rule applies only to vowels within the past-tense affix *-hin*.

The use of the symbol X to indicate that some extra phonemes might occur between the trigger of the change and the target (the element that will change) would also be useful for sibilant harmony in Chumash. Recall that, in this language, all sibilants in the word must have the same degree of palatality. Both [s] and [ʃ] cannot occur in the same word. If they would have co-occurred for some morphological reason, one of them changes to the other when the word is pronounced. Thus, /k + sunon + us/, which means "I obey him," remains as such: [ksunonus]. However, /k + sunon + ʃ/, which means "I am obedient," must change to [kʃunotʃ]. (The /n/ changes to [t] for other reasons.) Similarly, *I pay* is [saxtun], whereas *to be paid* is [ʃaxtunitʃ] (Poser, 1982). This rule may be written as follows:

$$[+sibilant] \rightarrow [\alpha \text{ palatal}]/\_\_\_\_X\begin{bmatrix} +sibilant \\ \alpha \text{ palatal} \end{bmatrix}$$

In other words, a sibilant will become as palatal as a sibilant that follows it, regardless of what appears between.

Clinical Implications
The most critical impact of generative phonology on clinical practice was the new emphasis placed on sound classes, sound changes, and phonological environments. A simple table can be made to keep track of these elements during the phonological analysis process:

Sound/Sound Class	Change	Environment
Affected elements	Feature difference	Position, surrounding sounds

The difference made by this approach at the segmental level can be highlighted by use of an example. Consider again the following data from the hypothetical child "Nathan" (discussed in Chapter 4). Table 4-14 is reproduced here as Table 5-5 for easy reference.

A traditional substitution analysis would yield an extremely long list of consonant substitutions. On the basis of these few data only, the report would look approximately as follows:

Initial position: d/b,[5] d/p, d/t, d/k, n/m, d/f, d/s, d/ʃ
Medial position: d/g, d/t, d/k, n/m, d/s, d/θ
Final position: d/g, n/ŋ, d/r
Clusters: d/str-, d/bl-, d/-sk-, n/-nst-, d/-rst

This analysis is not very satisfying—it does not provide a very good sense of what is going on here. It just seems to

---

[4]In fact, this rule still does not cover words that begin with liquids (illegal, irreverent, etc.). For it to do so, additional symbols would indicate that the nasal will agree in liquidity with the consonant following as well. If the consonant following is liquid, the nasal becomes liquid; otherwise, it remains nasal. For this purpose, an additional Greek letter (usually β) would be used.

[5]Note that *x/y* is used, as is common in clinical practice, to indicate that *x* is substituted for *y*.

TABLE 5-5.
"Nathan"'s Use of [d] and [n]

doggie	[dɔdi]
cookie	[dʊdi]
go	[do]
mom	[nɑn]
more	[nod]
no	[no]
butter	[dʌdʌd]
bye	[dɑɪ]
pig	[dɪd]
shoe	[du]
feather	[dedʊd]
sing	[dɪn]
string	[dɪn]
blue	[du]
basket	[dædæ]
monster	[nʌnʌd]
first	[dɪd]

TABLE 5-6.
Phonological Rule Table for "Nathan"

Sound/Sound Class	Change	Environment
Any non-nasal	d	Everywhere
Nasal	n	Everywhere

TABLE 5-7.
Phonological Rule Table for "Nathan"

Sound/Sound Class	Change	Environment
Any C	Alveolar	Everywhere
Any C	Voiced	Everywhere
Any C	Deleted	Immediately after any other C

be a big mess. Grouping these substitutions into sound classes to write phonological rules is far more helpful: All (presumed) target non-nasal consonants are changed to (pronounced as) [d], whereas all (presumed) target nasals become [n]. These patterns could be written in rule format as follows:

$$[-\text{nasal}] \rightarrow [\text{d}] \text{ everywhere}$$
$$[+\text{nasal}] \rightarrow [\text{n}] \text{ everywhere}$$

Alternatively, they could be written on a phonological rule table, as shown in Table 5-6. It is not really necessary to specify the environment in this case because this change occurs in all syllable and word positions; the use of the word *everywhere* makes the breadth of application explicit.

However, consideration of the features involved leads to the realization that all consonants, regardless of their place of articulation in the adult word, were produced by Nathan at the alveolar place of articulation. Both [d] and [n] share the place of articulation [+alveolar] or,

$$\begin{bmatrix} +\text{anterior} \\ +\text{coronal} \end{bmatrix}$$

and both are considered to be stops ([−continuant]). Nasality features ([−nasal] or [+nasal]) were not changed by the child. Nasality is the only feature distinction that Nathan consistently maintained; when the adult consonant was nasal, Nathan always produced a nasal. Thus, nasality is not actually relevant to the rule, as it does not change. With this insight, the rule can be written as follows:

$$[+\text{consonantal}] \rightarrow \begin{bmatrix} +\text{anterior} \\ +\text{coronal} \\ +\text{continuant} \end{bmatrix}$$

or described on the table as:

Sound/Sound Class	Change	Environment
Any C	Noncontinuant alveolar	Everywhere

That is, Nathan produced all consonants as alveolar (nasal *or* oral) stops, in all positions, regardless of surrounding sounds. Note that those consonants that were not voiced already became voiced as well. This voicing can be added to the rule:

$$[+\text{consonantal}] \rightarrow \begin{bmatrix} +\text{anterior} \\ +\text{coronal} \\ -\text{continuant} \\ +\text{voice} \end{bmatrix}$$

A rule that states that consonant clusters are reduced to one element also needs to be written. It is not difficult to see that Nathan reduced all clusters to one consonant and that that consonant always was alveolar, regardless of the elements of the cluster in adult speech. (This was, of course, in keeping with Nathan's general pattern of producing all consonants as [d] or [n].) Thus, the following rule, using ∅ to represent *nothing*, will suffice:

$$[+\text{consonantal}] \rightarrow \emptyset / [+\text{consonantal}]\_\_\_$$

This last piece of information can be added to a complete table of Nathan's phonological rules, shown as Table 5-7.

In other words, any consonant was deleted if it appeared immediately after another consonant. This rule reapplied until only one consonant remained. At that point, the rule became irrelevant (vacuous), as no remaining consonant immediately followed another. Note that it must be the *first* element of the cluster that was preserved because the nasality associated with the [n] remained in *monster* but not in *picnic*. In each case, the first target consonant determined the nasality of the consonant actually produced. In all other

TABLE 5-8.
Phonological Derivations for "Nathan"

Rule	monster	picnic
Target form	/mɑnstɚ/	/pɪknɪk/
Cluster reduction	[mɑnsɚ]	[pɪkɪk]
Cluster reduction	[mɑnɚ]	Not applicable
Alveolarization	[nɑnɚ]	[tɪtɪt]
Vowel changes	[nʌnʌ]	Not applicable
Voicing	Not applicable	[dɪdɪd]

TABLE 5-9.
Amahl's Consonant-Vowel Interactions

pedal	[bɛgu]
beetle	[bi:gu]
bottle	[bɔgu]
lazy	[de:di:]
horses	[ɔ:tid]
sometimes	[fʌmtaɪmd]

Note: Colon indicates vowel lengthening.
Source: Adapted from NV Smith. *The Acquisition of Phonology: A Case Study.* Cambridge, MA: Cambridge University Press, 1973.

TABLE 5-10.
Phonological Rule Table for Amahl

Sound/Sound Class	Change	Environment
l	u	Final position
Alveolar	Velar (back)	Before u (back vowel)

Source: Adapted from NV Smith. *The Acquisition of Phonology: A Case Study.* Cambridge, MA: Cambridge University Press, 1973.

respects, the choice of preserved consonant did not matter because they all ended up as [d] or [n] anyway, owing to the other rules.

These three rules could have occurred in any order. Voicing could have occurred at any time without affecting the other two rules. Either the alveolarization rule would have changed all consonants to [d, t, n] and then the cluster reduction rule would have eliminated the second consonant in any cluster, or the cluster reduction rule would have ensured that only one consecutive consonant occurred and then the alveolarization rule would have fixed the place of articulation of whatever consonants might have been left. This latter derivation is shown in Table 5-8. Note that an additional rule, the details of which are ignored here, had to be added to the derivation to account for the fact that some vowels changed as well.

A final rule that had to be considered for Nathan was his treatment of fricatives and liquids. These, like all other non-nasal consonants, were reduced to [d]. A general rule can be written easily because [d] and [n] are both stops: [d] is an oral stop, and [n] is a nasal stop. In contrast to liquids and fricatives, they are not continuant.

$$[+continuant] \rightarrow [-continuant]$$

This rule, too, should be added to the list.

Sound/Sound Class	Change	Environment
Any continuant	Stopped	Everywhere

Thus, phonological rules can enhance the clinician's understanding of sound classes as they are affected by sound changes in certain environments.

Smith's case of consonant-vowel assimilation later in phonological development (Smith, 1973; Macken, 1979; Table 5-9) is another case in point. The phonology of Smith's son included a rule of vowelization of final [l]. Amahl ([ǽməl]) pronounced lateral liquids in final position as [u]. Recall that final [l] typically is velarized (dark), produced with the tongue backed in a fashion more similar to the production of [u], even in adult speech. In Amahl's speech, alveolars became velar (i.e., back) before the resulting [u]s. This was a physiology-based change: The [u] is a back vowel, so the consonant assimilated to it. This consonant feature change could have appeared to be

backing (substitution of velars for alveolars), but alveolars remained alveolar in all other contexts. Without a consideration of the effect of the vowels, nothing could explain why this velarization of alveolars happened only before [u] and not in other word-medial environments.

Clearly, these alveolar consonants were affected by the place of articulation of the vowels following. In generative phonological notation, one could write:

$$\begin{bmatrix} +liquid \\ +anterior \end{bmatrix} \rightarrow \begin{bmatrix} +vocalic \\ +back \\ +high \end{bmatrix} / \_\_\_\# \quad (/l/ \rightarrow [u] \text{ in final position})$$

$$\begin{bmatrix} +consonantal \\ -continuant \\ +coronal \end{bmatrix} \rightarrow [+back] / \_\_ \begin{bmatrix} V \\ +high \\ +back \end{bmatrix}$$

(alveolar stops → velar before [u])

The use of the feature [back] in the change as well as in the environment highlights the nature of the change (i.e., the fact that it was assimilatory). The list of sound changes would appear as shown in Table 5-10. Note that the rules must have applied in this order. If /l/ had not changed to [u], the second rule would not have been applicable.

Harmony, as well as assimilation, can be expressed in rule format. A child who had velar harmony, for example, and said such words as *body* in an adult manner but produced *doggie* as [gɔgi] could be said to have had the following rule:

$$[+alveolar] \rightarrow [+velar] / \_\_\_\_ X[+velar]$$
or
$$[+coronal] \rightarrow [+dorsal] / \_\_\_\_ X[+dorsal]$$

In other words, an alveolar (or coronal) consonant was pronounced as velar (dorsal) before a velar (dorsal), regardless of what else came between. If, instead, the child produced *body* as [dɔdi] and *copy* as [pɑpi], this rule would have been the following:

$$[+\text{consonantal}] \rightarrow [\alpha \text{ place}] \; / \; \underline{\hspace{1cm}} \; X[\alpha \text{ place}]$$

This rule states that any consonant agrees in place of articulation with a following consonant, regardless of intervening material.

One of the advantages—and disadvantages—of generative phonology was that rules of this sort could be written so easily. Very few actual limits governed the elements, the environments, or the changes that could be included in any rule. Such symbols as X and α gave the rule writer a great deal of flexibility. Therefore, writing rules about changes that never occur in any language in the world was almost as easy as writing rules about changes that are quite common. More important, both probable and improbable rules fell within the guidelines of the theory.[6] Phonologists saw this as a drawback and as an indicator that the theory was too broad. An ideal theory will fit "just the facts, ma'am": no more, no less.

Another disadvantage of generative phonology was that it did not facilitate the description of rules affecting an entire syllable, word, or phrase. The use of X to represent "any intervening elements" (i.e., the rest of the word) was awkward, inelegant, and unrevealing. This disadvantage was particularly striking to child phonologists and clinical phonologists, who often had to deal with just such patterns. Often, whole-word patterns were ignored clinically, which undoubtedly reduced the effectiveness of intervention.

Despite the fact that writing rules seemed too easy (i.e., too broadly defined) to theoretical phonologists, the long lists of features to be remembered and the detailed, abstract notation often seemed too cumbersome to speech-language pathologists. They wanted an easier way to capture the same generalizations without writing phonological rules. Natural phonology provided such a shortcut.

Summary

Generative phonology had an important impact on child phonological theory and also on child phonological intervention. It called attention to the importance of looking for patterns affecting classes of sounds in a systematic manner. However, it suffered in one sense from too much breadth, as it allowed nonexistent phonological rules as well as common ones. In another sense, it suffered also from too little scope, as seen in the difficulty in describing patterns that apply to more than a single segment or an adjacent pair of segments. Describing or explaining word-level patterns within this theory was very awkward.

---

[6]Typically, elements or environments that fall into natural classes can be described more succinctly. It is easier to express a rule that applies to all sibilants in final position, for example, than to express a rule that applies to /f/, /k/, and /o/ (three quite different phonemes) before /u/, /t/, and /r/ (also three quite different phonemes). However, a rule that describes an element's becoming more similar to an adjacent element (a common occurrence) is no easier to write than is one that describes a highly unexpected change, such as a vowel's changing to a velar stop before a labial fricative.

Natural Phonology: Processes

Overview

Natural phonology was an attempt by Stampe and Donegan (e.g., Donegan, 1979; Stampe, 1969; Stampe, 1979; for a historical overview, see Grunwell, 1997) to emphasize the universal phonetic bases of phonology. They proposed that all phonological patterns have their basis in human physiological limitations on speech production. Such physiological limitations were described as *natural processes*. For example, the physical difficulty of producing three consonants within a cluster leads to the tendency among humans to reduce such lengthy clusters. This natural process of *cluster reduction* is seen in the speech of children learning such languages as German and English. Some languages, such as Japanese, avoid temptation by excluding these difficult sequences altogether. However, for a language to be phonetically diverse enough to permit efficient communication, it must make a trade-off and permit *other* difficult elements or sequences (such as multisyllabic words). Thus, different languages require speakers to overcome different limitations or, in Stampe's terms, different languages allow different processes to apply to different extents (Stampe, 1969, 1979). For example, cluster reduction is given free rein in Japanese, but syllable reduction is not.

Overcoming a physiological limitation to produce the sound patterns of a language is termed *suppression* of a natural process. Infants do not know how to overcome these limitations to produce speech sounds. Their mission, then, is to learn to suppress those processes that are not permitted to apply in their language. If the language has many clusters (e.g., German), they must suppress the process of cluster reduction. If the language has many multisyllabic words (e.g., Japanese), they must suppress syllable deletion, and so on.

It is important to note that many processes are neither totally suppressed nor totally applied in a language. Recall that, in American English, for example, speakers may neglect to pronounce word-final [t] as such. Often, it is substituted by [ʔ] (e.g., "I've [gɑʔ] a [koʔ]" rather than "I've [gɑtʰ] a [kotʰ]"). The point at which this occurs typically depends on sociolinguistic factors, such as the formality of the situation and the status and dialect of the speaker. The glottal stop [ʔ] also routinely substitutes for [t] in the medial position of certain words with a strong-weak stress pattern, such as *curtain* ([kɚʔən]) and *button* ([bʌʔən]), except in very formal speech or citation contexts (e.g., reading a word list). Stops from other places of articulation, however, are very rarely replaced with glottals. Thus, the natural process of glottalization is permitted to apply in certain phonological contexts (e.g., word-finally and word-medially if the stress pattern is appropriate), to certain phonemes (/t/), under certain sociolinguistic circumstances. In cases that do not meet these criteria, the process is suppressed.

It is important to note that process theory is grounded strongly in phonetic reality. Therefore, phonological patterns that do not have a clear physiological basis or are not well attested among the languages of the world are not considered to be natural. Sometimes, they are termed *deviant processes*.

Clinical Implications

From a very practical clinical standpoint, the theory of natural phonology provided convenient labels for many of the phonological rules that had been noted in the speech of young children and children with nonfunctional phonology (NFP). Phonological processes are far easier to reference either in writing or aloud than are generative rules. On the one hand, a certain basic set of processes came to be known and agreed on by most people. On the other hand, however, the principles of the theory, especially the principle of phonetic naturalness, were not always followed. It was easy to give a name to almost any phonological rule that could be written. In addition, names that were too general could be confusing. For example, does *backing* refer to producing *any* consonant farther back in the oral cavity, or specifically to producing alveolars as velars? So-called deviant (non-natural) processes proliferated, and they were not necessarily either phonetically natural or in keeping with universal tendencies.

Some proponents of the theory attempted to maintain the theoretical rigor of Stampe's original proposal by arguing for a specific set of natural processes and a strict order of naturalness. Shriberg and Kwiatkowski's (1980) *Natural Process Analysis* is one example of this attempt. Within this analysis procedure, each of the child's error productions is assigned to a small set of the most natural or basic processes with a predetermined hierarchy of naturalness. The problem with this approach is that different children appear to have different tendencies, many of which are not in keeping with the proposed hierarchies. For example, one child might have frequent use of assimilation. Those assimilations that resulted in a velar's being pronounced as alveolar (e.g., [dɔdi] for *doggie*), however, would have to be credited as velar fronting because this process must be assigned first (before assimilation) to all possible errors, according to the *Natural Process Analysis* guidelines. Thus, this scoring procedure would result in a loss of generalization for that particular child. Also, many children demonstrate patterns that cannot be described using such a small set of processes (e.g., backing, voicing changes, glottal replacement, and reduplication). Thus, strict adherence to the theory appears to reduce the usefulness of the analysis.

Whatever their viewpoint, most developers of process tests or analyses agree in dividing processes into certain types: syllable-structure processes, assimilation processes, and substitution processes.

SYLLABLE STRUCTURE PROCESSES. Syllable structure processes are those that affect the shape of the word or the syllable. In other words, they are phonotactic patterns. Many of these processes result in a reduction in the number of elements within a syllable or word. They include the following processes:

- *Syllable reduction* (also known as *unstressed syllable deletion*): This process refers to the omission of a syllable that is present in the adult form of the word. Often the omitted syllable is unstressed, especially in sequences of a weak syllable followed by a strong one. Of course, in most cases, it is difficult to know with any certainty whether

this syllable is included within the child's underlying representation of the word. Because unstressed syllables have lower salience, some children may not be processing them perceptually as relevant linguistic units. In other words, children may be omitting the unstressed syllables in their underlying representations because they are not prominent acoustically or because they do not match the immature structures of their phonological systems. Therefore, the term *deletion* may not always be appropriate. The more neutral *omission* may be more fitting. In any case, one or more syllables of the adult form are not produced by the child with syllable reduction.

- *Final consonant deletion*: This process occurs when the final consonant of a word is not produced. Again, sometimes it is difficult to determine whether the child is unaware of the segment or is aware of the segment but does not produce it.

- *Initial consonant deletion*: This process occurs when the initial consonant of a word is not produced. Initial consonant deletion generally is considered a deviant process—one that is neither phonetically natural nor in keeping with phonological universals. In fact, many languages have constraints against word-initial vowels; they require words to begin with consonants. No known language requires words to begin with vowels, as children with initial consonant deletion appear to do.

- *Consonant cluster reduction*: Consonant cluster reduction involves production of fewer consecutive consonants than are present in the adult form of the word. In some cases, none of the consonants may be produced; in others, two of three or one of two may be preserved.

- *Coalescence*: Coalescence is an alternative strategy for children who have difficulty with clusters. It consists of preserving one or more of the features of each consonant in a cluster, merging these features into one distinct consonant. A common example exemplified by "Martin" (Grunwell, 1982) is the combination of frication from the [s] and labialization from the [w] in an *sw-* cluster into a single [f], yielding [fɪmɪŋ] for *swimming*, [fit] for *sweet*, and so on. When this process occurs, it can be generalized further by the child, who then produces [f] for a variety of other consonant clusters that may not share features with [f].

- *Metathesis and migration*: These processes involve movement of elements from their locations within the adult word. In metathesis, elements are interchanged (as in [ækst] for *asked* or [gʌbi] for *buggy*). In migration, one element moves elsewhere, usually owing to distribution requirements (as in [nos] for *snow*). One child, "W," who exhibited this process was reported by Leonard and McGregor (1991). She consistently put initial fricative sounds in final position, even when this practice resulted in final consonant clusters, as shown in Table 5-11 (repeated from Table 2-13). Fricatives migrated to final position, apparently to avoid appearing in initial position.

ASSIMILATION AND HARMONY PROCESSES. **Assimilation** and **harmony** processes are those in which two elements within

TABLE 5-11.
Fricative-Final Migration Pattern

fall	[ɑf]
fine	[ɑɪmf]
school	[kus]
soup	[ups]
zoo	[uz]
sheep	[ips]
shoe	[us]

Source: Adapted from LB Leonard, KK McGregor. Unusual phonological patterns and their underlying representations: A case study. *Journal of Child Language* 1991;18:261–272.

the word (or phrase or utterance) become more alike. Typically, they result in a reduction in articulatory effort because fewer oral motor transitions need to be made within the word. Contrast within the word is also reduced, of course. Recall that assimilation occurs when adjacent elements become more alike, and harmony occurs when the elements are separated by at least one other element. Assimilation and harmony processes include consonant and vowel harmony and reduplication.

Consonant or Vowel Harmony.   **Consonant** and **vowel harmony** are processes that occur when the consonants (or vowels) within a word become alike or more alike. Child phonological systems often exhibit a specific harmony pattern in which all consonants within a word assimilate to a particular feature if it is present anywhere in the word. For example, many children show velar harmony: All consonants within the word become velar if a velar occurs anywhere within the word. Often this harmony is directional: The harmony will change consonants preceding (or after) the velar but will not change other consonants.[7]

The terms *progressive harmony* (left to right), *regressive harmony* (right to left), and *bidirectional harmony* can be used to describe well what is happening with respect to the direction of the harmony. For example, [bɑbəl] for *bottle* would be an example of progressive labial harmony, [gɔgi] for *doggie* of regressive velar harmony, and [mɪm] for *wing* of bidirectional harmony (labiality spread to the right or end of the word and nasality spread to the left or beginning of the word).

In some cases, however, the harmony affects only certain types of consonants (e.g., coronals) or vowels (e.g., high vowels). In other words, only one certain type of consonant or vowel may change under the influence of another. In these instances the process name is too broad; it is misleading to say that the child has velar harmony, for example, if only alveolars harmonize with velars. More specific descriptions should be given in these cases (e.g., regressive velar harmony affecting alveolars).

Reduplication.   **Reduplication** is, in a sense, total harmony. It involves repetition of the same syllable (or, in some examples from adult languages, the same foot). Examples from Menn (1978a) are repeated here:

down	[doʊdoʊ]
around	[wæwæ]
handle	[hɑhɑ]

The process name is quite descriptive, albeit a bit redundant, with appropriate implications about the breadth of its application.

SUBSTITUTION PROCESSES.   Substitution processes are those that result in one element substituting for another when assimilation is *not* the source of the change. They are classified (e.g., by Hodson & Paden, 1991) according to the type of change that occurs:

1. Place changes: The place of articulation of the phoneme changes.[8] The following examples are taken from Hodson and Paden (1991):
   a. Fronting (typically, velars are fronted to alveolar position)
   b. Backing (typically, alveolars are backed to velar position)
   c. Palatalization (alveolars are palatalized, as when /s/ is pronounced as [ʃ])
   d. Depalatalization (palatals fronted to alveolar position, as when /ʃ/ is pronounced as [s] or /tʃ/ as [ts]).
   e. Place shifts affecting /θ/ (fronting to [f], backing to [s], etc.)
   As these descriptions illustrate, much confusion results from the fact that such terms as fronting and backing could have many different interpretations. Some people attempt to use them only to refer to very specific changes, whereas others use them more broadly. It is important to specify the meanings of these terms when using them (e.g., fronting of /θ/ to [f]).
2. Manner changes: The manner of articulation of the phoneme changes:
   a. Stopping (typically, fricatives are stopped at the closest stop place of articulation)
   b. Gliding (typically, liquids are produced as glides)
   c. Vowelization (vowels substitute for liquids in medial or final position)
   d. Affrication (fricatives are incompletely stopped, as in [tʃu] for *shoe*)
   e. Deaffrication (affricates are produced either without a stop portion, yielding [ʃiz] for *cheese*, or without a fricative portion, yielding [tiz] for *cheese*).
   Again, many variations of these processes are possible and must be specified. These include stopping of

---

[7]According to Stoel-Gammon (1996), velar harmony occurs most often when the velar is in final position.

---

[8]The use of the word *changes* implies that the child's underlying representation is adultlike (i.e., that the phoneme is changing as it makes its way from underlying to surface levels of the phonology). Typically, this assumption is made by those who advocate natural process analysis, but it is not made by this author.

glides, gliding of fricatives, and affrication of stops. Specification is necessary also in the case of deaffrication to indicate the portion omitted.

3. Voicing changes: The voicing of the element changes:
   a. Voicing of initial consonants (e.g., [bɪg] for *pig*)
   b. Devoicing of final consonants (e.g., [pɪk] for *pig*)
   It is important to recall, however, that the apparent voicing of stops that results from cluster reduction in *sC*- clusters actually is appropriate. English speakers tend to think of the stops [b, d, g] as voiced, but actually they are voiceless unaspirated, just as are stops that follow [s] in a cluster. Thus, a child who produces *ski* as what an American would transcribe as [gi] is guilty of cluster reduction but *not* really of voicing a voiceless stop. Note also that so-called deviant voicing processes do occur, such as voicing of final consonants.

Many commercial process analyses are available for clinical use. Alternatively, for a structured list of a child's processes, Form 5-1 can be used. This form includes a list of likely processes and allows the user to indicate those that occur in a particular child's speech. For more experienced users, Form 5-2, which provides a clinician-generated overview of the child's processes, will provide more flexibility albeit less structure. This form allows the user to list those processes that have been noted in the child's speech, with frequency indicated.

A process analysis of Nathan's speech (see foregoing) would be likely to yield the following list:

- Fronting (of velars)
- Backing (of labials)
- Initial consonant voicing
- Stopping of fricatives
- Stopping of liquids
- Consonant cluster reduction
- Consonant harmony (alveolar)
- Reduplication

These elements are listed on Forms 5-1 and 5-2, as Examples 5-1 and 5-2, for illustration. Although these terms may be less intimidating than are the phonological rules generated for Nathan earlier, they also are clearly less general, as more of them are needed to describe the same phonological patterns.

Of all of them, the one process that seems to describe the largest number of Nathan's words is alveolar consonant harmony. This appears to be quite appropriate for such words as *butter* ([dʌdʌ]) and *feather* ([dɛdʊ]). However, this description would not be helpful at all with such words as *go* ([do]), *more* ([no]), *bye* ([daɪ]), *shoe* ([du]), and *blue* ([du]). Yet, the child did seem to be treating the /b/ in *butter* in the same way as the /b/ in *bye* (producing them both as [d]), so it would be appropriate to have one way to describe both. Unfortunately, as harmony is inappropriate for several cases, no one process will cover all of the pattern. A variety of processes seem to be responsible for Nathan's productions of these words. Furthermore, some of the

processes appear to be contradictory. For example, fronting and backing both occurred. The clinician is left with a long list of processes to address in therapy and little idea of where to start.[9]

Of course, Nathan is a hypothetical child, and the data were selected purposely to illustrate the possible disadvantages of traditional procedures, such as substitution analysis, generative analysis, and process analysis. However, the general problems identified here are common results of process analysis, especially the findings of an overabundance of processes to treat and contradictory processes operating within the same child's speech. In fact, process analysis was the inspiration for the subtitle of this book. The author's clinical colleagues have come to her many times with long lists of processes that have been found in a child's speech, posing the question, "What do I do first?"

The long-term result of natural process theory for clinical phonology has been a positive change toward more general statements being made about children's phonologies and toward addressing *classes* of sounds and *patterns* of errors rather than individual segmental substitutions. However, this new focus has been accompanied by a great deal of confusion in deciding which processes are natural and which are deviant and in deciding which processes to address first. Also, the convenient shorthand of process names has discouraged clinicians from learning to distinguish different children's patterns more specifically. It has led also to a tendency to ignore phonological patterns that do not fit these pre-existing labels. Ironically, despite their grounding in phonetic naturalness, the easy (even careless) use of process labels by a great many people appears to have reduced many clinicians' awareness of the physiological bases for phonological patterns.

Summary
Natural process theory provided convenient labels for many of the common phonological patterns seen in the languages of the world and in early or disordered phonologies. The efficiency and clarity of these labels made phonological theory appear far more clinically accessible and increased many clinicians' awareness of phonological patterns. Also, the consideration of syllable structure and harmony processes heightened the interest in patterns affecting entire syllables, words, or even phrases. However, these very labels have also proved to be susceptible to careless (nonspecific) use. Furthermore, the theory provides little guidance for prioritizing goals, as many diverse processes may appear to account for a child's phonological profile.

---

[9]Hodson and Paden (1991) do make lengthy recommendations regarding intervention of phonological processes. Other authors (Shriberg & Kwiatkowski, 1980; Weiner, 1979) include briefer discussions of this topic. However, many children's profiles do not fit even Hodson and Paden's extensive recommendations because of the many possible variations, combinations, and interactions of processes.

Process Summary

Name: Age:
Date: Examiner:
Source of sample: Size of sample:

Process	Context/example/frequency
Syllable structure	
Syllable reduction	_____
Final consonant deletion	_____
Initial consonant deletion	_____
Cluster reduction	
Liquid clusters	_____
/s/ clusters	_____
Coalescence	_____
Metathesis/migration	_____
Epenthesis	_____
Other	_____
Harmony/assimilation	
Harmony (specify feature)	
Consonant	_____
Vowel	_____
Reduplication	_____
Other	_____
Substitution	
Fronting	
Velar	
/ʃ/ → [s]	_____
/θ/ → [f]	_____
Backing	
Alveolar to velar	_____
Palatalization	_____
Depalatalization	_____
Stopping	
All fricatives	_____
/v ð ʒ tʃ dʒ/ only	_____
Other place changes	_____
Gliding	
/l/	_____
/r/	_____
Vowelization	
/l/	_____
/ɚ/	_____
Affrication	_____
Deaffrication	_____
Voicing	
Voice initial consonants	_____
Devoice final consonants	_____
Denasalization	_____
Vowel deviations	_____
Other	_____

FORM 5-1.
Process summary.

Process Analysis

Name: Age:
Date: Examiner:
Source of sample: Size of sample:

Process type	Adult phoneme/sound class	Process(es)	Frequency
Example: *Substitution*	*All fricatives*	*Stopping*	*Predominant (90%)*

FORM 5-2.
Process analysis.

Process Summary

Name: *Nathan*   Age: *4*
Date: *12/12/2012*   Examiner: *SLV*
Source of sample: *hypothetical*   Size of sample: *18 words*

Process	Context/example/frequency
Syllable structure	
Syllable reduction	
Final consonant deletion	
Initial consonant deletion	
Cluster reduction	
Liquid clusters	[du] *for blue; 100%*
/s/ clusters	[dɪn] *for string; 100%*
Coalescence	
Metathesis/migration	
Epenthesis	
Harmony/assimilation	
Harmony (specify feature)	
Consonant	*Alveolar (e.g.,* [dɔdi] *for doggie); 100%*
Vowel	
Reduplication	*E.g.,* [dʌdʌd] *for butter; 3/7 (43% of 2-syllable words)*
Substitution	
Fronting	
Velar	*To alveolar (e.g.,* [dʊdi] *for cookie)*
/ʃ/ → [s]	
/θ/ → [f]	
Backing	
Alveolar to velar	
Other	*Labial to alveolar (e.g.,* [daɪ] *for bye)*
Palatalization	
Depalatalization	
Other place changes	
Stopping	
All fricatives	*E.g.,* [du] *for shoe; 100%*
/v ð ʒ tʃ dʒ/ only	
Other	*Liquids (e.g.,* [nʌnʌd] *for monster); 100%*
Gliding	
/l/	
/r/	
Vowelization	
/l/	
/ɚ/	
Affrication	
Deaffrication	
Voicing	
Voice initial consonants	*E.g.,* [dʊdi] *for cookie*
Devoice final consonants	
Other voice changes	*Voice final Cs (e.g.,* [dædæd] *for basket)*
Denasalization	
Vowel deviations	*E.g.,* [nʌnʌd] *for monster*

EXAMPLE 5-1.
Process summary.

Process Analysis

Name: *Nathan*
Date: *12/12/2012*
Source of sample: *hypothetical*

Age: *4*
Examiner: *SLV*
Size of sample: *18 words*

Process type	Adult phoneme/sound class	Process(es)	Frequency
Syllable structure	*All CC*	*CC reduction, first C omitted*	*100%*
Harmony	*Nonalveolars*	*C harmony (alveolar)*	*100%*
Substitution	*Velars*	*Fronting (to alveolar)*	*100%*
	Labials	*Backing (to alveolar)*	*100%*
	Fricatives	*Stopping*	*100%*
	Liquids	*Stopping*	*100%*
	All consonants	*Voicing*	*100%*

EXAMPLE 5-2.
Process analysis.

Phonological Avoidance: Constraints

Overview

The idea of **phonological constraints** was actually included in generative phonology (in which constraints sometimes were termed *conspiracies* [e.g., Branigan, 1976; Kenstowicz & Kisseberth, 1977]). This approach is also not untrue to the basic principles of natural phonology. Basically, a constraint is another way of expressing a phonological rule or process, using negative rather than positive terms. Rather than saying that in Japanese all consonant clusters are reduced to single consonants, for example, one can say that Japanese has a *constraint against* consonant clusters. In other words, clusters are not allowed in this language. This constraint is written with an asterisk to indicate an "illegal" (or nonpreferred) pattern[10]:

$$*[+consonantal][+consonantal]$$

or

$$*CC$$

Japanese also has a constraint against non-nasal final consonants; only nasal consonants can occur in final position. Using # to indicate a word boundary (in this case, the end of the word), this constraint is written as follows:

$$*\begin{bmatrix} -nasal \\ +consonantal \end{bmatrix}\#$$

A consonant that is not nasal may not occur in final position.

Such constraints are very common in the languages of the world. In English, for instance, [ŋ] does not occur in word-initial position. This constraint may be written:

$$*\#ŋ$$

This constraint states that the dorsal nasal may not appear immediately after (to the right of) a word boundary. In fact, [ŋ] is not even allowed at the beginning of a syllable, a fact that may be represented by using $ to represent a syllable boundary:

$$*\$ŋ$$

A restriction also governs the vowels that can occur in word-final position—that is, in open syllables at the ends of words. English [ɪ] and [ɛ] are not permitted in word-final position, whereas [i] (*knee*) and [e] (*neigh*) are permitted. The low front vowel [æ] is marginal; it occurs mostly in slang or colloquial and baby-talk contexts (e.g., *yeah* for *yes*, *nah* for *no*, *dada* for *daddy*). This constraint against word-final front lax vowels can be written as follows[11]:

$$*\begin{bmatrix} +vocalic \\ +front \\ -tense \end{bmatrix}\#$$

More specific consonant cluster constraints also occur. Spanish provides an example of an initial consonant cluster constraint. This language does not allow *initial* sequences of [s] + stop, although it does allow them in medial position (where the [s] may close one syllable while the stop opens the next). Such words as *steak*, *scare*, and even *Spanish* are not allowed. The constraint may be written as follows:

$$*\#[s]\begin{bmatrix} +consonantal \\ -continuant \end{bmatrix}$$

Constraints are less all-or-nothing than are generative phonological rules. The set of constraints with which the speaker must deal is seen as a ranked list of preferences. Thus, unlike rules and processes, constraints are not totally inviolable. Some are violated frequently; others are violated when the situation requires it. Those at the top of the ranking (*constraint hierarchy*) are very strong and rarely or never violated. The lower the constraint is in the hierarchy, the more likely the speakers of the language are to violate it when this is called for, to avoid violating a more highly-ranked constraint.

For example, Japanese has a very highly ranked constraint against consonant clusters. It is never violated. English may be said to have a very weak constraint against consonant clusters. Speakers prefer not to use them and will reduce them when the linguistic or social situation allows (e.g., in casual speech in a redundant context) or the physiological situation requires (e.g., when very tired or drunk). However, this constraint is violated very frequently. English speakers often produce most or all the consonants within a cluster.

Clinical Implications

Although the germ of the idea has been around for decades in various forms, constraint theory in and of itself is relatively new—only a few years old. Applications for clinical diagnosis and treatment are in their infancy. However, the idea of looking at children's phonology from the point of view of what those children are *not* doing rather than what they *are* doing is highly appealing and efficient. The line from constraints (the roadblocks in the phonological system) to goals is much more direct than that from rules or processes to goals.

---

[10]The constraint labels and other jargon associated with optimality theory are deliberately avoided in this section to the extent possible. Some of these terms and conventions are introduced in the "Optimality Theory" section of the chapter. This avoidance of jargon should not be seen as the author's attempt to rename common constraints nor to develop her own constraint system. Rather, it is an attempt to explain the basic concepts as simply as possible without immersing the reader in the complications of competing sets of theoretical labels.

---

[11]The actual constraint is somewhat more complicated because [ʊ] (as in *book*) also is disallowed but [ɔ] (as in *law*) is permitted.

A reconsideration of Nathan's phonology, for example, makes clear that the most general possible description of what actually was nonfunctional about this child's phonology is a very simple statement about his *phonetic* repertoire: He had only two consonants, [d] and [n], and he used them everywhere! Various processes or rules conspired to substitute these two consonants for all others. From an efficiency point of view, however, the actual processes involved were far less important to intervention planning than is this simple phonetic generalization.

This generalization can be written using a set of generative phonological rules, as discussed. However, the use of these rules implies that Nathan had all consonant features in his underlying representations—that is, the rule is based on the assumption that complete information about each adult word was stored in Nathan's mental lexicon. Many child phonologists are uncomfortable with this claim. They believe that children are likely to store only those features that are salient and useful phonologically to them at any time. It is possible to circumvent this issue and to arrive at a far simpler and more goal-related statement of Nathan's problem by using a constraint rather than a rule.

$$* \begin{bmatrix} -\text{alveolar} \\ +\text{consonantal} \end{bmatrix} \quad or \quad * \begin{bmatrix} -\text{coronal} \\ -\text{anterior} \\ +\text{consonantal} \end{bmatrix}$$

A simple statement that Nathan had this constraint implies no assumptions about his underlying representations. It is *only* a statement that he did not produce nonalveolar consonants. Therefore, it is a claim about his *output forms* only. Information about other places of articulation may or may not have been stored in his underlying representation, but the output form really was the only information available.

As discussed in the generative phonology section, Nathan had a constraint against continuant consonants (fricatives, liquids, and glides) as well. He produced only oral ([d]) and nasal ([n]) stops. This constraint, also, is fairly simple:

$$*[+\text{continuant}]$$

Note that this constraint is separate. If the list of features in the first constraint simply is increased, the constraint will have a meaning that is actually too specific. That is,

$$* \begin{bmatrix} -\text{coronal} \\ -\text{anterior} \\ +\text{continuant} \\ +\text{consonantal} \end{bmatrix}$$

means that nonalveolar continuants are not allowed. It implies that nonalveolar stops would occur, which is not accurate in this (hypothetical) child's speech.

Nathan's constraint against consonant clusters can also be written simply as *CC. These constraints are simple and pervasive: three general principles that summarize his entire phonological disorder.

Children's constraints, divided into word and syllable structure versus feature constraints, can be organized using Form 5-3, as illustrated for Nathan in Example 5-3. On this form, the indexing (subscripts) indicates whether two elements are the same or different. For example, C_1VC_1V indicates that the two consonants are the same (harmonized); C_1VC_2V indicates that they are different. Similarly, $\sigma_1\sigma_2$ indicates two different (nonreduplicated) syllables.

Simple statements about constraints clarify the issue of the appropriate place to intervene. One need not choose among all those processes or rules that may be attributable to this child. All that is needed is to persuade Nathan to weaken his constraints. Clinical goals will be for Nathan to produce nonalveolar consonants, to produce continuant consonants, and to produce consonant clusters.

At this point, the *choice* of the specific nonalveolar consonants, continuant consonants, or consonant clusters that he will produce is a fairly minor question, as is the issue of word position. *Any* nonalveolar consonant in *any* word position (initial, medial, or final) would represent a significant breakthrough and would be likely to trigger massive changes in Nathan's phonology as a whole. Production of any continuant or any cluster also would signal significant progress, although they might represent less pervasive changes in his phonological system. A *cycles approach* (Hodson & Paden, 1991), in which various classes of consonants would be intensively modeled, each for short periods, might be the most reliable way to break this logjam. If Nathan appears to be receptive to a particular class of consonants or a particular word position—even if it be [θ] in final clusters, a developmentally very unexpected direction—a more specific short-term objective will have emerged.

Summary
Constraint theory facilitates the expression of more basic phonological truths by considering those phonological possibilities that do not occur in the (child's) phonology. The use of this approach can permit the clinician to write more general goals that address the heart of the problem and thereby avoid skirting issues.

RELATIONSHIPS AMONG PATTERN TYPES

Within constraint theory, each language's use of what may be referred to as *repair strategies* is also studied. When faced with the possible violation of a constraint, what do the speakers do about it? Consistent preferences for particular repairs are evident in different languages. The most clear-cut cases appear in words borrowed by one language from other languages, in which the constraint hierarchy is different. The Japanese tendency to epenthesize (to add a vowel to break up a consonant cluster) has already been noted. This repair strategy occurs occasionally in English as well. For example, Vietnamese names beginning with [ŋ] (especially those beginning with an ŋg- cluster) are sometimes modified to better fit English phonotactics by epenthesiz-

Summary: Phonological Constraints

Name: Age:

Date: Examiner:

Source of sample: Size of sample:

Use a check mark to indicate the occurrence of a constraint or a percentage to indicate its frequency of occurrence. Make appropriate specifications and comments. All sequences of Cs and Vs are assumed to be within the same word.

Note: C = consonant
        V = vowel
        # = word boundary
        σ = syllable (e.g., $\sigma\sigma$ = disyllabic word)
        x_1x_2 = x_1 and x_2 are different from each other
        * = disallowed form

I. Phonotactic constraints

Constraint	Age equivalence	Restrictions/comments
Syllable shapes	Expected up to:	
*C#_____	3;0_____	
*#C_____	<u>Not expected</u>	
*#CC_____	4;0_____	
*VCCV_____	_____	
*CC#_____	_____	
Word shapes		
*#$\sigma\sigma$#_____	2;0_____	
*#$\sigma\sigma\sigma$#_____	_____	
Harmony/assimilation		
*$\sigma_1\sigma_2$_____	2;0_____	
*C_1VC_2V_____	2;0_____	
*C_1VC_2_____	2;0_____	
*CV_1CV_2_____	2;0_____	

Note: Age equivalences are approximate. They are based on Grunwell (1985), Chin & Dinnsen (1992), Smit et al. (1990), and Stoel-Gammon (1987). "Not expected" indicates a constraint not found in normally developing children. A blank indicates that norms are not available on this measure.

Comments:

FORM 5-3.
Summary: phonological constraints.

II. Specific feature restrictions

Restricted feature	Restricted word position	Comments
Examples: *Velar*	*Final*	*Omitted*
Fricative	*All*	*No fricatives anywhere ever*

FORM 5-3.

Summary: Phonological Constraints

Name: *Nathan*   Age: *4*
Date: *12/12/2012*   Examiner: *SLV*
Source of sample: *hypothetical*   Size of sample: *18 Words*

Use a check mark to indicate the occurrence of a constraint or a percentage to indicate its frequency of occurrence. Make appropriate specifications and comments. All sequences of Cs and Vs are assumed to be within the same word.

Note: C = consonant
        V = vowel
        # = word boundary
        σ = syllable (e.g., $\sigma\sigma$ = disyllabic word)
        $x_1x_2 = x_1$ and x_2 are different from each other
        *: = disallowed form

I. Phonotactic constraints

Constraint	Age equivalence	Restrictions/comments
Syllable shapes	Expected up to:	
*C#	3;0	
*#C	Not expected	
*#CC ✔	4;0	*No clusters*
*VCCV ✔		*No clusters*
*CC# ✔		*No clusters*
Word shapes		
*#$\sigma\sigma$#	2;0	
*#$\sigma\sigma\sigma$#		
Harmony/assimilation		
*$\sigma_1\sigma_2$ ✔	2;0	*Occasional apparent reduplication*
*C_1VC_2V ✔	2;0	*Occasional apparent harmony*
*C_1VC_2 ✔	2;0	*Occasional apparent harmony*
*CV_1CV_2	2;0	

Note: Age equivalences are approximate. They are based on Grunwell (1985), Chin & Dinnsen (1992), Smit et al. (1990), and Stoel-Gammon (1987). "Not expected" indicates a constraint not found in normally developing children. A blank indicates that norms are not available on this measure.

Comments: *Feature constraints result in apparent reduplication and harmony.*

EXAMPLE 5-3.
Summary: phonological constraints.

II. Specific feature restrictions

Restricted feature	Restricted word position	Comments
Nonalveolar	*All positions*	
Continuant (fricative, liquid, glide)	*All positions*	

EXAMPLE 5-3.

TABLE 5-12.
Constraint on Fricative Occurrence

cap	[kæf]
fish	[pɪʃ]
stupid	[tufɪz]
dog	[dɔx]

ing a vowel at the beginning of the word. Thus, *Nguyen* may be pronounced as [əŋgujɛn]. In this way, the [ŋ] is bumped to the *end* of the first syllable, and the [g] initiates the second syllable rather than participating in an initial cluster with [ŋ]. More often, one of the consonant cluster consonants simply may be omitted altogether (yielding, for example, [nujɛn] or [gujɛn]). The same repairs may be used for such African names as *Njeri.*

Consonant cluster reduction (e.g., [nɛk#stap] rather than [nɛkst#stap] for *next stop*) is a repair strategy more common than epenthesis in English, however. Glottal replacement of alveolar stops, especially in final position, is also allowed. In some dialects in New York City and surrounding areas, glottal replacement is more frequent in medial position (e.g., [baʔəl] for *bottle*). Syllable reduction, either to [ə] or total deletion of the syllable, is also acceptable in English. These repair strategies together yield such reduced phrases as [dʒiʔjɛʔ] ("Did you eat yet?").

The Spanish initial consonant cluster constraint tends to cause Spanish speakers to resort to epenthesis when attempting English words that violate the constraint. By epenthesizing a vowel before such clusters when they encounter them in English, Spanish speakers move the cluster from initial position to medial position, where it is allowed. This leads to stereotypical productions, such as "I a-speak a-Spanish" ([aɪ əspik əspænɪʃ]; Hyman, 1975).

In a way, the fact that a repair strategy is used by speakers is the information needed to determine that a constraint exists in that language or dialect. The contrapositive[12] of the principle "If it ain't broke, don't fix it" implies that the person trying to fix it must have thought it was broken. Thus, if speakers use a repair strategy (e.g., deletion of one consonant from a cluster), they must consider the form to need fixing for some reason (e.g., it contains a cluster). Thus, the tendency for American English speakers to delete elements of clusters, for example, is the basis for the claim that English has a constraint (albeit a weak one) against clusters.

One can easily see that these constraint repair strategies are exactly the same as the rules discussed in generative phonology and the processes discussed in natural phonology. Thus, constraint theory does not contradict the patterns identified within these earlier perspectives. Instead, it focuses on the reasons for the occurrence of these rules or processes rather than on the rules or processes themselves. Within this perspective, rules or

processes are pointers to some limitation that the speaker is attempting to circumvent in the phonological system. For example, careful consideration of Nathan's long list of processes reveals his underlying constraint against any nonalveolar consonants. This constraint is the heart of the matter; the processes are his superficial attempts to cope with the constraint.

It is important to keep in mind also the focus of each approach. Specifically, generative rules and natural phonology have been used clinically to focus primarily on comparing child productions to adult productions so as to identify error patterns. Phonological processes, the patterns with which most speech-language pathologists are most familiar, have been used exclusively for relational analysis. The child's production is compared to the adult production of the word, and the difference is described as a process. For example, if a child says [dɔ] for *dog*, it is noted as an instance of final consonant deletion. The function of the process is comparative only. Phonological rules have been used mostly for the same purpose. In the case just cited, for instance, the child would be credited with a rule that states that consonants are deleted in final position. These approaches highlight the respects in which the child's system is deficient in comparison to an adult English phonological system but do not clarify the manner of functioning of the child's system itself.

Phonological rules can be used for independent analysis as well as for relational analysis. An independent analysis phonological rule is a statement about the child's system only, without reference to the adult standard. For example, a child might have an allophonic alternation between fricatives and stops, with stops occurring only in initial position and fricatives occurring in medial and final positions, as shown in Table 5-12. Then this child has a set of rules that state that obstruents (stops and fricatives) in the system are produced as stops in initial position and as fricatives in medial and final position ("elsewhere"). Using the relevant phonological features ([+consonantal] and [−sonorant] for obstruents, [−continuant] for stops, and [+continuant] for fricatives), the following rules emerge:

$$\begin{bmatrix} +consonantal \\ -sonorant \end{bmatrix} \rightarrow [-continuant]/\#\underline{\quad}$$

(Nonsonorant Cs are stops in initial position.)

$$\begin{bmatrix} +consonantal \\ -sonorant \end{bmatrix} \rightarrow [+continuant] \text{ elsewhere}$$

(Nonsonorant consonants are fricatives in noninitial position.)

These rules may or may not apply to the adult language. In this case, they do not; however, that information is irrelevant. For independent analysis, the only concern is the patterns that are active *in the child's own system.*

Constraints are used also to describe the child's own system. They describe patterns that are not allowed in the child's system: those that do not occur or occur only very rarely. Many of the patterns that can be described as inde-

---

[12]For further information about contrapositives, see DJ Velleman (1994).

pendent phonological rules can be written even more simply as constraints. For example, a constraint against final consonants can be written as *C#.

The constraint is actually far more general than either a phonological rule or a process label (final consonant deletion) would be. It will account both for cases in which children fail to produce final consonants at all and for the choice of other possible strategies that could allow them to be more faithful to the adult representation without producing a consonant in final position. For example, recall that "Molly" (Vihman & Velleman, 1989) went through a stage in which she produced words idiosyncratically, including some words with correct final consonants. After systematizing her phonology, however, she ceased to produce final consonants in final position. Instead, she added a vocalic offset to final obstruents and nasals (vowel epenthesis in final position). This allowed her to produce the adult final consonants somewhere in the word, without actually producing consonants *in final position* in her own word forms. This pattern is illustrated in Table 5-13. Thus, Molly had the same constraint as a child who uses final consonant deletion to avoid final consonants, but her strategy for coping with the *C# constraint differed.

This example highlights the importance of the flexibility and changeability of constraint priority orders within constraint theory. Change over time is expected in the priority order of constraints within a certain phonological system (that of a language, a dialect, or even that of an individual child). In other words, a constraint that exhibits prominent effects at one time might cease to have a visible impact on the phonology at another time as other constraints become more important. This viewpoint is useful with respect to Molly's phonology. The constraint against final consonants was not weighted heavily at an extremely early stage in her phonology[13] but was prioritized shortly after systematization. Her phonological response (rule or process) to this constraint was to epenthesize vowels in final position so as to preserve the final consonants without having to produce them as such.

In other cases, the same child might omit final consonants part of the time but use epenthesis, migration, or some other strategy another part of the time, all with the same purpose of avoiding final consonants. Several processes or rules would have to be identified to account for these strategies. Unlike a phonological process or rule, the simple constraint *C# (no final consonants) will cover all those cases. It is a direct and explicit statement about the child's phonological limitations rather than about her strategies for dealing with those limitations. As such, the constraint provides a more direct route to determining therapy goals. In Molly's case, the appropriate goal (if she were delayed or disordered, rather than merely young) clearly would be to increase production of consonants in final position. Once the child's phonology will tolerate final consonants, she no longer will need to use the epenthesis strategy (or any other strategy) to cope

[13]Or, more likely, phonological constraints were irrelevant before phonological systematization.

TABLE 5-13.
"Molly"'s Vocalic Offsets

bang	[pɑnⁿə]
around	[wɑnə]
Brian	[pɑnə]
down	[tænə]
clock	[kɑkkɪ]
teeth	[tɪttʰi̥]
peek	[pekxe]
squeak	[kʰʊkʰʌ]
tick	[tɪtʰə]

Source: Adapted from MM Vihman, SL Velleman. Phonological reorganization: A case study. *Language and Speech* 1989;32:149–170.

with adult final consonants. Note that the goal for Molly *cannot* be to decrease final consonant deletion because she does *not* delete final consonants—she merely buries them within the word.

The foregoing set of rules describing one child's use of fricatives and stops in complementary distribution can also be written as constraints:

$$*\#[+\text{continuant}]$$

$$*V[-\text{continuant}]$$

These constraints state that continuant sounds (fricatives) may not occur in initial position and that noncontinuant sounds (stops) may not occur after vowels (in medial or final position). Again, the therapy goals are clear: to break down these constraints so that stops and fricatives stand in contrast instead of in complementary distribution. In other words, the goal is to encourage the child to do exactly what the constraint states she currently does not do: produce fricatives in initial position and produce stops in other positions.

The constraints do not indicate actually how the child accommodates these phonological limitations. She happens to stop initial fricatives and to fricate medial and final stops. However, this information actually is largely irrelevant to setting therapy goals. If the child becomes able to produce initial fricatives and medial and final stops, the stopping and the frication will cease. If a process approach is used and the stopping and frication are eliminated without the ability to produce initial fricatives and medial and final stops, new strategies (processes) will crop up to help her to continue to avoid these productions. She may begin to delete or affricate initial fricatives, for example. Then the clinician will have to start from scratch, eliminating the new processes.

Another case in which constraints may have explanatory value broader than that of processes or even rules is that of consonant clusters. Again, children whose phonological systems do not include the possibility of consonant clusters have many options for dealing with this problem. Cluster reduction is one possibility, but coalescence (e.g., [fɪm] for *swim*), migration (e.g., [nos] for *snow*), and epenthesis of a vowel between the two consonants (e.g., [bəlu] for *blue*) also are common strategies. A list of four processes or phonological rules affecting clusters may daunt the clinician. A constraint sums the situation up very concisely: *CC (no clusters). The goal is now clear: to facilitate production of two consecutive consonants. This approach will have the consequence of reducing all of the child's strategies, thereby decreasing the incidence of all of the processes (cluster reduction, coalescence, migration, and epenthesis). Thus, the question of choosing which process to address first becomes moot.

Constraints may also render goal setting clear in cases in which a child is using a less common process or using a common process in an unusual manner. The foregoing examples from Leonard and McGregor (1991), in which the child moved all initial fricatives to final position, are a case in point. Migration of fricatives to final position is not likely to be found in the typical phonological processes therapy kit. Rephrasing of the pattern into constraint form renders it far less formidable: *#[+continuant].

The constraint simply states that fricatives are not produced in initial position. Although the constraint is not specific with respect to this child's strategy for avoiding initial fricatives (it does not indicate that they migrate to final position), that information actually is irrelevant for setting therapy goals. Simply reducing the child's use of migration might only induce the child to use some other, equally inappropriate strategy, such as stopping or gliding of initial fricatives. However, facilitating the child's production of fricatives in initial position—directly addressing the constraint itself—will cause the child to discontinue the use of this inappropriate strategy because it no longer will be needed.

In summary, rules and processes can be seen as the strategies that children (and languages) use to cope with words that otherwise would violate their phonological constraints. In the case of children with NFP, the constraint is the more basic statement of the actual impediment to functional phonology. The rules and processes may help to highlight the limits of the child's phonological system, or they may obscure them. This is especially true if the clinician focuses only on relational analysis, comparing the child's productions to the adult target words. Independent analysis of the child's system, especially of elements or structures that are or are not permitted within the system, is necessary to identify accurately the actual source of the difficulty.

OPTIMALITY THEORY

Optimality theory (OT; as described by Archangeli & Langendoen, 1997; Bernhardt & Stemberger, 1998; McCarthy & Prince, in press; Prince & Smolensky, in press; Stemberger, 1996) is the formalization of the ideas presented in the two previous sections as constraint theory. It posits the existence of a universal set of phonological constraints with human phonetic limitations (and possibly perceptual and cognitive limitations as well) as their foundation.

These constraints are not absolute. They represent those phonological elements, structures, and patterns that present greater articulatory difficulty and, perhaps in some cases, more perceptual or cognitive difficulty. To communicate a wide range of ideas, a linguistic community must violate some (but not all) these constraints. Some languages choose to include consonant clusters, others multisyllabic words, others more challenging segments, and so on. In each language, a unique balance is struck between ease of production, ease of perception, and possibly other types of processing ease. Formally, this is expressed as a ranking of the universal phonological constraints. In other words, each language is believed to have the same constraints as every other language but to prioritize (i.e., never violate) some and to tolerate (i.e., violate) others. Each language has its unique *constraint hierarchy*.

Thus, the OT view of phonology is that all languages have the same constraints. They are part of the human apparatus.[14] However, each language has its own prioritization of these constraints. In one language (e.g., Japanese or Hawaiian), the constraint against consonant clusters may be clear because it is prioritized so highly that no clusters whatsoever occur in the language. In another (e.g., English or German), this constraint may be ranked so low that finding evidence of its existence is very difficult (McCarthy & Prince, 1994). Language change may involve reranking of constraints so that different ease of production or ease of perception factors are prioritized and pronunciations change. Languages that are similar have similar rankings. Dialects may differ only in a few differences in rankings.

In some respects, these ideas are similar to those expressed by proponents of natural phonology. As stated earlier, however, natural phonology formalized the repair strategies that may be used to avoid violating a constraint. For example, fronting might be used in a language with a constraint against velars. Similarly, epenthesis or cluster reduction might be used in a language with a constraint against consonant clusters. OT sees these processes as responses to the more basic phonological truths: the constraints themselves. In other words, the processes used by a language (or a child with NFP) reveal the language's (or the child's) constraints by pointing out the types of structures being avoided.

OT, then, addresses the following goals:

- To identify and verify the universal constraints
- To identify and verify the rankings of the constraints within each language
- To demonstrate that related languages have similar constraint rankings
- To demonstrate that language change can be identified as reranking of constraint hierarchies over time

In addition, clinical linguists have taken on the mission of validating OT by demonstrating that it can account for the phonological patterns of young children and of children (and adults) with NFP.

---

[14]How and why they are a part of the human apparatus (i.e., whether innate phonological *knowledge* of constraints exists) are still debated.

Technical Background of Optimality Theory

The constraints of OT have technical names, many of which may seem obscure to the reader. Furthermore, at least two sets of names are in use by different groups in the field (i.e., the original terminology used by such linguists as Archangeli & Langendoen [1997] and McCarthy & Prince [1994, 1995, in press] versus the newer terms coined by such clinical linguists as Bernhardt & Stemberger [1998] and Stemberger & Bernhardt [1997]). Furthermore, these constraint names are in flux because the theory is being developed. Thus, only those technical labels that refer to basic concepts and are in fairly general use are used here. Sometimes, as in the preceding section, the constraint is termed simply *X (to be read as *not X*), with the X replaced by the name of the element (or type of element) that is not allowed. When technical terms must be used, they are defined as carefully as possible, and alternative labels also are given where applicable.

One important distinction in OT is that between **markedness constraints** and **faithfulness constraints**. Markedness constraints are those that, like Stampe's natural processes (1969, 1979), reflect ease of production or ease of perception limitations. Restrictions on consonant clusters, final consonants, unusual segments, and so on have a basis in the physiological capacities of the human species. Those that create more difficulty in production or perception are marked and are less common in the languages of the world.

As discussed at the beginning of this section, however, some of these limitations must be overcome in each language in order for its phonology to include enough contrast for efficient communication. To avoid all physiological difficulty in speaking, humans would have to restrict themselves to the most basic syllables ([bɑ], perhaps) or not speak at all. To include a diverse lexicon, markedness must be overcome. To communicate effectively, humans' spoken words must be recognizably related to our mental representations of the words (or to the pronunciations of the words that other speakers of the language use). For example, if a speaker pronounces the word *unspoken* as [bɑ], eliminating the difficult consonant cluster, the final consonant, and the unstressed syllables, this word may as well have been literally unspoken, as communication will not have occurred.

This need to be true to the distinctive mental representation of the word is what is meant by *faithfulness*. It is easy to see that faithfulness and markedness are opposing forces. The former, like ease of perception, encourages the speaker to pronounce every element or structure without any changes. The latter, like ease of production, encourages the speaker to reduce each word to its simplest output form. In adult phonologies, faithfulness typically has the upper hand (McCarthy & Prince, 1994). Adults produce difficult words with relatively little simplification. Young children and those with NFP, on the other hand, often avoid producing marked forms, despite the loss of communicative effectiveness that results. Thus, markedness is prioritized over faithfulness in child phonology (Gnanadesikan, 1995) and in dysfunctional phonologies.

Seeing how constraints operate in adult languages requires considering words that are part of the language yet violate the language's constraints. How could such words ever occur? One source of examples is morphology. When an affix is added to a word, the combination of the particular stem plus the particular affix may result in a word that would be considered unpronounceable in that language.

Archangeli (1997) provides examples of the problems caused by suffixes that begin with consonants. If the stem of the word ends in a consonant cluster, the result of suffixation will be occurrence of three consecutive consonants. Such a string of consonants violates the constraints of some languages. Archangeli (1997) describes several options for dealing with this problem:

- Allow the three consonants to occur consecutively. This faithfulness option is elected by English; thus, such complex words as *limpness* or *thankful* are produced with three medial consonants in English.
- Omit a consonant. Archangeli (1997) stated that this option is elected by Spanish; thus, when a Spanish stem, such as *esculp-* (from *esculpir*, meaning "to sculpt"), is combined with a suffix, such as *-tor* (meaning "one who does something"), the correct pronunciation is [ɛskultor] (*sculptor*). The [p] is lost to prevent a three-consonant cluster.
- Insert a vowel between the consonants to break up the cluster. This option is selected by Yawelmani, a Native American language from California, according to Acrhangeli (1997). When a Yawelmani stem, such as *logw-* (*pulverize*), is combined with a suffix, such as *-hin* (past tense), the cluster is broken up by the insertion of [i] between the consonants, yielding [logiwhin] (*pulverized*).[15]
- Allow one consonant to take a vocalic role. This option seems the most unusual to speakers of English, although English speakers actually do allow a nasal or a liquid to carry an entire unstressed syllable in such words as *button* ([bʌʔn̩]) and *bottle* ([bɑtl̩]) or such phrases as *dig 'em* ([dɪgm̩]). Berber (a Moroccan language) takes this practice to an extreme, according to Archangeli (1997): The third-person feminine singular prefix *t-* may be added to some consonant-cluster-initial words. This morpheme plays a role similar to the *-s* on the ends of such English verbs as *plays, kicks, eats*, and the like. The result may be three consecutive consonants. For example, the stem *-ldi* (*to pull*) may have the *t-* prefix added to express *(she) pulls*. The resulting pronunciation is a two-syllable word (with the two syllables marked off with a dot)—[tl̩.di]—of which the first syllable consists of two consonants. The [l], then, plays the role of a vowel.

Archangeli's (1997) examples can be summarized as choices among four constraints:

- Faithfulness (Vowels)[16]: Do not add or delete vowels (abbreviated as *FAITH(V)*).
- Faithfulness (Consonants)[16]: Do not add or delete consonants (abbreviated as *FAITH(C)*).

---

[15]Note that the [w] and [h] are pronounced as separate consonants, not together as [w] or [ʍ], as most Americans do with the digraph *wh* in such words as *when, where*, and the like.

[16]This constraint is called *Survived* by Bernhardt and Stemberger (1998).

Forms↓	Constraints→			
/skul/	*COMPLEX	PEAK	FAITH(C)	FAITH(V)
[skul]	*			
[s.kul]		*		
[sul]			*	
[kul]			*	
☞[əs.kul]				*

FIGURE 5-1.
Constraint tableau for /skul/, spoken by a Spanish speaker. (*COMPLEX = the markedness constraint against consonant clusters.)

- *COMPLEX[17]: Do not produce three consonants consecutively in the same syllable.
- PEAK[18]: Every syllable must include a vowel as its peak.

Each language listed earlier has all four constraints, but they are ranked differently in each. In English, speakers do not change the vowels or consonants (we are faithful), and we prefer that vowels serve as syllable peaks. Thus, *COMPLEX is the constraint that must be violated: It is the lowest-ranked of these four, so all three consonants are pronounced. In Spanish, *COMPLEX gets a higher ranking (three consonants may not occur consecutively), but FAITH(C) has lower priority (in medial position); therefore, it is violated, and one consonant is deleted. In Yawelmani also, *COMPLEX has a high ranking, but FAITH(V) is lowest ranked. Therefore, a vowel is inserted to break up the cluster. Finally, Berber grants low priority to PEAK and breaks up the cluster by allowing one of the consonants to act as a vowel in its own syllable.

Applications to Second-Language Learning

Some of the clearest examples occur in words borrowed from other languages. Borrowed words that violate the new language's strongest constraints are especially interesting.

Spanish has a fairly strong markedness constraint against word-initial *sC* clusters ([s] plus any other consonant, as in *school*—[skul]), a constraint that is a subtype of *COMPLEX. When Spanish speakers attempt to produce an English word with such a cluster, they have some of the choices discussed

earlier. They can add a vowel, omit a consonant, treat one consonant as a vowel, or simply produce the cluster.

As discussed, the highest-ranked constraint in Spanish is *COMPLEX; saying [skul] is out. Spanish also does not like to treat consonants as vowels, so [s.kul], with the [s] in a separate syllable all by itself, is not a possibility either. In this case (because it is a different word position), however, omitting a consonant (FAITH(C)) is not the lowest-ranked constraint. For this word position, adding a vowel (FAITH(V)) is the most violable constraint. Therefore, a vowel is added, rendering the first consonant in the cluster the last consonant in the first syllable instead. For example, /skul/ becomes [əs.kul] (the dot shows the syllable boundary).[19] This repair strategy preserves all the segments but changes the syllable structure so that the sequence of consonants will be acceptable.

In OT, this jockeying among various constraints is displayed in a table (or *tableau*), as illustrated in Figure 5-1. The constraints are listed across the top in order of priority. The highest-priority constraint is placed at the left, with more *violable* constraints placed toward the right. The target (input) form is indicated within phonemic slashes (//) at the top left. The possible pronunciations of the word (outputs) are listed vertically below the input form on the far left. Asterisks in the chart indicate forms that violate a particular constraint. The pronunciation that "wins" (i.e., is actually chosen by the speakers of the language) is indicated with a pointed finger. This preferred output is the

---

[17]This constraint is called *NotComplex* by Bernhardt and Stemberger (1998).
[18]This constraint is called *Not σ-Peak* (not syllable peak) by Bernhardt and Stemberger (1998).

[19]Even fairly fluent English speakers whose first language is Spanish may be thrown off by this difference in constraint ranking. This author heard one Spanish speaker speaking English with an otherwise almost completely undetectable accent talking about a person who "scaped" from prison. Obviously, she had confused the correct pronunciation of the English word with Spanish speakers' tendency to epenthenize vowels in other similar cases (e.g., [əskul]), and she had hypercorrected as a result.

Forms↓	Constraints→		
/nɛkst#stɑp/	*EPEN	*COMPLEX	*DELETE
[nɛkst#stɑp]		****	
[nɛkəsətu#sətɑp]	****		
☞[nɛk#stɑp]		**	**

FIGURE 5-2.

English constraint ranking for /nɛkst#stɑp/. (*EPEN = constraint against epenthesis of vowels; *COMPLEX = the markedness constraint against consonant clusters; *DELETE = the constraint against deletion of consonants.)

Forms↓	Constraints→		
/nɛkst#stɑp/	*COMPLEX	*DELETE	*EPEN
[nɛkst#stɑp]	****		
☞[nɛkəsətu#sətɑpu]			*****
[nɛk#stɑp]	**	**	

FIGURE 5-3.

Japanese constraint ranking for /nɛkst#stɑp/. (*COMPLEX = the markedness constraint against consonant clusters; *DELETE = the constraint against deletion of consonants; *EPEN = constraint against epenthesis of vowels.)

form with the fewest asterisks toward the left-hand side of the chart. The shaded boxes are those that are irrelevant to the final choice, because a violation of a high-ranked constraint has already eliminated that possible form.

In this tableau, the output form at the top of the list, [skul], violates the top-ranked constraint, *COMPLEX, and therefore is ruled out despite the fact that it does not violate the other three. The second form, [s.kul], violates PEAK and therefore is ruled out, although it is relatively true to the input and it avoids a violation of the important *COMPLEX. The third form eliminates the problem sequence of two consonants, but it violates FAITH(C). The same is true of the fourth form. The epenthesized form, [əs.kul], is better than all of those preceding, as the first constraint it violates is FAITH(V), the lowest-ranked of these choices in this case. The constraint it violates is less of a priority than are those it avoids violating, and [əs.kul] therefore is the *optimal form.*

Another example may be helpful. Consider an English speaker and a Japanese speaker riding on a bus in the United States. Both wish to debark as soon as possible and must therefore call out, "Next stop!" By definition, all languages have *COMPLEX, the markedness constraint against consonant clusters, but the constraint is ranked far higher in Japanese than it is in English. In the Japanese language, the only possible clusters occur when a nasal-final syllable is followed by a consonant-initial syllable (e.g., as in *Honda* [hon.da]). In English, consonant clusters may be reduced if too many occur consecutively, but otherwise they are acceptable. All languages also have faithfulness constraints against epenthesis and against deletion. They were grouped together as FAITH(V) (do not add or delete vowels) and FAITH(C) (do not add or delete consonants) in the preceding example from Archangeli (1997). However, it is sometimes necessary to separate the constraint against deletion from the constraint against epenthesis. For simplicity's sake, the constraint against deletion of consonants is termed **DELETE(C),* and the constraint against epenthesis of vowels is termed **EPEN(V)* in this example (idiosyncratically).[20] In English, *EPEN is ranked higher than is *DELETE. English speakers prefer to delete consonants rather than to add vowels. In Japanese, the reverse is true. The results are quite different for the two speakers, as illustrated in the tableaux in Figures 5-2 and 5-3.

---

[20]McCarthy and Prince (1995, in press) refer to *EPEN as *DEP I-O* (Output should DEPend on Input) and to *DELETE as *MAX I-O* (MAXimize the correspondence between Input and Output). Bernhardt and Stemberger (1998) refer to *EPEN as *LinkedDownwards* and to *DELETE as *Survived.*

Forms↓ Constraints→			
Molly at 16 mos /bæŋ/	*C#	*DELETE (C#)	*EPEN (V)
[baɪŋ]	*		
[baɪ‚pæ:]		*	
☞[panⁿə]			*

FIGURE 5-4.
"Molly"'s constraint tableau for /bæŋ/. (*C# = no final consonants; *DELETE (C#) = do not delete final consonants; *EPEN = constraint against epenthesis of vowels.)

The English speaker prefers to delete twice rather than to violate *COMPLEX four times, because *DELETE is ranked lower than is *COMPLEX.[21] Epenthesis in this type of situation is not a possibility because *EPEN(V) is ranked too highly in English. Therefore, the English speaker omits one -st- sequence and calls out [nɛk.stɑp] (causing one Japanese speaker to ask this author, "What does it have to do with a neck?").

The Japanese speaker, on the other hand, would rather epenthesize vowels five times (one of which avoids the final consonant, p#, as the result of another constraint) than produce even one sequence of two consonants or delete any consonants. *COMPLEX and *DELETE are given very high priority. Thus, the Japanese speaker calls out, "[nɛkəsətu#sətapu]!" (which may not be understood in the United States at all). The basic insight of OT is that the *same* constraints are operative in both languages but are ranked differently. Different rankings of the same constraints yield very different results.

Applications to Child Phonology

OT can shed some light also on child phonology. Consider Molly, for example, the 16-month-old described by Vihman and Velleman (1989) as epenthesizing vowels after final consonants (and whose data are repeated in Table 5-13). It has been shown that Molly had a high-ranked markedness constraint against final consonants; she avoided producing consonant-vowel-consonant (CVC) words. However, the faithfulness constraint that specifies that the features of a final consonant must also be preserved was high-ranked in her system at 16 months. This ranking was consistent with her phonological history. She was a child who often appeared to select words on the basis of their final consonants, showing unusual interest in this word position.

As discussed, at the presystematic phonology stage, she had produced some words with final consonants, until her final consonant constraint became prominent. The only way for her to reconcile her two constraints at 16 months was for her to violate a faithfulness constraint against epenthesis, which was ranked much lower in her phonological system at the same time. Thus, her constraints are listed in order of priority as follows:

1. *NOCODA*[22]: *C#; do not produce consonants in final position.
2. **DELETE(C#)*: Do not delete final consonants.
3. *EPEN(V)*: Do not add vowels.

The interactions among these constraints are illustrated in the tableau in Figure 5-4.

Thus, at 16 months, Molly no longer produced *bang* as [baɪŋ] because this would involve production of a final consonant. Her constraint against final consonants was too highly ranked at that time. However, deletion of the final consonant ([baɪ, pæ:]) also was unacceptable to her. Therefore, she violated *EPEN(V), which is ranked low, and she produced *bang* as [panⁿə].

Another child who also showed an interest in final consonants (especially final velars) handled them differently at 16 months. "Sean" (Vihman & McCune, 1994) agreed with Molly in trying not to delete final consonants, contrary to the more common pattern among young English-speaking children. However, his *EPEN(V) was ranked higher, and NOCODA was ranked lower. Therefore, Sean generally was more faithful to the (presumed) input word shapes. In fact, however, NOCODA was ranked so low that even some words that do not have a final consonant in the adult form (e.g., *moo*) did have final consonants in his form! This consonant epenthesis (as in [mæk] for *moo*) explains why *EPEN had to be specified as referring specifically to epenthesis of vowels in his case. *EPEN(C)

---

[21]Obviously, some details are being glossed over here, as *COMPLEX does not result in the English speaker's deleting three or four consonants.

[22]This constraint appears to be included in Bernhardt and Stemberger's *WordFinalMassiveness* (1998).

must have been much lower in his constraint hierarchy than was *EPEN(V). Sean's data (slightly simplified) are given in Table 5-14. The interactions among his constraints are illustrated for the production of *block* in the tableau in Figure 5-5. Note that *EPEN(V) and *DELETE are divided by a dotted line instead of a solid line, to indicate that both are ranked equally.

The first form, [bakə], which is undoubtedly the one that would have been preferred by Molly, is ruled out because of the epenthesized [ə]. The second, [ba], which is the form preferred by many children of this age, is ruled out because the final consonant is not preserved. Only the faithful [bak] is optimal for Sean at this stage.[23] Note, however, that Sean did more than simply always produce words correctly. For one thing, he clearly simplified consonant clusters. Furthermore, he added a final [k] to *moo*, which is certainly not an adult form that he would ever have heard.

Another type of constraint, the alignment constraint, accounts for cases in which a child preserves all the segments in the (presumed) target word but moves them around (migration or metathesis). Velleman (1996b) has illustrated the use of OT to account for child metathesis, migration, harmony, and default medial consonants with alignment constraints. For example, W, the child described by Leonard and McGregor (1991), consistently produced fricatives in final position, regardless of their position in the adult word. (W's data are repeated from Table 2-13 in Table 5-11.) W sacrificed syllable structure to achieve her goal of fricatives in final position. The constraint against onsetless (vowel-initial) syllables (called *ONSET*), and the constraint against consonant clusters (*COMPLEX*) are common in children's phonologies. In contrast, W tolerated these marked syllable structures, even when no other constraint made them necessary. For example, she used a consonant cluster in [geps] for *grapes* and allowed a word without an initial consonant in [ʊk]

---

[23]Some variability in Sean's productions is being ignored here for clarity's sake. Note also that he did omit final consonants at an earlier phonological stage.

TABLE 5-14.
"Sean"'s Final Consonants

block	[bɑk]
book	[bɑk]
truck	[tɛk]
bug	[bʌk]
monkey	[mək]
moo	[mæk]

Source: Adapted from MM Vihman, L McCune. When is a word a word? *Journal of Child Language* 1994;21:517–542.

for *look*. However, she would not permit fricatives except in final position, even if moving the fricative to final position left the word without an onset or created a cluster at the end of a word. Thus, W's fricative distribution requirement constraint (also known as a *melody constraint*) was ranked higher than were cluster and onset constraints in her system.

It is important to note that, in W's phonology, consonant features were moved rather than deleted. Both segments (i.e., the correct number of consonants and vowels) and features (i.e., the correct types of consonants and vowels) were maintained whenever possible. These facts of W's fricative-final pattern may be accounted for in OT using the following constraints:

- *ALIGN Fricative Right*: Fricatives must be word-final.
- *DELETE*: No deletion of segments can occur.
- *IDENTITY* (*Continuant*): Continuant feature must be preserved (i.e., fricatives remain fricatives).
- *COMPLEX*: No clusters are allowed.
- *ONSET*: Initial consonants are obligatory.

*DELETE prohibits deletion of segments, whereas IDENTITY prohibits changing features (e.g., changing a fricative to a stop; McCarthy & Prince, 1995). Thus, an output, such as [ops] for *soap*, can be represented as in the tableau in Figure 5-6.

Forms↓	Constraints→		
Sean at 16 mos /blɑk/	*EPEN (V)	*DELETE	*C#
[bɑkə]	*		
[bɑ]		*	
☞ [bɑk]			*

FIGURE 5-5.
"Sean"'s constraint tableau for /blɑk/. (*EPEN(V) = the constraint against epenthesis of vowels; *DELETE = the constraint against deletion ; *C# = no final consonants.)

Forms↓   Constraints→

W /sop/	ALIGN Fric. Right	IDENT(Cont)	*DELETE	*COMPLEX	ONSET
[sop]	*				
[top]	N/A	*			
[op]	N/A	N/A	*		*
[so]	*		*		
[os]			*		*
☞ [ops]				*	*

FIGURE 5-6.
W's constraint tableau for /sop/. NA = not applicable. (Adapted from SL Velleman. Metathesis highlights feature-by-position constraints. In Bernhardt B, Gilbert J, Ingram D [eds]. *Proceedings of the UBC International Conference on Phonological Acquisition.* **Somerville, MA: Cascadilla Press, 1996b, 173–176.)**

The forms [sop] and [so] are not possible; the fricative is not word-final in these productions. The fricative feature has been lost in [top],[24] although a segment still is marking its place, so this form is also unacceptable. Deletion has occurred in [op], [so], and [os], so they are ruled out. Only [ops] does not violate the three highest priority constraints: ALIGN Fricative Right, IDENTITY (Continuant), and *DELETE. It does violate *COMPLEX and ONSET, but these are of minor importance for this particular child. As her phonology matures, she must deprioritize ALIGN Fricative Right (as it is not ranked highly in English). IDENTITY and *DELETE should remain highly ranked, and *COMPLEX and ONSET will remain ranked relatively low, in keeping with the language that W was learning.

The foregoing description implies that W was on a straight course to the appropriate constraint ranking for her native language. This was not necessarily the case. Velleman (1996b) used a longitudinal example to illustrate two findings: Not all of children's rerankings are always appropriate to the language being learned, as temporarily inappropriate prioritizations may occur, and children may rerank in an appropriate way, then appear to regress with respect to their languages' rankings before acquiring the correct language-specific constraint ranking.

Molly (described earlier) illustrated the first of these findings. Initially, she produced appropriate final conso-

nants, as her language dictated. Presumably, NOCODA (*C#) was ranked fairly low at that point. As she systematized her phonology and reranked her constraints, she allowed NOCODA to rise to the top of the priority ranking and allowed *EPEN to fall, as exemplified by forms such as [panⁿə] for "bang." Her constraint hierarchy became less, not more, like that of the language she was learning. Thus, like the course of true love (to paraphrase Shakespeare), the course of phonological constraint acquisition does not always run smooth.

Clinical Implications

It has been stated that constraints are related more directly to therapy goals than are rules and processes. As discussed, it is more important to note, for example, that a child is avoiding fricatives than to note what specific avoidance strategies are being used (deletion, stopping, gliding, cluster reduction, etc.). The ultimate goal is to eliminate the inappropriate constraints (e.g., to get such a child to produce fricatives). Simply eliminating one process or rule (e.g., deletion of fricatives) may well lead to the use of another rule or process (e.g., stopping) that achieves the same purpose (no fricatives).

The *ranking* of constraints, a critical theoretical element in OT, also has direct clinical implications. Those constraints that are ranked high in many children's phonologies but low in a particular child's ambient language (e.g., NOCODA in English) are the most likely to interfere with intelligibility. However, they also are the

---

[24]Note that Fricative Right is irrelevant if no fricative is found in the output.

least violable, most central constraints in the child's system, and they may therefore be most resistant to intervention. The most workable strategy is likely to be to chip away at constraints ranked somewhat lower, those that the child is willing to violate on occasion. The clinician can gradually work up to those constraints that are ranked higher. In fact, as the child's phonology reorganizes as a result of other changes, those constraints that were initially resistant are likely to shift in their ranking order, becoming more vulnerable and thus more likely to change with the proper encouragement.

These clinical impressions remain to be verified empirically. The investigation of constraint-based intervention is likely to yield exciting results that will have an impact on phonological therapy for a long time. Readers who seek more information on OT should consult Archangeli and Langendoen (1997), a highly readable introduction to the theory as it applies to linguistics in general and to phonology in particular. Those who wish to know more about the applications of OT to clinical phonology are referred to Bernhardt and Stemberger (1998) and Stemberger and Bernhardt (1997).

CHAPTER SIX

Phonological Systems: A Longitudinal Case Study

What happens when a child's phonological system is analyzed as a whole and all of the pieces are examined in relation to each other? Not only can deficient aspects of each component be identified but the impacts of each difference or delay on every other component of the system also can be revealed.

Of course, to use every do-it-yourself form for a child evaluated clinically is an onerous task, especially if the forms are used quantitatively. This mission should be undertaken only by the rare speech-language pathologist with extra time on his or her hands. More typically, the following four forms are used to get a sense of other phonological aspects requiring further investigation:

- Form 2-1, Phonotactic Repertoire: Word and Syllable Shapes
- Form 2-2, Phonotactic Repertoire: Reduplication and Harmony
- Form 3-1, Consonant Repertoire
- Form 3-2, Vowel Repertoire

These four forms can be summarized on Form 5-3 (Phonological Constraints). As a set, these five forms give an excellent snapshot of a phonological system, although surprises sometimes do await the clinician who delves more deeply. Additional analyses should be carried out as appropriate, either for the initial assessment or within a period of diagnostic therapy.

In this chapter, the phonological system of one child with a nonfunctional phonology (NFP) is analyzed at two different times. The two analyses are discussed in their entireties, highlighting the functioning of the child's phonology as a system at each time. In each case, the functional and nonfunctional aspects of the system are identified, and some suggestions for possible remediation targets are made. Later data illustrate the different directions in which a phonological system may develop. For each period, all do-it-yourself forms for the child are provided and discussed. Some will not prove to be enlightening for this child at a particular time, as is typically the case in clinical phonology.

"ELLEN"

Time 1: Age 2 Years, 3 Months

"Ellen" is the pseudonym for a child who has been followed clinically by this author. At age 2 years, 3 months, she was becoming less and less intelligible, and everyone concerned was becoming frustrated. Her mother, a speech-language pathologist, was especially concerned because Ellen's older brother had received a diagnosis of dyspraxia. Although (as seen later) many of Ellen's patterns actually were not terribly unusual for a child of her age, the combination and effects of these patterns were devastating to her ability to communicate effectively. Therefore, although she may not have been far from developmental norms, this communication disorder had to be remediated.

TABLE 6-1.
"Ellen"'s Intelligible Words and Holophrases at Age 2 Years, 3 Months

[peɪ]	play, plate
[pʰi]	please
[boʊ]	bow
[baɪ]	bite
[bu]	blue
[mi]	me
[weɪ]	swing
[waɪ]	grapes
[wi]	three
[tʰu]	school, two
[tʰo]	cold
[tʰɪʔ]	kiss
[ni]	knee
[ja]	yeah
[aʊ]	out
[i]	eat
[ʌpʰ]	up
[gʌgʰ], [gʌk]	duck
[dʌpʰ], [dʌt]	gum
[buɸi], [bup]	poop
[pʌpi], [pap]	puppet
[woʊwoʊ], [wʌl]	roll
[wɔwə]	Laura
[momo], [mɔ]	more
[bubu], [pʰʊ]	spoon
[adədʌdʌ]	happybirthday
[wawa]	water
[ha], [haha]	hot
[dadə], [dædæ]	thankyou
[dadæ], [dada]	daddy
[nɛnɛnɛnɛnaɪ]	night-night
[ʌbʌbaɪbaɪ]	bye-bye
[tuʳwi], [i]	cookie
[ʌʔo]	uh-oh
[ʌno]	Idon'tknow
[ʌki]	yucky
[awaɪ]	allright
[ɔdɪd]	alldone
[bʌdə]	kitty
[badə]	panda
[pæpita]	patty-cake
[aɪdɪd]	Idid
[aɪtʰu], [aɪtʰ]	Ido

Ellen's speech data for age 2 years, 3 months, grouped into intelligible words and holophrases, intelligible phrases, and unintelligible utterances, are given in Tables 6-1 through 6-3. The distinction between holophrases (formulas, written without spaces—e.g., *alldone*) and phrases (e.g., *more cheese*) was made on the basis of context and prosody. Holophrases were treated as single words; phrases were treated as sequences of words.

Form 2-1 (reproduced here as Example 6-1) was used to determine Ellen's word and syllable shapes. At 2 years, 3 months, Ellen's favorite word shape was a monosyllabic consonant-vowel (CV) sequence. Form 2-1 identified 66% CV and 21% V syllables, with rare closed syllables (12% VC + CVC total). Clearly, she avoided final consonants. Words were monosyllabic 50% of the time, disyllabic 33% of the time, and only rarely longer, although

TABLE 6-2.
"Ellen"'s Intelligible Phrases at Age 2 Years, 3 Months

[aʊ wu]	my shoe
[aʊʔ dʒu]	out juice
[bu bubu]	dog boo-boo
[ba baba]	not bottle
[ʌ aʊ]	want out
[aʊ̃ aʊ]	not out
[ĩ ɪn]	not in
[wiʔ ĩ]	yes, in
[dɪ:: di]	not Stephen
[bi ti]	more cheese
[bʌdɪʔ]	blow it

Note: Colon represents vowel lengthening.

TABLE 6-3.
"Ellen"'s Unintelligible Words and Phrases at Age 2 Years, 3 Months

[bɔdə]
[bidə]
[bububu]
[bʌdə bʌ bʌdə]
[ʌbububibu]
[ɔdɔtʰ]
[bʊdɪvʊ]
[ʌdʌbabaɪ]
[aʔl]
[bʊdæ]
[bʌdʊ]
[bʌnəmaʊ]
[bʌdʌmbʌ]
[bʌdʌ]

words of up to five syllables did occur. Thus, she was capable of combining multiple syllables into a sequence but did not do so often.

When she produced a word with two syllables or more, Ellen reduplicated perhaps 38% of the time, as shown in Example 6-2. Typical productions included [dada] for *daddy* and [wawa] for *water*. A few target one-syllable words were extended to two syllables in Ellen's productions through reduplication: [bubu] for *spoon*, [woʊwoʊ] for *roll*, and [haha] for *hot*. Obviously, producing a two-syllable word was no great hardship for her as long as it was reduplicated.

Ellen harmonized consonants in 31% of the remainder of her two-syllable words, as in [pʌpi] for *puppet*[1] and [pæpita] for *patty-cake*. Overall, then, she produced two *different* consonants in a multisyllabic word only about a third of the time. Clearly, she had difficulty in maintaining two different sets of consonant features within the same word.

Vowels never were harmonized, but other patterns were evident when additional analyses (not on this form) were performed. For instance, among words with two (or more) different vowels, the first vowel was most likely to be one of [a, ʌ, ɔ], and the later vowels were most likely to be one of [ə, i, aɪ]. This pattern is in keeping with patterns in American English "motherese": The second vowel of the word is more likely to be higher than the first (as in *horsie, baby, doggie*, etc.).

Similar consonant harmony held for Ellen's monosyllabic CVC words as was noted for CVCV words, as illustrated in the bottom section of Example 6-2. Those few CVC words that Ellen did produce, such as [gʌgʰ] for *duck* and [dʌt] for *gum*, included two different[2] consonants less than a third of the time (29%).

An examination of Ellen's phrases illustrated that harmony had a strong hold there as well. Function words in these phrases took on the phonological characteristics of the accompanying content words at least 60% of the time.[3] *Not*, for example, was produced as [aʊ] before *out*, [ĩ] before *in*, [ba] before *bottle* ([baba]), and [dɪ] before *Stephen* ([di]). Clearly, Ellen had some difficulty in maintaining different consonants both within and across words in the same phrase.

Ellen did not demonstrate any significant C-V interactions, as shown in Example 6-3 (from Form 2-3). Labial and alveolar stops co-occurred with vowels from all corners of the English vowel space. Furthermore, some patterns one would expect in a child with consonant-vowel dependencies were not noted. For example, Davis and MacNeilage (1990) found that children used [u] with velars, as both involve a high back tongue position. Ellen produced [i, ʌ] with velars but did not produce [u] with velars. This form did reveal, however, that Ellen's most common syllable was [dʌ]. Her favorite vowels appeared to be [a, ʌ], those that require the least tongue shaping. Also, her favorite consonants apparently were [d, b].

Examples 6-4 and 6-5 reflect Ellen's stress patterns. She did not produce a large number of multisyllabic words. Furthermore, the majority of those that she did produce were reduplicated; therefore, judging them was difficult, as both syllables in reduplicated words appeared to get approximately equal weight. Other words, such as *all right* and *all done*, have variable stress patterns, including equal stress sometimes, in adult speech; therefore, judging them also was difficult in this young child. (It seems to be easier to detect an error than to detect the details of an appropriate production.) The remaining few words were trochaic in the adult model, and Ellen produced them as such. Among these were several two-syllable words, the three-syllable *patty-cake*, and the four-syllable *happy birthday*.

These forms lead to the conclusion that Ellen was able to produce trochaic stress patterns without error (see

---

[1]Recall that this analysis is independent, so the fact that the adult form also includes the same consonant twice is irrelevant. For production, Ellen may be selecting words that follow her preferred patterns, avoiding adult words that do not have the shapes that she likes.
[2]Recall that voicing is not considered a difference for these purposes. Thus, [dʌt] is considered to exemplify consonant harmony.

---

[3]It was difficult to gauge some examples; therefore, they were counted as not harmonized, to give Ellen the benefit of the doubt.

Phonotactic Repertoire: Word and Syllable Shapes

Name: *Ellen*   Age: *2;3 (27 months)*
Date: *10/12/94*   Examiner: *SLV*
Source of sample: *speech in play*   Size of sample: *76 words*

Note: C = consonant
        V = vowel
        # = word boundary
        Predominant: 61–100%
        Frequent: 41–60%
        Occasional: 16–40%
        Rare: 1–15%

	% or ✓	Frequency estimate: Circle appropriate word.				

Syllable types[a]: *115 total*

Incomplete						
C alone	0%	~~Predominant~~	~~Frequent~~	~~Occasional~~	~~Rare~~	Absent
V, V?, ?V	21%	~~Predominant~~	~~Frequent~~	Occasional	~~Rare~~	~~Absent~~
Open						
CV, CV?	66%	Predominant	~~Frequent~~	~~Occasional~~	~~Rare~~	~~Absent~~
Closed						
VC, ?VC	2%	~~Predominant~~	~~Frequent~~	~~Occasional~~	Rare	~~Absent~~
CVC[b]	10%	~~Predominant~~	~~Frequent~~	~~Occasional~~	Rare	~~Absent~~

Clusters[c]: *None*

Initial						
#CC-	0%	~~Predominant~~	~~Frequent~~	~~Occasional~~	~~Rare~~	Absent
#CCC-	0%	~~Predominant~~	~~Frequent~~	~~Occasional~~	~~Rare~~	Absent
Final						
-CC#	0%	~~Predominant~~	~~Frequent~~	~~Occasional~~	~~Rare~~	Absent
-CCC#	0%	~~Predominant~~	~~Frequent~~	~~Occasional~~	~~Rare~~	Absent
Medial						
-CC-	0%	~~Predominant~~	~~Frequent~~	~~Occasional~~	~~Rare~~	Absent
-CCC-	0%	~~Predominant~~	~~Frequent~~	~~Occasional~~	~~Rare~~	Absent

Word shapes[c]: *76 total*

# of syllables						
1	50%	~~Predominant~~	Frequent	~~Occasional~~	~~Rare~~	~~Absent~~
2	33%	~~Predominant~~	~~Frequent~~	Occasional	~~Rare~~	~~Absent~~
3	1%	~~Predominant~~	~~Frequent~~	~~Occasional~~	Rare	~~Absent~~
4+	4%	~~Predominant~~	~~Frequent~~	~~Occasional~~	Rare	~~Absent~~

[a]Out of all syllables.
[b]Includes CCVC, CVCC, etc.
[c]Out of all words.

Maximum # of syllables produced in any word: *5*

Notes:

EXAMPLE 6-1.
Phonotactic repertoire: word and syllable shapes.

Phonotactic Repertoire: Reduplication and Harmony

Name: *Ellen*   Age: *2;3 (27 months)*
Date: *10/12/94*   Examiner: *SLV*
Source of sample: *speech in play*   Size of sample: *76 words*

Note: C = consonant
       V = vowel
       Reduplication = same syllable repeated in word (*baba, deedee, gogo*, etc.)
       Harmony = same C repeated (*goggie, tootie*, etc.) or same V repeated (*daba, boogoo*)
       Predominant: 61–100%
       Frequent: 41–60%
       Occasional: 16–40%
       Rare: 1–15%

	% or ✓	Frequency estimate: Circle appropriate word.

Words of two syllables or more: *29 total*[a]

Reduplicated syllables	_38%_	~~Predominant~~	~~Frequent~~	[Occasional]	~~Rare~~	~~Absent~~
Harmonized vowels	_0%_	~~Predominant~~	~~Frequent~~	~~Occasional~~	~~Rare~~	[Absent]
Harmonized consonants	_31%_	~~Predominant~~	~~Frequent~~	[Occasional]	~~Rare~~	~~Absent~~

Monosyllabic words: *7 total*[b]

Harmonized consonants	_71%_	[Predominant]	~~Frequent~~	~~Occasional~~	~~Rare~~	~~Absent~~

[a]Out of all **multisyllabic** words.
[b]Out of all **monosyllabic** CVC words.

Notes:

Consonant harmony/reduplication applies at least 60% of the time across words within phrases (e.g., [bɑ bɑbɑ] = "not bottle").

EXAMPLE 6-2.
Phonotactic repertoire: reduplication and harmony.

Phonotactic Repertoire: Consonant-Vowel Dependencies

Name: *Ellen*   Age: *2;3 (27 months)*
Date: *10/12/94*   Examiner: *SLV*
Source of sample: *speech in play*   Size of sample: *76 words*

Indicate (✓ or %) combinations that do occur: *percentages*

C type	High front (i, ɪ)	Mid front (e, ɛ)	Low front (æ)	Mid central (ə, ʌ)	High back (u, ʊ)	Mid back (o, ɔ)	Low back (ɑ)
Stops							
Labial (b, p)	5	2	2	5	8		6
Alveolar (d, t)	3		5	13	3	2	8
Velar (k, g)	2			3			
Nasals							
Labial (m)						5	
Alveolar (n)		6					2
Glides							
Labial (w)	2	2		5		3	6
Palatal (j)							
Liquids							
Alveolar (l)							
Palatal (r)							
Fricatives							
Labial (f, v)							
Interdental (θ, ð)							
Alveolar (s, z)							
Palatal (ʃ, ʒ)							
Affricates (tʃ, dʒ)							
Glottals (h, ʔ)							5
Other							

Notes:

EXAMPLE 6-3.
Phonotactic repertoire: consonant-vowel dependencies.

Stress Patterns: Independent Analysis

Name: *Ellen*
Date: *10/12/94*
Source of sample: *speech in play*

Age: *2;3 (27 months)*
Examiner: *SLV*
Size of sample: *76 words*

For each stress pattern, list words that the child produces with that pattern, whether or not they are correct. Examples in parentheses are intended to facilitate the speech-language pathologist's recognition of varied stress patterns only. The child should not necessarily be required to attempt these words.

Note: S = strong syllable
W = weak syllable

Target stress pattern	Examples from child
SW (e.g., mónkey)	[pʌ́pi] *puppet* [wɔ́wə] *Laura* [túʸwi] *cookie* [bádə] *panda*
WS (e.g., giráffe)	
ŚWS̀ (e.g., télephòne)	[pǽpità] *patty-cake*
SWW/ŚS̀W (e.g., hámburger)	
WSW (e.g., spaghétti)	
WWS/S̀WŚ (e.g., kàngaróo)	
ŚWS̀W (e.g., cáterpìllar)	
WŚWS̀/S̀ŚWW (e.g., rhìnóceros)	
WWSW/S̀WŚW (e.g., dìsappóinted)	[àdədʌ́dʌ] *happy birthday*
Other 4-syllable words (SWWS, WSWS, WSSW)	
5+ syllables	

EXAMPLE 6-4.
Stress patterns: independent analysis.

Stress Patterns: Relational Analysis

Name: *Ellen*   Age: *2;3 (27 months)*
Date: *10/12/94*   Examiner: *SLV*
Source of sample: *speech in play*   Size of sample: *76 words*

For each stress pattern, list words that the child attempts with that pattern, indicating whether the word is produced correctly, with weak syllable(s) omitted, with strong syllables omitted, or with other outputs (e.g., coalescence of two syllables into one). Examples in parentheses are intended to facilitate the speech-language pathologist's recognition of varied stress patterns only. The child should not necessarily be required to attempt these particular words.

Note: S = strong syllable
        W = weak syllable

Target stress pattern	Correct	W omitted	S omitted	Other
SW (e.g., mónkey)	*Several (see Example 6-4)*			
WS (e.g., giráffe)				
ŚWS̀ (e.g., télephòne)	[pǽpità] *patty-cake*			
SWW/ŚS̀W (e.g., hámburger)				
WSW (e.g., spaghétti)				
WWS/S̀WŚ (e.g., kàngaróo)				
ŚWS̀W (e.g., cáterpìllar)				
WŚWS̀/S̀ŚWW (e.g., rhìnóceros)				
WWSW/S̀WŚW (e.g., dìsappóinted)	[àdədʌ́dʌ] *happy birthday*			
Other 4-syllable words (SWWS, WSWS, WSSW)				
5+ syllables				

EXAMPLE 6-5.
Stress patterns: relational analysis.

Example 6-5) in words up to four syllables in length.[4] Unfortunately, no statement can be made about her ability to produce iambic words at that time. Had this author been more aware of the clinical implications of metrical abnormalities at the time of Ellen's initial evaluation, Ellen's production of iambic words would have been probed. However, the seminal work of Shriberg et al. (1997a,b,c) on metrical patterns in children with speech delay versus developmental verbal dyspraxia had not yet been completed. Certainly, the ability to produce varied stress patterns was something that should have been watched in Ellen's case, as her brother did have the diagnosis of developmental verbal dyspraxia.

Forms 3-1 and 3-2, reproduced here as Examples 6-6 and 6-7, yielded consonant and vowel repertoires that were fairly age-appropriate. When consonants are collapsed across positions, one can see that nasals, glides, and voiced and voiceless bilabial and alveolar stops either were mastered by or were emerging in Ellen. A few velars and fricatives were occasionally produced, indicating that they may have been coming into her repertoire. Ellen had mastered more labial consonants than consonants from any other place of articulation in all positions. Thus, labial may have been a preferred place of articulation for her.

Ellen produced all English simple vowels, and the most common diphthongs ([ɑɪ] and [ɑʊ]). Rhotic vowels ([ɝ, iɚ, ɑɚ], etc.) were neither expected nor in evidence, given her relatively young age. Thus, by the criteria used in many public schools, Ellen was within normal limits at this point, and "not in need of services."

Form 4-3 (Word and Syllable Contrasts, reproduced here as Example 6-8) identified quite a few minimal pairs and near-minimal pairs in Ellen's speech. She appeared to use the majority of the consonants and vowels in her repertoire in a contrastive fashion to differentiate word pairs. She had many minimal pairs; Ellen appeared to produce very few actual homonyms, although *thank you* ([dɑdə, dædæ]) and *daddy* ([dɑdæ, dɑdɑ]) were very similar.

Despite her lack of homonymy and despite her age-appropriate consonant and vowel repertoires, however, intelligibility was a significant problem for Ellen (and for her family). What was the source of her problem? A couple of hints already have been provided. First, consonant harmony both in words and across words in phrases was a significant factor. Second, word recipes, such as using a lower vowel before a higher one, also were present. Additional analyses highlighted even more factors.

Filling out Forms 4-1 and 4-2 (Examples 6-9 and 6-10) confirmed the dysfunctionality of her system: Very few consistent substitution patterns seemed to exist. For example, [g] substituted for /d/ in initial position, but [d] also substituted for /g/ in the same position. Similarly, in medial position, [b] substituted for /d/ and vice versa. In fact, the phone [b] seemed to substitute for just about everything else! In initial position, it substituted for /d, p,

m, n/, and in medial position for /d, p, t/. In final position, its voiceless counterpart, [p], substituted for /m, t/.

With respect to vowel substitutions, some mysterious examples were also noted. This time, [ɑ] substituted for many other sounds (including [i, ɪ, æ, ʌ, ɚ]). The low front [æ] substituted for both high tense vowels ([i, u]), which is quite unusual. Further, some bidirectional substitutions were noted (e.g., [ɪ] substituted for [ʌ] and [ʌ] for [ɪ]). Sixty-nine percent of the time, the vowel that was actually produced was lower than the vowel that was assumed to be Ellen's target. Another 19% of the time, [æ] was backed to [ɑ]. In the same number of cases, a diphthong (e.g., [eɪ]) was replaced by a simple vowel (e.g., [ɑ]). Ellen, then, had a preference for low, back, simple vowels.

Overall, Ellen's substitution patterns did not seem to make much sense. Many phonemes had more than one substitute, often in addition to some correct productions. Some phonemes seemed to substitute for each other. Some pattern had to emerge from these replacements, but it was not clear from this analysis only. The substitution analysis did not give the big picture.

The most helpful aspect of these relational (substitution) analyses was a discovery made through identifying those phonemes that were crossed out in each position on the consonant substitution form. This procedure revealed those consonant phonemes that Ellen was attempting very rarely from the adult forms of words: fricatives. (Consequences of this finding for Ellen's later phonological development are revealed in the section on Ellen's speech at 4 years.) Also, this form highlighted the high functional load for [b] in Ellen's system, as it was a substitute for so many other consonant sounds. Similarly, the vowel substitution form revealed that Ellen rarely was attempting rhotic vowels and that she had a high functional load for [ɑ]. It appeared that Ellen's very favorite syllable was that universal favorite: [bɑ]. However, substitution analysis per se (what substitutes for what) did not help to answer the question of the source of the basic dysfunctionality of her system.

Ellen's process summary, another relational analysis that was based on the previous two forms and on the phonotactic harmony and reduplication form, confirmed the sense of confusion. Her list of intelligible words and holophrases is repeated in Table 6-4, with processes listed for each. (Process abbreviations used in Table 6-4 are given in Table 6-5.)

This list of processes as applied to each word was used to fill out Forms 5-1 (Example 6-11) and 5-2 (Example 6-12). The process analysis indicated that Ellen was attempting many final consonants, clusters, liquids, and vowels she could not (or did not choose to) produce. It confirmed that she frequently harmonized and reduplicated words. Alveolar harmony—in which all consonants in the word are pronounced as alveolars if there is one target alveolar—was especially common. This finding was somewhat surprising, given the relative rarity of alveolar harmony in English-speaking children (Stemberger & Stoel-Gammon, 1991) and Ellen's high functional load for [b]. Apparently, labials substituted for other consonants, but alveolars triggered harmony in her speech.

---

[4]In fact, stress is perhaps the only thing that is correct in her production of *happy birthday*!

Consonant Repertoire

Name: *Ellen*
Date: *10/12/94*
Source of sample: *speech in play*

Age: *2;3 (27 months)*
Examiner: *SLV*
Size of sample: *76 words*

Note: Phones circled are mastered (i.e., occurred at least ___3___ times in that position in any context, whether correct or not). Phones marked with an X did not occur in any context.

	Labial	Interdental	Alveolar	Palatal	Velar	Glottal	Other/notes:
Initial							
Stops	ⓑ		ⓓ		g¹		
	ⓟ		ⓣ		X		
Nasals	m²		n²				
Glides	ⓦ			j¹			
Fricatives	X	X	X	X			
	X	X	X	X		h¹	
Affricates				X, dʒ¹			
Liquids			X	X			
Medial							
Stops	ⓑ		ⓓ		X		
	p²		t²		k¹	ʔ²	
Nasals	ⓜ		ⓝ		X		
Glides	ⓦ			X			
Fricatives	v¹	X	X	X			
	φ¹,X	X	X	X		h¹	
Affricates				X, X			
Liquids			X	X			
Final							
Stops	X		d²		g¹		
	ⓟ		t²		k¹	X	
Nasals	X		X		X		
Fricatives	X	X	X	X			
	X	X	X	X			
Affricates				X, X			
Liquids			X				

Note: [r] not listed in final position as [ɚ] is a rhotic **vowel**. Medially, [r] should be counted only where it is consonantal (*around*), not vocalic (*bird*). φ is a voiceless bilabial (not labiodental) fricative.

EXAMPLE 6-6.
Consonant repertoire.

Vowel Repertoire

Name: *Ellen*   Age: *2;3 (27 months)*
Date: *10/12/94*   Examiner: *SLV*
Source of sample: *speech in play*   Size of sample: *76 words*

Note: Phones circled are mastered (i.e., occurred at least __3__ times in that position in any context, whether correct or not). Phones marked with an X did not occur in any context.

	Front	Central	Back
Simple vowels			
High			
Tense	ⓘ		ⓤ
Lax	ⓘ(ɪ)		(ʊ)
Mid			
Tense	(e)		(o)
Lax	(ɛ)		(ɔ)
Low		(ʌ) , (ə)	
	(æ)		(ɑ)
Diphthongs			
		X͟ɔɪ	
		(aɪ)	
		(aʊ)	
Rhotic vowels			
High			
Mid	X͟ɪ˞		X͟ʊ˞
	X͟ɛ˞		X͟ɔ˞
Low		X͟ʌ˞	
			X͟ɑ˞

EXAMPLE 6-7.
Vowel repertoire.

Word and Syllable Contrasts

Name: *Ellen*   Age: *2;3 (27 months)*
Date: *10/12/94*   Examiner: *SLV*
Source of sample: *speech in play*   Size of sample: *76 words*

Contrast	Minimal pair words	Minimal pair syllables	Near-minimal pairs
p - m - w - t - d - n	pʰi - mi - wi - ti - di - ni *please - me - three - cheese - Stephen - knee*		
p - w	pʰeɪ - weɪ *play, plate - swing*		
b - w	baɪ - waɪ *bite - grapes*		
p - w - t - d - j - h	wɑwɑ - dɑdɑ - hɑhɑ *water - daddy - hot* jɑ - hɑ *yeah - hot*	**pæpitɑ - bɑ**də *vs. those at left* *patty cake - panda*	**pɑp** *vs. those at left* *puppet*
p - b - d		**pʌpi - bʌ**də *puppet - kitty*	**dʌp, dʌt** *vs. those at left* *gum*
p - t			tʰu - pʰʊ *two - spoon*
i - other Vs	pʰi - peɪ *please - play, plate* wi - weɪ - waɪ *three - swing - grapes*	ʌki *vs. those at left and right* *yucky*	ti - tʰu - tʰɪ - tʰo *cheese - two - kiss - cold*
u - other Vs	bubu - baɪbaɪ *booboo - byebye*		tʰu - pʰʊ *two - spoon*

EXAMPLE 6-8.
Word and syllable contrasts.

Consonant Phoneme Substitutions (Relational Analysis)

Name: *Ellen*
Date: *10/12/94*
Source of sample: *speech in play*

Age: *2;3 (27 months)*
Examiner: *SLV*
Size of sample: *76 words*

Indicate substitutions beside (presumed) target phonemes (e.g., f^b). Mark phonemes that are not attempted with an X, and those that are omitted with Ø.

	Labial	Interdental	Alveolar	Palatal	Velar	Glottal	Other/notes:
Initial							
Stops	b^b		d^{d,b,g}		g^d		
	p^{p,b}		t^t		k^t		
Nasals	m^{m,b}		n^{n,d,b}				
Glides	w^w			j^j			
Fricatives	X	X	X	X			
	X	θ^d	X	ʃ^w		h^h	
Affricates				tʃ^t, dʒ^{dʒ}			
Liquids			l^w	r^w			
Medial							
Stops	b^{b,d,n}		d^{d,t,b}		X	ʔ^ʔ	
	p^{p,d}		t^{t,p,w}		k^{k,t,ɣ}		
Nasals	Xm		n^n		X		
Glides	Xw			X			
Fricatives	X	X	X	X			
	X	X	X	X		X	
Affricates				X, X			
Liquids			X	r^w			
Final							
Stops	X		d^d		X		
	p^p		t^{Ø,p}		k^{k,g}	X	
Nasals	m^{p,t}		n^{Ø,n,d}		ŋ^Ø		
Fricatives	X	X	z^Ø	X			
	X	X	s^{Ø,ʔ}	X			
Affricates				X, X			
Liquids			l^{Ø,l}				

Note: [r] not listed in final position as [ɚ] is a rhotic **vowel**. Medially, [r] should be counted only where it is consonantal (*around*), not vocalic (*bird*).

EXAMPLE 6-9.
Consonant phoneme substitutions (relational analysis).

Vowel Phoneme Substitutions (Relational Analysis)

Name: *Ellen*   Age: *2;3 (27 months)*
Date: *10/12/94*   Examiner: *SLV*
Source of sample: *speech in play*   Size of sample: *76 words*

Indicate substitutions beside (presumed) target phonemes (e.g., ʊᵊ). Mark with an X any phonemes not attempted.

	Front	Central	Back
Simple vowels			
High			
Tense	i^{i,ə,æ,a}		u^{u,ʊ,ə,æ}
Lax	ɪ^{ɪ,eɪ,ʌ,a}		ʊ^{u}
Mid			
Tense	e^{e,aɪ,ʌ}		o^{o,ʌ}
Lax	**X**		ɔ^{ɔ}
Low		ʌ,ə^{ʌ,ə,ɪ,a}	
	æ^{a,æ}		ɑ^{a}
Diphthongs			
			X
		ɑɪ^{aɪ,ɛ}	
		ɑʊ^{aʊ}	
Rhotic vowels			
High			
	X˞		**X**˞
Mid			
	X˞		ɔɚ^{ɔ,o,i}
Low		ɚ^{ʌ,a}	
			X˞

EXAMPLE 6-10.
Vowel phoneme substitutions (relational analysis).

TABLE 6-4.
"Ellen"'s Processes at 2 Years, 3 Months (Word by Word)

Production	Presumed Target Word	Processes Applied
[peɪ]	play, plate	CCR, FCD
[pʰi]	please	CCR, FCD
[baɪ]	bite	FCD
[bu]	blue	CCR
[weɪ]	swing	CCR, FCD, VDV
[waɪ]	grapes	CCR, FCD, GLD, VDV
[wi]	three	CCR, GLD
[tʰu]	school	CCR, FCD, FRNT
[tʰo]	cold	FCD, FRNT
[tʰɪʔ]	kiss	FRNT, FCD
[aʊ]	out	FCD
[i]	eat	FCD
[gʌgʰ], [gʌk]	duck	HRM/BCK, VOI
[dʌpʰ], [dʌt]	gum	FRNT, HRM, DNS
[bup]	poop	VOI
[pʌpi], [pap]	puppet	FCD, SRED, VDV
[woʊwoʊ], [wʌl]	roll	GLD, FCD, RDP
[wɔwə]	Laura	GLD, HRM?
[mɔmo], [mɔ]	more	VOW, RDP
[bubu], [pʰʊ]	spoon	FCD, RDP, VDV
[adədʌdʌ]	happybirthday	ICD, HRM, VDV
[wawa]	water	RDP, VOW
[ha], [haha]	hot	FCD, RDP
[dadə], [dædæ]	thankyou	HRM/RDP, VDV
[dadæ], [dada]	daddy	HRM/RDP, VDV
[nɛnɛnɛnɛnaɪ]	night-night	RDP, VDV, FCD
[ʌbʌbaɪbaɪ]	bye-bye	EP
[tuˠwi], [i]	cookie	FRNT, BCK, SRED, ICD
[ʌki]	yucky	ICD
[awaɪ]	allright	GLD, FCD
[ɔdɪd]	alldone	HRM, VDV
[bʌdə]	kitty	FRNT, VDV
[badə]	panda	CCR, VOI
[pæpita]	patty-cake	HRM, VDV

Note: Process name abbreviations are explained in Table 6-5.

TABLE 6-5.
Process Name Abbreviations

Abbreviation	Meaning
BCK	Backing
CCR	Consonant cluster reduction
COAL	Coalescence
DNS	Denasalization
EP	Epenthesis
FCD	Final consonant deletion
FRNT	Fronting
GLD	Gliding
GREP	Glottal replacement
HRM	Harmony
ICD	Initial consonant deletion
RDP	Reduplication
SRED	Syllable reduction
STOP	Stopping
VOW	Vowelization
VDV	Vowel deviation
VOI	Voicing-devoicing

Quite a few vowel deviations occurred, which was a cause for concern and for careful monitoring, as it is a common symptom of developmental verbal dyspraxia.

The frequency and nature of her harmony processes added one more piece to the puzzle of Ellen's unintelligibility and, in conjunction with Examples 6-1 and 6-2, highlighted the sources of her dysfunctionality: Ellen did produce a variety of consonant sounds but *not within the same word*. Her frequent use of reduplication and harmony, especially at the phrase level, significantly reduced the amount of contrast available within her system. Final consonants, which she used only 12% of the time in any case, were not able to add to the contrastive potential of her system because they harmonized with other consonants in the word more than 70% of the time. These patterns, plus her over-reliance on [b] and [a] in addition to her frequent vowel deviations, reduced the contrast in her speech significantly and thereby decreased her intelligibility.

The final piece of the puzzle came from a separate minianalysis of Ellen's unintelligible utterances (discussed in Chapter 4), which not only confirmed over-reliance on [b] and [a] and frequent reduplication and harmony but

also an additional word recipe. A [labial-V-alveolar-V] pattern (usually [bVdV]) had been noted in several unintelligible utterances. A review of her intelligible utterances revealed the same pattern in such words as *kitty* ([bʌdə]), *panda* ([badə]), *blow it* ([bʌdɪʔ]) and, somewhat less obviously, in *patty-cake* ([pæpita]). Such a word recipe, especially in combination with frequent reduplication and harmony and the extremely high functional load of [b] and [a], further reduced the interpretability of her speech. All of this information was summarized on Form 5-3, Phonological Constraint Summary, reproduced here as Example 6-13.

Phonotactic constraints that were noted included constraints against the use of final consonants, of consonant clusters, of two different syllables within the same word, and of two different consonants within the same word. The latter two constraints were present also at the phrase level. Phonetic constraints included wholesale constraints on fricatives, rhotic vowels, and velars. Position-specific phonetic constraints included alveolars in initial position, nasals in final position, and diphthongs and nonlow vowels in the first syllable of a word.

Although the occurrence of some of these patterns is not unusual in a child of Ellen's age, their frequency and combination were having a significant impact on her communicative effectiveness, and both mother and child were extremely frustrated. Therefore, remediation was appropriate (despite public school criteria). Deriving therapy goals for Ellen from Example 6-13 was easy. Where appropriate, process equivalences are given for constraint-based goals here. It is important to note, however, that use of a process perspective might cause the child merely to change processes (i.e., to use a different strategy for respecting the same constraint). In many cases, a change in process would not improve her intelligibility. For example, if she were to begin omit-

Process Summary

Name: *Ellen*   Age: *2;3 (27 months)*
Date: *10/12/94*   Examiner: *SLV*
Source of sample: *speech in play*   Size of sample: *76 words*

Process	Context/example/frequency
Syllable structure	
Syllable reduction	*2 (e.g.,* [pɑp] *for puppet)*
Final consonant deletion	*16 (e.g.,* [bɑɪ] *for bite)*
Initial consonant deletion	*2 (e.g.,* [ʌki] *for yucky)*
Cluster reduction	
Liquid clusters	*6 (e.g.,* [bu] *for blue)*
/s/ clusters	*2 (e.g.,* [tʰu] *for school)*
Other	*1 (* [bɑdə] *for panda)*
Coalescence	*1 (* [wɑɪ] *for grapes)*
Metathesis/migration	
Epenthesis	*1 (* [ʌbʌbɑɪbɑɪ] *for byebye)*
Harmony/assimilation	
Reduplication	*8 (e.g.,* [hɑhɑ] *for hot)*
Harmony (specify feature)	
Consonant	*5 alveolar, 1 labial, 1 velar, 1 glide (e.g.,* [dʌt] *for gum)*
Vowel	
Substitution	
Fronting	
Velar	*5 (e.g.,* [tʰo] *for cold)*
/ʃ/ → [s]	
/θ/ → [f]	
Backing	
Alveolar to velar	
Other	*1 (* [tuˠwi] *for cookie)*
Palatalization	
Depalatalization	
Stopping	
All fricatives	
/v ð ʒ tʃ dʒ/ only	
Gliding	
/l/	*1 (* [wɑwə] *for Laura)*
/r/	*3 (e.g.,* [wʌl] *for roll)*
Other	
Vowelization	
/l/	*4 (e.g.,* [wouwou] *for roll)*
/ɚ/	*2 (e.g.,* [wɑwɑ] *for water)*
Affrication	
Deaffrication	
Voicing	
Voice initial consonants	*2 (e.g.,* [bɑdə] *for panda)*
Devoice final consonants	
Other voice changes	*1 final C voiced (* [gʌgʰ] *for duck)*
Denasalization	*1 (* [dʌp, dʌt] *for gum)*
Vowel deviations	*10 (e.g.,* [weɪ] *for swing)*

EXAMPLE 6-11.
Process summary.

Process Analysis

Name: *Ellen*   Age: *2;3 (27 months)*
Date: *10/12/94*   Examiner: *SLV*
Source of sample: *speech in play*   Size of sample: *76 words*

Process type	Adult phoneme/ sound class	Process(es)	Frequency
Syllable structure	All consonants	Final consonant deletion	Frequent
		Consonant cluster reduction	Predominant (no CC occur)
Harmony/assimilation	Syllables	Reduplication	Frequent
	All consonants	Harmony	Frequent (especially alveolar)
Substitution	Velars	Fronting	Frequent
	Liquids	Gliding, vowelization	Predominant
	Vowels	Deviations (substitutions)	Occasional

EXAMPLE 6-12.
Process analysis.

Summary: Phonological Constraints

Name: *Ellen*   Age: *2;3 (27 months)*
Date: *10/12/94*   Examiner: *SLV*
Source of sample: *speech in play*   Size of sample: *76 words*

Use a check mark to indicate the occurrence of a constraint or a percentage to indicate its frequency of occurrence. Make appropriate specifications and comments. All sequences of Cs and Vs are assumed to be within the same word.

Note: C = consonant
        V = vowel
        # = word boundary
        σ = syllable (e.g., $\sigma\sigma$ = disyllabic word)
        $x_1 x_2$ = x_1 and x_2 are different from each other
        * = disallowed form

I. Phonotactic constraints

Constraint	Age equivalence	Restrictions/comments
Syllable shapes	Expected up to:	
*C# ✓	3:0	*Occur only 12% of the time; limited repertoire; often harmonized*
*#C	Not expected	
*#CC ✓	4:0	*No clusters*
*VCCV ✓		*No clusters*
*CC# ✓		*No clusters*
Word shapes		
*#$\sigma\sigma$#	2:0	*33%*
*#$\sigma\sigma\sigma$#		*Only 5% of words have more than two syllables (age-appropriate)*
Harmony/assimilation		
*$\sigma_1\sigma_2$ ✓	2:0	*Reduplication 38%; also applies at phrase level*
*C_1VC_2V ✓	2:0	*Harmony 31% in CVCV; see part II also; also applies at phrase level*
*C_1VC_2 ✓	2:0	*Harmony 71% in CVC; see part II also*
*CV_1CV_2	2:0	*No vowel harmony (except reduplication); see part II*

Note: Age equivalences are approximate. They are based on Grunwell (1985), Chin & Dinnsen (1992), Smit et al. (1990), and Stoel-Gammon (1987). "Not expected" indicates a constraint not found in normally developing children. A blank indicates that norms are not available on this measure.

Comments:

EXAMPLE 6-13.
Summary: phonological constraints.

II. Specific feature restrictions

Restricted feature	Restricted word position	Comments
C place of articulation: alveolar	#_____ (initial)	*Preference for labial-alveolar pattern, so alveolars less likely to occur in initial position*
Vowel place of articulation: nonlow	*First syllable*	*Preference for lower vowels to occur in first syllable*
Diphthongs	*First syllable*	*Preference for simpler vowels to occur in first syllable*
Fricatives	*All*	*Labiodental emerging in medial position*
Nasals	_____# (final)	
Velars	*All*	*Emerging in all positions*
Rhotic vowels	*All*	*Do not occur anywhere ever (age-appropriate)*

EXAMPLE 6-13.

ting consonants to avoid harmonizing them, understanding her would be even more difficult. The goals, then, were clear:

1. Increase use of words with two different consonants (i.e., reduce reduplication and harmony). For each objective within this goal, both CVCV words and CVC words should be attempted until they revealed clearly the pattern that was the easiest for Ellen to produce without harmony (as both appeared to have somewhat the same levels of harmony at that moment).
   a. Initially, words with a bilabial-V-alveolar(-V) pattern (beginning with bVd(V)) should be modeled. Variations on this word shape should be expanded with nasals, glides, and (if possible), fricatives. For example, mVnV (e.g., *money*), mVdV (e.g., *muddy*), fVʃV (e.g., *fishie*), would be appropriate CVCV word shapes to attempt. Once other types of bilabials were being produced within this pattern, words with initial [b] no longer should be targeted. Ellen appeared to seek and use these already, without any adult encouragement.
   b. Next, highly motivating, interesting words with other consonantal patterns should be modeled. Ellen produced one word ([tuˠwi] for *cookie*) with an alveolar-labial pattern. Thus, [alveolar]-V-[labial]-V might be a good place to begin this objective. Alternatively, she might be better able to produce patterns containing relatively new consonants, such as velars, which were just beginning to emerge in her speech, perhaps in a [velar]-V-[alveolar]-V pattern.
2. Increase the differentiation of words in phrases (i.e., reducing reduplication and harmony at the phrase level). Ellen might be best able to accomplish this with vowel-initial words (e.g., *out juice*) so that the tendency for consonant harmony would be short-circuited. Likely pivot words should be selected (i.e., words that are combined easily with a variety of nouns or verbs) and should be modeled in many combinations. For example, *ow* could be used in conjunction with various body parts in doll-play (e.g., putting plastic bandages on dolls), or *out* could be used with various food names while pretending to unpack grocery bags.
3. Increase production of final consonants (i.e., reducing final consonant deletion). Initially, this would be achieved most easily by using words that have harmonized consonants in the target (e.g., *pop*). Given that Ellen preferred a labial-alveolar consonant pattern, a likely second step would be to target labial-vowel-alveolar words (e.g., *pot*), as suggested in the foregoing harmony goal.
4. Increase accuracy of vowel production. Initially, target vowels should be low, back, or simple (her preferred features) and should occur in her preferred word shapes (CV, or CVCV with harmonized consonants). For words with two different vowels, the first words to target were those in which the first vowel is lower and simpler (i.e., not a diphthong) than the second. Then, the process could expand to other patterns.
5. Increase the production of emerging consonant features: nasals in final position, velars in any position for

which Ellen was stimulable, and fricatives in any position for which she was stimulable.

Many child phonologists suggest addressing one phonotactic goal (e.g., final consonants) and one phonetic goal (e.g., vowel or consonant features) at the same time, although this recommendation has not been verified through research. Some of Ellen's goals were not clearly assignable to one or another of those categories: For example, is reduction of harmony a phonotactic goal because it has to do with word shapes, or is it a phonetic goal because it relates to producing consonant features? The point on which to focus was simply addressing goals that differed from each other so that the child would not confuse them. Goals should be rotated (cycled, á la Hodson & Paden, 1991), as determining the specific goal for which a child's system may be ready is very difficult. If she or he gives evidence of being ready for a particular goal, that goal may be addressed as long as the child is making steady progress on it, or it may be cycled after a fixed period (typically, a month or two), at the clinician's discretion.

Achievement of the previously listed goals, especially the reduction of harmony and reduplication, required only 6 weeks of intensive therapy in this case. This therapy made a significant difference in Ellen's intelligibility. Given her good phonetic repertoires, additional therapy was not needed for another 18 months once these goals were achieved.

Time 2: Age 4 Years

Phonological Systems Over Time

Repeated independent analyses of a child's phonological system (or of portions thereof) reveal the functioning and growth of that system over time. In very young children or those with severe NFP, often it is possible to observe the emergence of the system itself. Sometimes, organization suddenly emerges from the random phonological variation that exists between a child's first word and perhaps the fiftieth word. In other cases, the system expands slowly but surely. Often, progress can be identified in areas that normally are not assessed using an "artick" test or even a process analysis. Sometimes, at later stages of development, one can discern in the child's system continuities that persist in different forms as the phonology expands. Examples of some of these types of phonological change were observed in Ellen as her intelligibility decreased once more in the preschool years. At 4 years, she returned for another phonological evaluation, and a comprehensive analysis of her phonological system again was carried out.

Reports in the child language literature (Lleó, 1990; Vihman, 1978, 1996) indicate that strategies children use in their early phonologies may reappear as they attempt more difficult forms later in development. Harmony is often cited in this respect. Clinically, many older children with NFP still use harmony in multisyllabic words, with pronunciations such as [əlumɪmə fɔɪjə] for *aluminum foil*, [ri:fɪdʒədʒɛʔɚ] for *refrigerator*, or [hɪpopɑmənɪs] for *hip-*

TABLE 6-6.
"Ellen"'s Speech Sample at 4 Years

[æwijĩ]	ambulance	[noʊgʰ]	nose
[bækɪt]	basket	[ɔf]	off
[beɪdi wuʔ]	bathing suit	[peɪdʒ]	page
[bifɔ]	before	[pweɪn]	plane
[bʊdeɪ]	birthday	[wɛd]	red
[bwæk]	black	[wɑk]	rock
[botʰ]	boats	[wæntə kwɔg]	Santa Claus
[kændəl]	candle	[kwudwaɪvʊ]	screwdriver
[tʃɛʊ]	chair	[hi]	see
[kɑʊbɔɪhæt]	cowboy hat	[wɛvɪn]	seven
[kweɪjɑŋg]	crayons	[ʃʊgʰ]	shoes
[ɛʊvwɪnt]	elephant	[wɪk], [wɪg], [ʃɪk]	six
[fwɛdʊ]	feather	[faɪd]	slide
[wil]	feel	[hmoʊk]	smoke
[fwɪk]	fish	[sneɪk]	snake
[ʃɑʊwʊ]	flower	[woʊpʰ]	soap
[βɔk]	fork	[pʰʊn]	spoon
[wʊ]	four	[pwɪŋkʊd]	sprinkles
[gwækɪgʰ]	glasses	[kwɛʊ]	square
[gwʌp]	glove	[tʰɑ]	star
[gwin]	green	[nɛfʊmi]	Stephanie
[gʌm]	gum	[divɪn]	Steven
[hænz]	hands	[twɪŋ]	string
[hæŋgʊ]	hanger	[fwɛdʊ]	sweater
[hævə]	hafta	[tɛwəbɪgɪn]	television
[hæg], [hæ]	have	[ðæ]	that
[hɑʊk]	horse	[ðə], [də], [ə]	the
[aɪkjub]	ice cubes	[den]	then
[ɪk]	if	[ðeɪ]	they
[ɪg]	is	[fwi]	three
[dʒɛfi]	Jeffy	[wʌm]	thumb
[dʒɛkɪkə]	Jessica	[tivi]	TV
[dʒɪmi]	Jimmy's	[tutʰbwʌtʃ]	toothbrush
[dʒɑn]	John	[twʌk]	truck
[dʒʌmpwoʊp]	jump rope	[ʌk]	us
[wif]	leaf	[wʊgə]	uses
[wi]	leave	[beɪk]	vase
[mækʰ]	mask	[watĩ]	washing
[mɪki mɑʊk]	Mickey Mouse	[waʔʃ]	watch
[mɑʊkʰ]	mouth	[jɛwə]	yellow
[mjugɪk bɑkʰ]	music box	[joʊjoʊ]	yoyo
[neɪkɪn]	Nathan	[dʒɪpʊ]	zipper
[nɑɪ]	nice		

popotamus. This pattern, or even a history of consonant harmony, in a child with NFP can be used clinically to help the child to master a difficult class of sounds by using harmonized stimuli first. This use of familiar patterns was, in fact, the strategy that was used for Ellen when she returned for therapy.

Ellen's Speech at 4 Years

Ellen's speech sample at age 4, taken from the *Assessment of Phonological Processes, Revised* (APP-R; Hodson, 1986) and supplemented by 41 spontaneous words, is given in Table 6-6. Although her phonological process score on the APP-R only rated a moderate severity level,[5] Ellen was extremely unintelligible. Clearly, more than process analysis was required. As usual, the phonological analysis began

with phonotactics, considering Ellen's syllable and word-shape repertoires and looking for evidence of reduplication or harmony. The results on Form 2-1 are shown as Example 6-14.

In contrast to her previous results, Ellen now had quite a few final consonants: Fully 45% of her syllables were closed (VC or CVC). Open syllables had decreased correspondingly. Use of consonant clusters now had improved as well; Ellen produced initial two-element clusters on 39% of her words and medial two-element clusters 8% of the time. The proportion of multisyllabic words had not changed very much; monosyllabic words still were the most frequent, with occasional bisyllabic words and rare longer words.

Form 2-2, reproduced here as Example 6-15, indicated that Ellen's use of harmony had decreased markedly in all contexts. From 38% reduplication and 31% consonant harmony in disyllables and 71% consonant harmony in

---

[5]Specific APP-R results are given later, when phonological processes are discussed.

Phonotactic Repertoire: Word and Syllable Shapes

Name: *Ellen*   Age: *4;0*
Date: *6/28/96*   Examiner: *SLV*
Source of sample: *APP-R + speech in play*   Size of sample: *91 words*

Note: C = consonant
       V = vowel
       # = word boundary
       Predominant: 61–100%
       Frequent: 41–60%
       Occasional: 16–40%
       Rare: 1–15%

	% or ✓	Frequency estimate: Circle appropriate word.				

Syllable types[a]: 141 total

	% or ✓					
Incomplete						
C alone	_0%_	~~Predominant~~	~~Frequent~~	~~Occasional~~	~~Rare~~	Absent
V, V?, ?V	_3%_	~~Predominant~~	~~Frequent~~	~~Occasional~~	Rare	~~Absent~~
Open						
CV, CV?	_52%_	~~Predominant~~	Frequent	~~Occasional~~	~~Rare~~	~~Absent~~
Closed						
VC, ?VC	_6%_	~~Predominant~~	~~Frequent~~	~~Occasional~~	Rare	~~Absent~~
CVC[b]	_39%_	~~Predominant~~	~~Frequent~~	Occasional	~~Rare~~	~~Absent~~

Clusters[c]: 91 total words

Initial						
#CC-	_39%_	~~Predominant~~	~~Frequent~~	Occasional	~~Rare~~	~~Absent~~
#CCC-	_0%_	~~Predominant~~	~~Frequent~~	~~Occasional~~	~~Rare~~	Absent
Final						
-CC#	_1%_	~~Predominant~~	~~Frequent~~	~~Occasional~~	Rare	~~Absent~~
-CCC#	_0%_	~~Predominant~~	~~Frequent~~	~~Occasional~~	~~Rare~~	Absent
Medial						
-CC-	_8%_	~~Predominant~~	~~Frequent~~	~~Occasional~~	Rare	~~Absent~~
-CCC-	_0%_	~~Predominant~~	~~Frequent~~	~~Occasional~~	~~Rare~~	Absent

Word shapes[c]: 91 total

# of syllables						
1	_59%_	~~Predominant~~	Frequent	~~Occasional~~	~~Rare~~	~~Absent~~
2	_31%_	~~Predominant~~	~~Frequent~~	Occasional	~~Rare~~	~~Absent~~
3	_9%_	~~Predominant~~	~~Frequent~~	~~Occasional~~	Rare	~~Absent~~
4+	_1%_	~~Predominant~~	~~Frequent~~	~~Occasional~~	Rare	~~Absent~~

[a]Out of all syllables.
[b]Includes CCVC, CVCC, etc.
[c]Out of all words.

Maximum # of syllables produced in any word: ___4___

Notes:

EXAMPLE 6-14.
Phonotactic repertoire: word and syllable shapes.

Phonotactic Repertoire: Reduplication and Harmony

Name: *Ellen*
Date: *6/28/96*
Source of sample: *APP-R + speech in play*

Age: *4;0*
Examiner: *SLV*
Size of sample: *91 words*

Note: C = consonant
V = vowel
Reduplication = same syllable repeated in word (*baba*, *deedee*, *gogo*, etc.)
Harmony = same C repeated (***goggie***, ***tootie***, etc.) or same V repeated (***daba***, ***boogoo***, etc.)
Predominant: 61–100%
Frequent: 41–60%
Occasional: 16–40%
Rare: 1–15%

	% or ✓	Frequency estimate: Circle appropriate word.				

Words of two syllables or more: *28 total*[a]

Reduplicated syllables	_4%_	~~Predominant~~	~~Frequent~~	~~Occasional~~	[Rare]	~~Absent~~
Harmonized vowels	_14%_	~~Predominant~~	~~Frequent~~	~~Occasional~~	[Rare]	~~Absent~~
Harmonized consonants	_3%_	~~Predominant~~	~~Frequent~~	~~Occasional~~	[Rare]	~~Absent~~

Monosyllabic CVC words: *55 total*[b]

Harmonized consonants	_2%_	~~Predominant~~	~~Frequent~~	~~Occasional~~	[Rare]	~~Absent~~

[a]Out of all **multisyllabic** words.
[b]Out of all **monosyllabic** CVC words.

Notes:

EXAMPLE 6-15.
Phonotactic repertoire: reduplication and harmony.

monosyllabic CVC words at 27 months, she had now reduced all of these patterns to the rare level. All occurrences of total consonant harmony were now velar (e.g., [gwækɪg] for *glasses*). Some examples of possible *partial* harmony also were noted but were not included in the quantitative data on the form. These examples were cases in which consonants agreed in labial place of articulation but not in manner of articulation. When Ellen said [wif] for *leaf* and [woʊp] for *soap*, for example, the initial and final consonants agreed in labiality.

Form 2-3, which forms the basis for Example 6-16, revealed no particular pattern of consonant-vowel interactions. Ellen's most frequent immediately prevocalic consonant,[6] [w], co-occurred with every possible vowel. Stops also co-occurred with vowels from all parts of the vowel triangle. Furthermore, some of the expected patterns of consonant-vowel dependencies seen in younger children were absent. For example, coarticulation would predict that velars would be preferred before high back vowels (Davis & MacNeilage, 1990). Yet, high front vowels were the most common vowels following velar stops. High back vowels were more common following labial and alveolar stops than following velars. Thus, as in the earlier session, no evidence of any consonant-vowel constraint was seen.

This form did reveal that Ellen's most common syllable was [wi], followed by [we] and [ki]. She used the high front vowels ([i, ɪ]) most often, followed by the mid front vowels ([e, ɛ]). Her favorite immediately prevocalic consonant appeared to be [w], probably owing in part to her frequent stop + glide consonant clusters. This most common consonant was followed at some distance by the alveolar and velar stops. Thus, her system had changed from her former preference for [ɑ, ʌ] and [d, b]. Her new preferences called for far more articulatory precision than did the old and probably reflected articulatory maturation.

Consideration of Ellen's stress patterns via Forms 2-4 and 2-5 (Examples 6-17 and 6-18) was next. She produced only one iambic word (*before*). This lack of iambs is in keeping with the language; English has far more trochaic than iambic words. The presence of one iambic word did provide some reassurance, but these and her previous stress analyses (in which she had no iambic forms at all) made it clear that this child had a strong preference for trochaic words.

The relational analysis made available in Form 2-5 (as Example 6-18) indicated only one potential syllable omission. A weak syllable may have been omitted from a SWS sequence ([ɛʊvwɪnt] for *elephant*, from which the medial weak [lə] syllable was either omitted or replaced with [ʊ]). This pattern is exactly what has been reported for young children who are developing normally (Gerken, 1991, 1994a,b; Gerken & McIntosh, 1993; Kehoe, 1995, 1996, 1997; Kehoe & Stoel-Gammon, 1997a,b; Schwartz & Goffman, 1995). Thus, although Ellen did not appear to be extremely adventurous with

respect to stress patterns, she did not seem to be in deep trouble either.

In summary, Ellen's phonotactic repertoire had improved markedly over the 21-month period between assessments. Both closed syllables and clusters now were fairly frequent. Even more important, reduplication and harmony had ceased to be a major factor in reducing her intelligibility. Furthermore, her labial-alveolar consonant word recipe and her low-high vowel word recipe were no longer in evidence. Therefore, some other level in the phonological system had to be responsible for her current extreme unintelligibility. The next place to investigate was her phonetic repertoire.

Ellen's consonant repertoire at 4 years (Example 6-19) included velar and voiceless stops mastered or emerging in all positions (both of which had been emerging in most positions before). She produced slightly more fricatives than she had at 2 years, 3 months, but not many. Only the following were mastered at age 4: [ð, ʃ, h, dʒ] in initial position, [v, f] in medial position, and none in final position. The majority of fricative tokens produced were [f] or [v] (a pattern that was even more marked if clusters were included). Clearly, labial was a preferred fricative place of articulation for Ellen. This preference was not a great surprise, given her previous profile. At 2 years, 3 months, she had shown a strong preference for labials in general. She had mastered more labial consonants than consonants from any other place of articulation in all positions. She had produced very few fricatives: [h, dʒ, v, ɸ] each once. However, of these four, two were labial.

Although Ellen now was producing far more final consonants, consonant features still remained the most restricted in final position. For instance, the fewest fricatives were found there. However, final position was the only place at which a liquid was noted ([l]). Generally, Ellen now seemed to prefer labials in medial position and alveolars in final position. Velars occurred more often in medial and final than in initial position.

Very little had changed with respect to Ellen's vowel repertoire, as shown in Example 6-20 (Form 3-2). Her vowel repertoire had been age-appropriate before but had been fairly static in the meantime. Rhotic vowels remained completely absent. One more diphthong—[ɔɪ]—was found to be emerging.

As shown in Example 6-21, most of Ellen's initial consonant clusters consisted of stop or [f] + [w]. Some consonants ([g, k, f]) occurred more often in combination with [w] than as initial singletons. In addition to these obstruent + glide clusters, two fricative + nasal clusters (*sn-* and *hm-*) each occurred once. The latter was produced in a manner not totally unlike the voiceless nasals sometimes produced by children with cleft palate (and produced as contrastive phonemes in such languages as Burmese). However, the [h] component was more distinct (i.e., temporally separate) than is the voicelessness of a voiceless nasal, and the *hm-* therefore was considered to be a cluster. Only one final cluster (*-nz*) occurred (once) in the sample (Example 6-22).

Thus, Ellen's phonetic repertoire at 4 years represented some progress with respect to velar stops, voiceless stops, fricatives, and [ɔɪ], but changes were not very sig-

---

[6]Recall that, in the case of a cluster, the consonant that comes immediately before the vowel is the one used for this form. The purpose of the form is to identify potential cases of consonant-vowel dependencies or assimilations, and these most likely will happen in strictly adjacent sequences.

Phonotactic Repertoire: Consonant-Vowel Dependencies

Name: *Ellen*
Date: *6/28/96*
Source of sample: *APP-R + speech in play*

Age: *4;0*
Examiner: *SLV*
Size of sample: *91 words*

Indicate (✓ or %) combinations that do occur: *percentages given*

C type	V type						
	High front (i, ɪ)	Mid front (e, ɛ)	Low front (æ)	Mid central (ə, ʌ)	High back (u, ʊ)	Mid back (o, ɔ)	Low back (ɑ)
Stops							
Labial (b, p)	2	2	1		2	2	1
Alveolar (d, t)	3	2		2	2		1
Velar (k, g)	6		1			1	2
Nasals							
Labial (m)	2		1			1	2
Alveolar (n)		2				1	1
Glides							
Labial (w)	9	6	2	4	4	2	3
Palatal (j)	1	1			2	2	1
Liquids							
Alveolar (l)							
Palatal (r)							
Fricatives							
Labial (f, v)	3			1	2	2	1
Interdental (θ, ð)		1	1	1			
Alveolar (s, z)							
Palatal (ʃ, ʒ)	1				1		1
Affricates (tʃ, dʒ)	2	2		1			1
Glottals (h, ʔ)	1		5				1
Other							

Note: Numbers add up to more than 100% due to rounding (e.g., 0.7 is rounded up to 1).

EXAMPLE 6-16.
Phonotactic repertoire: consonant-vowel dependencies.

Stress Patterns: Independent Analysis

Name: *Ellen*   Age: *4;0*
Date: *6/28/96*   Examiner: *SLV*
Source of sample: *APP-R + speech in play*   Size of sample: *91 words*

For each stress pattern, list words that the child produces with that pattern, whether correct or not. Examples in parentheses are intended to facilitate the speech-language pathologist's recognition of varied stress patterns only. The child should not necessarily be required to attempt these particular words.

Note: S = strong syllable
         W = weak syllable

Target stress pattern	Examples from child
SW (e.g., mónkey)	[bǽkɪt] *basket*, [búdeɪ] *birthday*, [kǽndəl] *candle*, [ɛúvwɪnt] *elephant*
WS (e.g., giráffe)	[bifɔ́] *before*
ŚWS̀ (e.g., télephòne)	[ǽwijì̃] *ambulance*, [beídi wù?] *bathing suit*, [míki mɑùk] *Mickey Mouse*
SWW/ŚS̀W (e.g., hámburger)	[dʒékɪkə] *Jessica*, [kwúdwɑìvʊ] *screwdriver*
WSW (e.g., spaghétti)	
WWS/S̀WŚ (e.g., kàngaróo)	
ŚWS̀W (e.g., cáterpìllar)	[téwəbìgɪn] *television*
WŚWS̀/S̀ŚWW (e.g., rhìnóceros)	
WWSW/S̀WŚW (e.g., dìsappóinted)	
Other 4-syllable words (SWWS, WSWS, WSSW)	
5+ syllables	

EXAMPLE 6-17.
Stress patterns: independent analysis.

Stress Patterns: Relational Analysis

Name: *Ellen*   Age: *4;0*
Date: *6/28/96*   Examiner: *SLV*
Source of sample: *APP-R + speech in play*   Size of sample: *91 words*

For each stress pattern, list words that the child attempts with that pattern, indicating whether the word is produced correctly, with weak syllable(s) omitted, with strong syllables omitted, or with other outputs (e.g., coalescence of two syllables into one). Examples in parentheses are intended to facilitate the speech-language pathologist's recognition of varied stress patterns only. The child should not necessarily be required to attempt these particular words.

Note: S = strong syllable
       W = weak syllable

Target stress pattern	Correct	W omitted	S omitted	Other
SW (e.g., mónkey)	[bǽkɪt] *basket, etc.*			
WS (e.g., giráffe)	[bifɔ́] *before*			
ŚWS̀ (e.g., télephòne)	[ǽwɪjǐ] *ambulance, etc.*			
SWW/ŚS̀W (e.g., hámburger)	[dʒékɪkə] *Jessica, etc.*	[ɛúvwɪnt] *elephant*		
WSW (e.g., spaghétti)				
WWS/S̀WŚ (e.g., kàngaróo)				
ŚWS̀W (e.g., cáterpìllar)	[téwəbìgɪn] *television*			
WŚWS̀/S̀ŚWW (e.g., rhìnóceros)				
WWSW/S̀WŚW (e.g., dìsappóinted)				
Other 4-syllable words (SWWS, WSWS, WSSW)				
5+ syllables				

Note: See Example 6-17 for further examples.

EXAMPLE 6-18.
Stress patterns: relational analysis.

Consonant Repertoire

Name: *Ellen*   Age: *4;0*
Date: *6/28/96*   Examiner: *SLV*
Source of sample: *APP-R + speech in play*   Size of sample: *91 words*

Note: Phones circled are mastered (i.e., occurred at least ___3___ times in that position in any context, whether correct or not). Phones marked with an X did not occur in any context.

	Labial	Interdental	Alveolar	Palatal	Velar	Glottal	Other/notes:
Initial							
Stops	ⓑ		ⓓ		g^1		
	p^2		ⓣ		k^2		
Nasals	ⓜ		ⓝ				
Glides	ⓦ			j^2			
Fricatives	X̶, β^1	ð̄	X	X			
	f^1	X̶	s^1	ʃ̄		ⓗ	
Affricates				tʃ^1, d̄ʒ			
Liquids			X̶	X			
Medial							
Stops	b^2		ⓓ		ⓖ		
	p^1		t^1		ⓚ	X	
Nasals	ⓜ		X̶		X̶		
Glides	ⓦ			ⓙ			
Fricatives	ⓥ	X̶	X	X			
	ⓕ	X̶	X	X		h^1	
Affricates				X̶, X̶ʒ			
Liquids			X	X			
Final							
Stops	b^1		ⓓ		ⓖ		
	ⓟ		ⓣ		ⓚ	ʔ^1	
Nasals	m^2		ⓝ		ŋ^1		
Fricatives	X̶	X̶	X	X̶			
	f^1	X̶	X	ʃ^1			
Affricates				tʃ^1, dʒ^1			
Liquids			l^2				

Note: [r] not listed in final position as [ɚ] is a rhotic **vowel**. Medially, [r] should be counted only where it is consonantal (*around*), not vocalic (*bird*).

EXAMPLE 6-19.
Consonant repertoire.

Vowel Repertoire

Name: *Ellen*   Age: *4;0*
Date: *6/28/96*   Examiner: *SLV*
Source of sample: *APP-R + speech in play*   Size of sample: *91 words*

Note: Phones circled are mastered (i.e., occurred at least __3__ times in any context, whether correct or not). Phones marked with an X did not occur in any context.

	Front	Central	Back
Simple vowels			
High			
Tense	ⓘ		ⓤ
Lax	Ⓘ		ⓤ
Mid			
Tense	ⓔ		ⓞ
Lax	ⓔ		ⓞ
Low		Ⓐ ,ⓐ	
	ⓐ		ⓐ

Diphthongs

$\mathrm{ɔɪ}^1$

ⓐɪ

ⓐʊ

Rhotic vowels
High

❌˞   ❌˞

Mid

❌˞   ❌˞

Low

❌

❌˞

EXAMPLE 6-20.
Vowel repertoire.

Initial Consonant Clusters

Name: *Ellen*   Age: *4;0*
Date: *6/28/96*   Examiner: *SLV*
Source of sample: *APP-R + speech in play*   Size of sample: *91 words*

Indicate with a check mark, specific number or specific percentage those clusters that occur in the child's speech. (If the child produces an "illegal" cluster that does not normally occur in English, list it under "other.")

Two-element clusters

Obstruent + liquid

pr___	pl-___	pj-___		br-___	bl-___	bj-___	
tr-___		tj-___	tw-_2_	dr-___		dj-___	dw-___
kr-___	kl-___	kj-___	kw-_3_	gr-___	gl-___	gj-___	gw-_3_
						mj-___	
						nj-___	

fr-___	fl-___	fj-___
θr-___	θj-___	θw-___
	sl-___	sj-___	sw-___
ʃr-___		

hj-___
vj-___
lj-___

[s] + obstruent

sp-___   st-___   sk-___   sm-___   sn-_1_

Other: *pw-: 2, bw-: 1, fw-: 3, hm-: 1*

Note: The glide [j] occurs far more often in initial clusters in British than in American English.

Three-element clusters: *None*

spr-___	spl-___	spj-__	
str-___		stj-___	
skr-___	skl-___	skj-___	skw-___

Other:

EXAMPLE 6-21.
Initial consonant clusters.

Final Consonant Clusters

Name: *Ellen*　　　　　　　　　　　　Age: *4;0*
Date: *6/28/96*　　　　　　　　　　　Examiner: *SLV*
Source of sample: *APP-R + speech in play*　　Size of sample: *91 words*

Indicate with check mark, specific number, or specific percentage those clusters that occur in the child's speech. (If the child produces an "illegal" cluster that does not normally occur in English, list it as "other.")

Two-element clusters

Nasals

-mp___　-mt___　　　　　-md___　-mf___　-mθ___　　　　　　　　　-mz___

　　　-nt___　　　　　　-nd___　　　　-nθ___　-ns___　-ntʃ___　-ndʒ___　-nz *1*

　　　　　　-ŋk___　　　-ŋd___　　　　　　　　　　　　　　　　　-ŋz___

Stops

　　　-pt___　　　　　　-bd___　　　　-pθ___　-ps___　　　　　　-bz___

　　　　　　　　　　　　　　　　　-tθ___　-ts___　　　　　　-dz___

　　　-kt___　　　　　　-gd___　　　　　　　　-ks___　　　　　　-gz___

Fricatives

　　　-ft___　　　　　　-vd___　　　　-fθ___　-fs___　　　　　　-vz___

　　　-θt___　　　　　　-ðd___　　　　　　　　-θs___　　　　　　-ðz___

-sp___　-st___　-sk___　-zd___　-zm___

　　　-ʃt___　　　　　　-ʒd___

　　　-tʃt___　　　　　-dʒd___

Liquids

-lp___　-lt___　-lk___　　-ld___　-lm___　-ln___

　　　　　　　　　　-lv___　-lf___　-lθ___　-ls___　-ltʃ___　-ldʒ___　-lz___

Other:

Three-element clusters

-mps___

　　　-nts___　　　　　　　　　　　　-nst___　-ntʃt___　-ndʒd___

　　　　　　-ŋks___　　　　　　　　　　-ŋst___

-lps___　-lts___　-lks___　　　　　　　　-lst___　-ltʃt___　-ldʒd___

Other:

EXAMPLE 6-22.
Final consonant clusters.

TABLE 6-7.
"Ellen"'s APP-R Results at 4 Years

Process	Percentage of Occurrence
Consonant cluster reduction	34
Omission and stopping of stridents	60
Gliding and omission of liquids	
/l/	73
/r/	100
Process average	27
Phonological deviancy score	37
Severity interval rating	Moderate

APP-R = *Assessment of Phonological Processes, Revised* (Hodson, 1986).

nificant in these areas. Clusters, a new phonotactic possibility for Ellen, were restricted mostly to obstruent + glide. However, producing [w] as the second element in a cluster appeared to facilitate Ellen's production of certain obstruents ([g, k, f]). This contextual facilitation was important to note for goal planning: Introducing new consonants in clusters rather than (or as well as) in singletons could be a useful strategy for her.

At 4 years, Ellen continued to demonstrate many word and syllable contrasts in her vocabulary, as she had done at 2 years, 3 months. Example 6-23 includes a variety of consonant and vowel minimal pair words and syllables and a few near-minimal pairs.

A comparison of Example 6-9 (Ellen's consonant substitutions at 2 years, 3 months) to Example 6-24 (her consonant substitutions at 4 years) revealed the most visually striking finding: that she was attempting a much wider variety of consonants in all positions at the later age. Very few consonants were not even attempted at 4 years, and those failed to appear mostly in final position (her least favorite position). Also, those that were not attempted at age 4 were mostly less common consonants, such as /ʒ/ and /dʒ/ in all positions, /ʔ/ in medial position, /ð/ in final position, and the like.

In particular, at 2 years, 3 months, Ellen was not attempting many fricatives or affricates, especially in medial position. Those she did attempt were substituted in initial position and omitted in final position (and, in the latter case, perhaps should not even be counted as attempted, as there is no evidence that Ellen was trying to produce a consonant in that position). Although she did produce four fricative sounds and one affricate (see the foregoing Phonetic Repertoire) at 2 years, 3 months, only the [h] and the affricate were produced in a context in which those were the actual target sounds (i.e., correctly). All of the other fricatives she had produced at the younger age were produced in unidentifiable words and so had not been included in Example 6-9. At 4 years, she attempted most fricatives and affricates and got some of them right, especially in initial or medial position.

Another visually striking aspect of Example 6-24 was the number of substitutes listed for various fricatives. Inconsistency was especially noticeable for /f/ and /s/ in initial position, /f/ in medial position, and /z/ in final position.

Unusual substitutions were noted for singleton /f/; it was replaced by *fw-* in initial position and *vw-* in medial position.

Another unusual aspect of Ellen's phonology at 4 years as revealed by this example was her substitutions of velars for fricatives, especially in medial and final position. Voiceless velar [k] replaced voiceless fricatives /f, θ, s/, and voiced velar [g] replaced voiced fricatives /v, z, ʒ/. Thus, Ellen was taking care to preserve the voicing quality of the fricative while changing its place and manner of articulation. This substitution pattern was loud and clear in cases in which the alveolar fricatives [s, z] represented morphological markers (plural, possessive) as well as in other instances. Sometimes, Ellen even aspirated the final velar, apparently to emphasize her morphological marking (as in [gwækɪgʰ] for *glasses* and [ʃugʰ] for *shoes*). Thus, the velar stops carried a heavy morphological functional load as well as a heavy phonological functional load. These hard-working velars represented a shift; previously, [b] had carried the heaviest consonantal functional load.

Though *fw-* and *vw-* sometimes substituted for singleton /f/, coalescence of clusters also was noted. In particular, [ʃ] substituted for *fl-* and [f] for *sl-* in initial position ([ʃɑʊwʊ] for *flower*, [faɪd] for *slide*). Also, [n] substituted for *st-* ([nɛfʊmi] for *Stephanie*).

In short, Ellen's adult phoneme-child production mapping was a mess, especially with respect to fricatives. Although now she was attempting most fricatives in most positions, her phonological bravery had not had a positive effect on the functionality of her phonological system. Certain fricative phonemes, especially [f, s], exhibited great inconsistency in their substitution patterns. Often the substitute was very unlike those chosen by other young children, including those with NFP. Replacement phones included velar stops and glides (especially [w]). Clusters substituted for singletons and vice versa. How could the listener possibly guess the intended fricative?

In contrast to her consonant phoneme substitutions, Ellen's vowel phoneme substitutions had decreased markedly at 4 years in comparison with age 2 years, 3 months, as shown in Example 6-25. Very few vowels were substituted at all. Other than the rhotics, those that were substituted (/u/, /ə/) were right more often than wrong. For example, /u/ was produced correctly (i.e., [u] produced for a target /u/) five times and was substituted with [i] only once. The only possible sources of confusion for the listener were the vowelization of the rhotics and the substitution of [ʊ] for the rhotics and occasionally for /ə/.

One could be overwhelmed easily by Example 6-26, Process Summary. Ellen demonstrated many varied and unusual processes, including coalescence, epenthesis, fronting, backing, stopping, and gliding. Many of these processes applied to unusual sound classes (e.g., gliding and backing of *fricatives*). The same was true of the APP-R (Hodson, 1986) results, given in Table 6-7. In addition to the processes listed on the front summary page of the test was a notation that Ellen exhibited quite frequent stopping, backing, and vowelization of liquids.

The next form, Example 6-27 (from Form 5-2), with its emphasis on the sound classes affected by various

Word and Syllable Contrasts

Name: *Ellen*
Date: *6/28/96*
Source of sample: *APP-R + speech in play*

Age: *4;0*
Examiner: *SLV*
Size of sample: *91 words*

Contrast	Minimal pair words	Minimal pair syllables	Near-minimal pairs
k - g	ɪk - ɪg *if - is*		
f - l	wɪf - wɪl *leaf - feel*		
h - w	hi - wi *see - leave*		
h - m	haʊk - maʊk *horse - mouth, mouse*		
w - fw-	wɪk - fwɪk *six - fish*		
k - v		neɪkɪn - wɛvɪn *Nathan - seven*	
b - n - kw-		**beɪ**diwuʔ - **neɪ**kɪn - **kweɪ**jaŋ *bathing suit - Nathan - crayons*	
b - sn-			beɪk - sneɪk *vase - snake*
æ - aʊ	mæk - maʊk *mask - mouth, mouse*		
i - ʊ	wi - wʊ *leave - four*		
ɪ - ʌ	ɪk - ʌk *if - us*		
æ - ə - eɪ	ðæ - ðə - ðeɪ *that - the - they*		

EXAMPLE 6-23.
Word and syllable contrasts.

Consonant Phoneme Substitutions (Relational Analysis)

Name: *Ellen*   Age: *4;0*
Date: *6/28/96*   Examiner: *SLV*
Source of sample: *APP-R + speech in play*   Size of sample: *91 words*

Indicate substitutions beside (presumed) target phonemes (e.g., f^b). Mark phonemes that are not attempted with an X, and those that are omitted with ∅.

	Labial	Interdental	Alveolar	Palatal	Velar	Glottal	Other/notes:
Initial							
Stops	b^b		d^d		g^g		
	p^p		t^t		k^k		
Nasals	m^m		n^n				
Glides	w^w			j^{j,w}			
Fricatives	v^b	ð^{ð,d}	z^{dʒ}	X			
	f^{f,w,fw,β}	θ^f	s^{w,s,f,ʃ,h}	ʃ^ʃ		h^h	
Affricates				tʃ^{tʃ}, dʒ^{dʒ}			
Liquids			l^w	r^w			
Medial							
Stops	b^{b,w}		d^d		g^g	X	
	p^p		t^t		k^k		
Nasals	m^m		n^n		ŋ^ŋ		
Glides	w^w		j^j				
Fricatives	v^{v,b}	ð^d	z^g	ʒ^g			
	f^{f,v,vw}	θ^f	s^{w,k}	ʃ^t		h^h	
Affricates				tʃ^{tʃ}, dʒ			
Liquids			l^{w,l,j}	r^w			
Final							
Stops	b^b		d^d		g	X	
	p^p		t^t		k^k		
Nasals	m^m		n^n		ŋ		
Fricatives	v^{p,g}	X	z^{g,z,d}	X			
	f^{f,k}	θ^k	s^k	X			
Affricates				tʃ, dʒ^{dʒ}			
Liquids			l^l				

Note: [r] not listed in final position as [ɚ] is a rhotic **vowel**. Medially, [r] should be counted only where it is consonantal (*around*), not vocalic (*bird*). Substitutes are listed in order of frequency of occurrence. *The first consonant in an initial cluster (e.g., [f] from fw-) and the last consonant in a final cluster (e.g., [z] from -nz) are counted here. Coalescence of clusters is noted: [ʃ] substitutes for fl- and [f] for sl- in initial position; also [n] and [d] substitute for -st in final position.*

EXAMPLE 6-24.
Consonant phoneme substitutions (relational analysis).

Vowel Phoneme Substitutions (Relational Analysis)

Name: *Ellen*   Age: *4;0*
Date: *6/28/96*   Examiner: *SLV*
Source of sample: *APP-R + speech in play*   Size of sample: *91 words*

Indicate substitutions beside (presumed) target phonemes (e.g., $\upsilon^{\eth}$). Mark with an X any phoneme not attempted.

	Front	Central	Back
Simple vowels			
High			
Tense	i^i		$u^{u,i}$
Lax	$\textsci^\textsci$		**X**
Mid			
Tense	e^e		o^o
Lax	ε^ε		$\textopeno^\textopeno$
Low		$\Lambda^\Lambda, \vartheta^{\vartheta,\textsci,\upsilon}$	
	$\ae^{\ae}$		α^a
Diphthongs			
			$\textopeno\textsci^{\textopeno\textsci}$
			$\alpha\textsci^{\alpha\textsci}$
			$\alpha\upsilon^{\alpha\upsilon}$
Rhotic vowels			
High			
	$\cancel{\textsci}^{\upsilon}$		$\cancel{\textsci}^{\upsilon}$
Mid			
	$\varepsilon\textrhookschwa^{\varepsilon\upsilon}$		$\textopeno\textrhookschwa^{\textopeno,\upsilon}$
Low		$\textrhookschwa^{\upsilon}$	
		$\cancel{\textrhookschwa}^{\upsilon}$	

EXAMPLE 6-25.
Vowel phoneme substitutions (relational analysis).

Process Summary

Name: *Ellen*
Date: *6/28/96*
Source of sample: *APP-R + speech in play*

Age: *4;0*
Examiner: *SLV*
Size of sample: *91 words*

Process	Context/example/frequency
Syllable structure	
Syllable reduction	*Rare (e.g., [ɛʊvwɪnt] for elephant)*
Final consonant deletion	*Occasional (e.g. [naɪ] for nice)*
Initial consonant deletion	
Cluster reduction	
Liquid clusters	
/s/ clusters	*Frequent (e.g., [pʰun] for spoon; [mæk] for mask)*
Other	*Occasional ([æ̃wiji̇̃] for ambulance)*
Coalescence	*Occasional ([ʃaʊwʊ] for flower; [faɪd] for slide)*
Metathesis/migration	
Epenthesis	*Occasional w/f,v ([fwɪk] for fish; [ɛʊvwɪnt] for elephant)*
Harmony/assimilation	
Reduplication	
Harmony (specify feature)	
Consonant	*Velar total ([dʒɛkɪkə] for Jessica); labial partial ([nɛfʊmi] for Stephanie)*
Vowel	
Substitution	
Fronting	
Velar	
Fricative	*f/s ([fwɛdʊ] for sweater); w/j ([wʊgə] for uses [juzəz])*
/θ/ → [f]	*Occasional (e.g., [fwi] for three)*
/ʃ/ → [s]	
Backing	
Alveolar to velar	*s, z to k,g (e.g., [haʊk] for horse; [noʊgʰ] for nose)*
Other	*g/v ([hæg] for have); h/s ([hi] for see)*
Palatalization	*Rare (e.g., [ʃɪk] for six)*
Depalatalization	*Rare (e.g., [wati̇̃] for washing)*
Other place changes	*Glottal replacement (e.g., [wuʔ] for suit)*
Stopping	
All fricatives	*See "Backing," above (Note: preserves voicing)*
/v ð ʒ tʃ dʒ/ only	*v, ð (e.g., [gwʌp] for glove; [bʊdeɪ] for birthday)*
Gliding	
/l, r/	*100% ([wif] for leaf; [gwin] for green)*
Other	
Vowelization	
/l/	*Rare (e.g., [ɛʊvwɪnt] for elephant)*
/ɚ/	*100% (e.g., [tʃɛʊ] for chair)*
Affrication	*Rare (e.g., [tutʰbwʌtʃ] for toothbrush)*
Deaffrication	
Voicing	
Voice initial consonants	
Devoice final consonants	
Denasalization	
Vowel deviations	*Rare (e.g. [æ̃wiji̇̃] for ambulance)*

EXAMPLE 6-26.
Process summary.

Process Analysis

Name: *Ellen*
Date: *6/28/96*
Source of sample: *APP-R + speech in play*

Age: *4;0*
Examiner: *SLV*
Size of sample: *91 words*

Process type	Adult phoneme/sound class	Process(es)	Frequency
Syllable structure	Initial /s/ clusters	Cluster reduction	Frequent
	Fricative clusters	Coalescence	Occasional
	Final fricatives	Final consonant deletion	Occasional
	Labial fricative singletons	Epenthesis of [w]	Occasional
Harmony/assimilation	Fricatives	Velar harmony	Occasional
	Fricatives, liquids (rarely glides)	Partial labial harmony	Occasional
Substitution	Alveolar fricatives	Fronting	Occasional
	/θ/	Fronting	Occasional
	Alveolar fricatives	1. Backing (velar; rarely glottal) 2. Stopping (velar)	Frequent (Note: voicing preserved)
	Other fricatives	Stopping	Occasional (Note: voicing not preserved)
	Fricatives	Gliding	Frequent
	Liquids	1. Gliding 2. Vowelization	Predominant (vowelization rare for /l/)

EXAMPLE 6-27.
Process analysis.

TABLE 6-8.
"Ellen"'s Fricative Substitutions

Pattern	Example	Word Position	Fricative Affected	Percentage of Occurrence
Sometimes correct		Initial	ð, dʒ, ʃ, tʃ	
		Medial	f, v	
		Final	f, tʃ, dʒ	
Velar replacement	[ʃug] for *shoes*	Medial	θ	20
			s	40
			z	100
			ʒ	100
		Final	f	50
			v	25
			s	44
			z	50
Omission	[twiŋ] for *string*	Initial	ð	10
			s (in s + stop clusters)	100
		Medial	θ (before another C)	20
			s (in s + stop clusters)	100
		Final	v	25
			s (in stop + s clusters; in singletons)	100
				11
			z (third-person singular)	50
Stopping to closest place of articulation	[beɪs] for *vase*	Initial	v	100
			ð	20
		Medial	v	25
			ð	100
			θ	33
			ʃ	100
		Final	v	25
			s (singletons)	11
Gliding	[wæntə] for *Santa*	Initial	θ	33
			s (singletons)	67
Epenthesis of [w]	[fwɪk] for *fish*	Initial	f	71
		Medial	f	50
Palatalization	[ʃɑʊwʊ] for *flower*	Initial	f	29
			s (singletons)	17
Affrication	[brʌtʃ] for *brush*	Initial	z	100
		Final	ʃ	100
Nasal emission		Initial	s (s + nasal clusters)	100
Cluster coalescence	[fɑɪd] for *slide*	Initial	s (s + liquid/glide clusters)	100
Glottalization	[hi] for *see*	Initial	s (singleton)	20

processes, provided some illumination. Those processes that applied occasionally or more frequently were listed here. A glance down the Sound Class column clearly revealed that 11 of the 12 listed processes applied to fricatives. One of the fricative processes applied to liquids as well (partial labial harmony, in which two consonants agreed in place but not manner of voicing), and another pair of processes applied to liquids only. Thus, the vast majority of the phonological patterns having a significant impact on Ellen's speech related specifically to fricatives, with liquids as the runner-up category. Furthermore, the main processes that applied to liquids (gliding and vowelization of liquids) were not unusual at all. As most listeners are accustomed to young children who say [wɛd] for *red* or [bɑdʊ] for *bottle*, that these processes caused Ellen's extreme unintelligibility seemed unlikely.

Yet, what is to be done with a child with 11 processes affecting fricatives? Which should be addressed first, and how? Mostly, these processes were sufficiently unusual to convince this clinician that process therapy kits likely would not address them. Where was one to start, then? An attempt was made to figure out Ellen's fricative system by listing all the substitution patterns that were noted. The result is given as Table 6-8; this list, too, was overwhelming and confusing.

The Phonological Constraint Summary (Example 6-28), plus a consideration of all that had been learned to this point about Ellen, helped to clarify the situation. The first page of Example 6-28 was almost blank. Ellen had very few residual phonotactic constraints, with the exception of a restriction against /s/-initial consonant clusters. The feature constraints page was far more enlightening. From this form, the crux of the problem was clear: Ellen had a constraint against fricatives (and one against liquids). Therefore, she simply was doing everything possible to avoid or simplify fricatives. All the many listed processes shared that one goal in her system.

The solution was not necessarily simple but was evident: Help Ellen to learn to produce fricatives. Several factors, mostly gleaned from her consonant repertoire (indepen-

Summary: Phonological Constraints

Name: *Ellen* Age: *4;0*
Date: *6/28/96* Examiner: *SLV*
Source of sample: *APP-R + speech in play* Size of sample: *91 words*

Use a check mark to indicate the occurrence of a constraint or a percentage to indicate its frequency of occurrence. All sequences of Cs and Vs are assumed to be within the same word.

Note: C = consonant
V = vowel
# = word boundary
σ = syllable (e.g., σσ = disyllabic word)
x_1x_2 = x_1 and x_2 are different from each other
* = disallowed form

I. Phonotactic constraints

Constraint	Age equivalence	Restrictions/comments
Syllable shapes	Expected up to:	
*C#_____	3;0_____	
*#C_____	Not expected	
*#CC __✓__	4;0_____	*sC(C) (Strategy: Omit [s]).
*VCCV __✓__	_____	*sC(C) (Strategy: Omit [s]).
*CC# __✓__	_____	*sC(C) (Strategy: Omit [s]).
Word shapes		
*#σσ#_____	2;0_____	
*#σσσ#_____	_____	
Harmony/assimilation		
*$σ_1σ_2$_____	2;0_____	*Very rare reduplication*
*C_1VC_2V_____	2;0_____	*Rare harmony*
*C_1VC_2_____	2;0_____	*Very rare harmony*
*CV_1CV_2_____	2;0_____	*Rare harmony*

Note: Age equivalences are approximate. They are based on Grunwell (1985), Chin & Dinnsen (1992), Smit et al. (1990), and Stoel-Gammon (1987). "Not expected" indicates a constraint not found in normally developing children. A blank indicates that norms are not available on this measure.

Comments:

EXAMPLE 6-28.
Summary: phonological constraints.

II. Specific feature restrictions

Restricted feature	Restricted word position	Comments
Manner of articulation: *Liquids* r, ɚ l	 *All* *#__, V__V (initial, medial)*	*Strategies used:* *Gliding* *Vowelization*
Manner of articulation: *Fricatives*	*All*	*Strategies used:* *Backing + stopping (to velar)* *Gliding (to* [w]*)* *Cluster reduction* *Cluster coalescence* *Final consonant deletion* *Epenthesis* *Velar harmony* *Partial labial harmony* *Fronting*

EXAMPLE 6-28.
Continued.

dent analysis) and from her consonant phoneme substitutions (relational analysis), suggested possible directions
for therapy:

- She was able to produce certain fricatives in certain specific
contexts. Labial fricatives were especially good, although
they did tend to trigger epenthesis of [w]. Other fricatives that she produced sometimes (regardless of the target) included [ʃ] in initial and final position, [ð] in initial
position, [v] in medial position, and [s] in initial position
(only once).
- Sometimes, the affricates [tʃ, dʒ] were also produced in
initial and final positions.
- Labial fricatives appeared to be facilitated by the glide
[w], perhaps because of its labiality. This glide was a
consistent substitute for the liquid [r] and sometimes
also was epenthesized after [f, v].
- Ellen had a history of consonant harmony and of a
labial-alveolar place of articulation word recipe.
- Ellen's strategies for dealing with her constraint against
liquids were common ones and likely would not have as
great an impact on her intelligibility as did her complex
and unusual strategies for dealing with her constraint
against fricatives.
- The phonotactic level of Ellen's phonological system
now appeared to be functioning fairly well. She was able
to produce (nonfricative) final consonants, multisyllabic
words, and two-element (non-[s]) initial consonant clusters with little problem.
- Ellen's strategy for dealing with initial s- clusters was to
delete the /s/.
- Velars appeared to be playing both a morphological and
a phonological role in final position, marking plural
and third-person singular morphemes. (Sometimes,
possessive was implied but was not marked morphologically.) Thus, velars had an extremely heavy functional
load, especially in final position.

The last of these factors served as an important warn-
ing: If therapy appeared to be threatening Ellen's ability
to mark morphology, she might become resistant and
make little progress. Plural and third-person singular
markers should not be targets of therapy until she had
more phonological knowledge of and phonetic control
over the alveolar sibilants ([s, z]) in other contexts. Only
then should her strategy of using velars to mark these morphological meanings be addressed. The penultimate factor also suggested something to avoid: If initial s- clusters
were used, Ellen would simply delete the /s/. Thus, targeting these clusters would likely not be helpful.

The fact that Ellen's liquid strategies most likely were
far less damaging to her intelligibility than were her fricative strategies suggested that this (liquid) sound class
could be ignored for the moment. Phonotactic goals also
were unnecessary.

Knowledge of Ellen's history was very helpful. It seemed
likely that her learning of fricatives could be facilitated if
they were presented in words with either consonant harmony or a labial-alveolar consonant pattern. The fricatives
she already produced sometimes could be used as a start-

ing point. The clusters fr-, vr-, and fl- might be helpful, as
Ellen likely would produce them as fw- and vw-, and the latter were clusters for which she had shown a preference
(even over singleton labial fricatives). Also, the affricates
might be helpful, as they contain a fricative element.

For these reasons, the following sequence of goals was
proposed:

1. Ellen will produce continuance (frication) in both initial and final positions of appropriate words.
A relevant first suggestion would be for the clinician to
target words with initial and final fricatives, preferably
the same fricative (or voicing cognates) in both positions. This redundancy would take advantage of Ellen's
preference for words with consonant harmony. As she
never had shown any consonant-vowel interactions, any
vowel could be used in the medial position without fear
of contaminating her production of the fricative.
Unfortunately, the English language is not rich in
appropriate preschool-level words, especially if plurals
and possessives must be avoided. Some are available,
however. Age-appropriate harmonized words that could
be modeled in play therapy and semiformal therapy sessions[7] included five, sis, sass, sauce, zoos, shush, and the
like. In some cases, either the initial or the final consonant might be an affricate instead. In other cases, the
initial fricative actually might be an fr-, a vr-, or an fl-
cluster (e.g., fluff).
The goal was to produce continuance in both positions, regardless of the accuracy of the place of articulation or even of voicing. If the word were fish, for
example, and Ellen produced [vwɪf], this production
would be considered to have met the objective.
Fricatives that sometimes were produced correctly were
targeted first, in their best word positions. Descriptive
imagery (e.g., "windy sounds") seemed to facilitate production of continuance in this bright child. Speech
discrimination-type tasks also appeared to be helpful
despite the fact that quite likely Ellen did have adultlike underlying representations. These tasks seemed to
heighten her conscious awareness of the fricative class.
2. Ellen will produce two different fricatives (or a fricative
and an affricate) in the same word.
Initially words were chosen in which the final fricative
was one that Ellen was able (and willing) to produce in
this position some of the time (e.g., [f, tʃ, dʒ]). These
choices took advantage of her reduced tendency to
replace these final fricatives, at least, with velar stops.
a. The initial objective within this goal was to produce
any two different fricatives in the word, regardless of

---

[7]Although the purpose of this book is not to discuss specific therapy
techniques, this author's strong preference is to render each therapy
session as naturalistic and meaningful for the child as possible. As the
goal is for the child to use the new phonological patterns in real contexts, reason mandates that they be taught in realistic contexts whenever feasible. However, this is not meant to imply that language
therapy will remediate phonological disorders. Specific patterns must
be targeted in specific ways. Making phonology therapy both effective
and fun is hard work for the clinician, but the trick is to make the
child think that the session is play.

their accuracy. As long as the places of articulation of the two fricatives differed, the production was counted as meeting the goal.

b. The second objective was to produce a front fricative in initial position and a farther back fricative in final position, regardless of the actual accuracy of production. This second pattern mimicked Ellen's old labial-alveolar pattern. Thus, labial fricatives were targeted (with or without /r/ or /l/) in words ending with a (nonmorphological) alveolar fricative. Words targeted for this pattern, then, included *face, fast, floss, fuzz, fizz, freeze, froze(n)* and so on. This pattern was eventually extended to labial-palatal words (*fresh, fish,* etc.). As long as the first fricative was farther front than the second, the production was considered to be a success.

c. Once this pattern had been mastered, words with the reverse pattern were targeted (back to front). Hand cues (and those tactile cues that Ellen would tolerate) to place of articulation became helpful at this stage.

If Ellen had been unable to achieve the latter portion of the second goal, an alternative approach would have been to target place of articulation and to ignore manner temporarily. In other words, Ellen would have continued to attempt words with two different target fricatives. However, the goal would have been her production of the appropriate *places* of articulation, even if she stopped or glided one or both of the fricatives. For example, [jud] would have been accepted for *shoes*, as [j] is palatal (as is [ʃ]), and [d] is alveolar (as is [z]). Hand cues or tactile cues to place of articulation again could have been used. Once this goal had been achieved, objective 2c could have been tackled again.

As it turned out, sidetracking to 2c was unnecessary. By the time she had completed 2b, Ellen was producing most fricatives distinctly. Not all fricatives were produced accurately (e.g., [s] was distorted in some positions), but each was produced in a manner that easily differentiated them. At this time, very little work was required to convince Ellen to switch her plural and possessive morphemes from velar stops to alveolar fricatives. Her intelligibility improved dramatically as these changes came about, of course.

CONCLUSION

Followed over time, the case of Ellen illustrates the usefulness of considering all aspects of a child's phonology in planning treatment. The patterns that increase or decrease the functionality of a child's phonological system at a certain time must be identified to set efficient, achievable therapy goals. One level of phonology (e.g., phonotactics) may be critical at one point and unimportant at another. Knowledge of previous patterns can help the clinician to plan facilitative intervention strategies.

Determining that which is not possible in the system as it is (i.e., the constraints) is far more useful than only identifying the strategies that the child is using to avoid violating those constraints (i.e., rules or processes). Once the constraints have been identified, goal setting is relatively easy: Remove the constraint. If the child is using harmony, reduplication, and deletion because she has a constraint against producing two different consonants in a word or phrase, she must learn to do so. Addressing deletion alone merely will increase her use of harmony and vice versa, if the constraint has not been removed. If the child is using stopping, fronting, backing, gliding, deletion, and coalescence to avoid fricatives, she must learn to produce fricatives. Addressing any one of the strategy patterns in isolation merely will increase the use of the others until the child learns to produce fricatives.

Ellen is a particularly bright child with a devoted speech-language pathologist mother; therefore, she may have benefited more quickly from therapy than do other children with similar patterns. However, the intervention issues raised by her phonological system, as unusual as it was at both points, are common to many other children. The approaches and solutions applied to her case have broad applicability.

It was only by analyzing Ellen's system thoroughly and from a primarily independent analysis perspective that these goals could be derived. As the analysis delved deeper, the workings—and roadblocks—of her phonological system were revealed. This understanding of the nonfunctional aspects of her phonology facilitated direct, efficient intervention.

Imagine the intriguing phonological puzzles and superefficient intervention approaches that await speech-language pathologists as more and more children with NFP are assessed in this way!

APPENDIX A

Commercial Assessment Material

ARTICULATION TESTS

Some examples of articulation tests include (in alphabetic order) Arizona Articulation Proficiency Scale (AAPS; Fudala & Reynolds, 1991); Goldman-Fristoe Test of Articulation (GFTA; Goldman & Fristoe, 1986); Photo Articulation Test, Second Edition (PAT; Pendergast et al., 1984); and Test of Minimal Articulation Competence (T-MAC; Secord, 1981).

These tests typically include a set of pictures (which may or may not be demographically, geographically, or culturally appropriate) for the child to label. The consonant sounds of English, which are distributed throughout the target words, are to be scored as correct or incorrect. Often, a set of /s/, /r/, and /l/ blends are also assessed. Vowels are included less commonly in the analyses. In all cases, the sounds are to be produced in words; in some cases, these words are embedded within specific sentences that children are to produce or repeat.

The data collected usually take the form of a list of sound substitutions by word position (initial, medial, final). The children's actual phonetic repertoires (i.e., the set of sounds that they actually produce in each position, whether correct or not) rarely are determined in this type of assessment. The purported sampling of all sounds in all positions may be compromised by the words selected (e.g., medial [n] assessed in the consonant cluster *window* on the GFTA instead of in a truly medial position, as in the word *winnow*). Phonological and morphological production variables may also be confounded in morphologically complex words (such as plurals). For example, test words with stops typically are simpler (fewer syllables, fewer consonant clusters, etc.) than are those intended to assess later developing sounds, such as fricatives (Shriberg & Kwiatkowski, 1980). As a result, children may be even more likely to err in their productions of later-developing sounds.

Some articulation tests yield a severity rating or score. In a few cases, the severity of individual errors is weighted according to the frequency of occurrence of the target sounds in written or spoken English. Sometimes, word position is considered as a factor in developmental appropriateness but, more commonly, productions of the same sound in initial, medial, and final position are considered together. At times, procedures are suggested for rank-ordering errors to determine treatment priorities.

Most of these tests do an adequate job of sampling the consonant repertoire of English. However, they differ greatly with respect to their inclusion of a variety of syllable and word shapes. Table A-1 lists several articulation tests, indicating each one's status with respect to several phonotactic sampling factors, including the number of words (Number of Words), the number of initial consonant clusters (#CC) and final consonant clusters (CC#), the number of multisyllabic words (Number of Multisyllabic Words), and the range of word lengths in syllables (Number of Syllables) sampled. In addition, whether the test includes stimuli that are longer than single words (>Single Words) is indicated for each test.

PROCESS TESTS

A few examples of process tests are The ALPHA Test of Phonology–Revised (ALPHA-R; Lowe, 1995); Assessment of Phonological Processes, Revised (APP-R; Hodson, 1986); Bankson-Bernthal Test of Phonology (BBTOP; Bankson & Bernthal, 1990); Khan-Lewis Phonological Analysis (KLPA [to be used in conjunction with the GFTA]; Khan & Lewis, 1986); and Phonological Process Analysis (PPA; Weiner, 1979).

In selecting a process test, one must choose between those that facilitate the identification of only a small number of processes, either for theory's sake or convenience's sake (e.g., BBTOP), and those that offer a far more comprehensive but atheoretical view of the child's process use (e.g., APP-R). The former are simpler to use, and typically they do identify the most common processes; however, they can be frustrating or confusing when some of the patterns identified cannot be credited. The latter take more time and can be overwhelming but allow the clinician to identify most processes that occur ever in children's phonologies.

Other factors include the number of words elicited, the manner of elicitation (e.g., objects rather than pictures are suggested for the APP-R; delayed imitation verbal stimuli are provided for the PPA and the ALPHA-R), sentence versus word elicitation, and the nature of the target words. For example, the ALPHA-R elicits entire sentences (in imitation) and, because of this approach, many more of the target words are verbs or adjectives (*sad*, *hide*, *sick*, *cry*, etc.). However, many of the words also are more advanced lexical items (e.g., *thorn*, *ditch*, *leash*) that would be unfamiliar to younger children.

TABLE A-1.
Phonotactic Factors on Articulation Tests

Test Name	Number of Words	#CC	CC#	Number of Multisyllabic Words	Number of Syllables (Range)	>Single Words
AAPS	50	6	6	13	1–4	Yes
GFTA	44	11	3	24	1–3	Yes
PAT	79	9	14	32	1–3	No
SPAT-D	53	20	7	25	1–3	No
T-MAC	107	27	5	39	1–4	No

AAPS = Arizona Articulation Proficiency Scale (Fudala & Reynolds, 1991); GFTA = Goldman-Fristoe Test of Articulation (Goldman & Fristoe, 1986); PAT = Photo Articulation Test (Pendergast et al., 1984); SPAT-D = Structured Photographic Articulation Test featuring Dudsberry (Kresheck & Werner, 1989); T-MAC = Test of Minimal Articulation Competence (Secord, 1981).

TABLE A-2.
Phonotactic Factors on Process Tests

Test Name	Number of Words	#CC	CC#	Number of Multisyllabic Words	Number of Syllables (Range)	>Single Words
ALPHA-R	50	10	3	7	1–3	Yes
APP-R	50	20	6	19	1–4	No
BBTOP	80	10	3	22	1–3	No
KLPA	43	11	3	24	1–3	Yes
PPA	136	31	14	50	1–4	Yes

ALPHA-R = The ALPHA Test of Phonology–Revised (Lowe, 1995); APP-R = The Assessment of Phonological Processes, Revised (Hodson, 1986); BBTOP = Bankson-Bernthal Test of Phonology (Bankson & Bernthal, 1990); KLPA = Khan-Lewis Phonological Analysis (used in conjunction with the GFTA; Khan & Lewis, 1986); PPA = Phonological Process Analysis (Weiner, 1979).

Table A-2 rates various process tests by using the same criteria used for rating articulation tests in Table A-1. Table A-3 lists the phonotactic (whole-word) processes sampled by the various process tests. Figure A-1 is a *Consumer Reports*–style chart with ratings on various measures for the articulation and process tests discussed here and in the previous section.

COMPREHENSIVE PHONOLOGICAL ANALYSIS PROCEDURES

More comprehensive analysis manuals include *Procedures for the Phonological Analysis of Children's Language* (Ingram, 1981); *Phonological Assessment of Child Speech* (PACS; Grunwell, 1985); and *Natural Process Analysis* (NPA; Shriberg & Kwiatkowski, 1980).

In-depth analysis procedures spring from two major theoretical sources: natural process theory and generative phonology. Process analyses typically are relational; generative analyses include both independent and relational analyses. Components of generative analyses, and some process analyses, may include phonotactic repertoire (syllable or word shapes produced), phonetic repertoire (sounds that the child produces, correctly or not), phonemic repertoire (sounds used contrastively), distinctive features (use of contrastive places and manners of production), substitutions, substitution patterns (processes/rules), selection-avoidance patterns, and homonymy. The size of the sample recommended ranges from 124 to 1,288 words. Such sample sizes in themselves represent a major disadvantage of such procedures for many clinicians; the time required to obtain and analyze such a sample often is prohibitive.

In-depth analysis of natural processes is exemplified by NPA (Shriberg & Kwiatkowski, 1980), which facilitates the identification of eight "natural" processes from a child's spontaneous speech sample. *Natural* processes are considered to be those that involve simplification of adult forms and that occur frequently in the languages of the world. Among a set of processes that might be considered natural by this definition, Shriberg and Kwiatkowski (1980) further selected those that are seen frequently in young (preschool and school-age) children with delayed speech and can be scored reliably by speech-language pathologists. These selection procedures reduced the set of processes to eight. Only those eight processes are identi-

TABLE A-3.
Phonotactic Processes on Process Tests

Process	ALPHA-R	BBTOP	KLPA	PPA	APP-R
Initial consonant deletion	X*				X
Final consonant deletion	X*	X	X	X	X
Syllable deletion	X	X	X	X	X
CC reduction	X	X	X	X	X
Voicing	X		X	X	X
Assimilation		X	X	X	X
Glottal replacement		X			X
Coalescence					X
Migration			X		
Epenthesis					X
Metathesis					X
Reduplication					X

ALPHA-R = The ALPHA Test of Phonology–Revised (Lowe, 1995); BBTOP = Bankson-Bernthal Test of Phonology (Bankson, & Bernthal, 1990); PPA = Phonological Process Analysis (Weiner, 1979); KLPA = Khan-Lewis Phonological Analysis (used in conjunction with the GFTA; Khan & Lewis, 1986); APP-R = The Assessment of Phonological Processes, Revised (Hodson, 1986).
*Initial and final consonant deletion are combined into one "consonant deletion" process on the ALPHA-R.

fied, and they must be assessed in the order given. The processes described are very specific (e.g., velar fronting and palatal fronting are considered to be separate patterns; they are not lumped together vaguely as "fronting"). The phonotactic processes included are final consonant deletion, unstressed syllable deletion, progressive (left-to-right) and regressive (right-to-left) assimilation, and initial and final cluster reduction. The clinician is encouraged to consider additional factors that may be influencing the child's process use, such as the word shape (CV versus VC versus VCV, etc.), the position of the sound in the word (for segmental processes), the length of the word, the stress pattern of the word, and the syntactic, pragmatic, and semantic functions of the word.

The advantages of this procedure are twofold. First, it can be learned relatively easily, as a small number of very specific processes are scored in the same order for every child. Second, the procedure does facilitate the identification of the most common processes that speech-language pathologists encounter in phonologically delayed children. One major disadvantage of NPA is that the manual provides little help to the clinician facing additional phonological

	Number of words	Vowels tested?	Phonetic variety	Independent phonetic repertoire	Relational phonetic repertoire	>Single words	Number and variety of consonant clusters	Multisyllables	Number of phonotactic processes	Number of segmental processes	Norms provided?
Traditional articulation tests											
SPAT-D	53	N	⇓	N	Y	N	▽	▽			Y
T-MAC	107	Y	▽	Y	Y	N	▽	▽			Y
PAT	79	Y	▽	N	Y	N	▽	▽			Y
AAPS	50	Y	▽	N	Y	Y	⇓	⇓			Y
GFTA	44	N	⇓	N	Y	Y	⇓	▽			N
Process tests											
ALPHA-R	50	N	▽	N	Y	Y	⇓	⇓	▽	▽	Y
BBTOP	80	N	♥	N	Y	N	⇓	▽	▽	▽	Y
PPA	136	N	♥	Y	N	Y	♥	♥	▽	▽	N
KL	43	N	⇓	Y	N	Y	⇓	▽	▽	▽	Y
APP-R	40	Y	♥	Y	N	N	▽	▽	♥	♥	Y

FIGURE A-1.
Strengths and weaknesses of articulation and process tests. (Y = yes; N = no; ♥ = very good; ▽ = average; ⇓ = below average; SPAT-D = Structured Photographic Articulation Test featuring Dudsberry [Kresheck & Werner, 1989]; T-MAC = Test of Minimal Articulation Competence [Secord, 1981]; PAT = Photo Articulation Test [Pendergast et al., 1984]; AAPS = Arizona Articulation Proficiency Scale [Fudala & Reynolds, 1991]; GFTA = Goldman-Fristoe Test of Articulation [Goldman & Fristoe, 1986]; ALPHA-R = The ALPHA Test of Phonology–Revised [Lowe, 1995]; BBTOP = Bankson-Bernthal Test of Phonology [Bankson & Bernthal, 1990]; PPA = Phonological Process Analysis [Weiner, 1979]; KLPA = Khan-Lewis Phonological Analysis [used in conjunction with the GFTA; Khan & Lewis, 1986]; APP-R = The Assessment of Phonological Processes, Revised [Hodson, 1986].)

patterns that do not fit within those assessed, such as nasalization or frication of stops, initial consonant deletion, movement processes (metathesis and migration), and the like. In addition, the order specification may diminish inappropriately the number of errors credited to a specific process (e.g., both the "fronting" and the "liquid simplification" processes are coded before the "assimilation" process, so that such errors as [dɔdi] for *doggie* and [jɛjo] for *yellow* will not be credited to consonant harmony). If the instructions are followed, the clinician is not given the liberty to examine other productions to determine the processes to which such errors should be attributed.

Broader phonological analyses are provided by *Procedures for the Phonological Analysis of Children's Language* (Ingram, 1981) and by *Phonological Assessment of Child Speech* (Grunwell, 1985). These manuals lead the clinician through several aspects of in-depth phonological analysis, including those that have been described in the later chapters of this book. The procedures are exhaustive. The level of detail that they provide is quite appropriate for establishing baselines in particular areas of phonology before the start of remediation. However, the amount of time required to complete the entire procedures typically is prohibitive for an initial evaluation or for setting general goals. An excellent way to learn the procedures one section at a time is to use any subsection repeatedly for establishing baselines for several children or for assessing the same child's progress over time. Eventually, one is comfortable with all these types of analyses. If time allows, a thorough evaluation of this sort of every child's phonology should be undertaken before therapy is initiated.

APPENDIX B

Examples of Stress Patterns

SW

cookie
bottle
monkey
apple
window
wagon
chicken
zipper
scissors
yellow
vacuum
matches
shovel
pencil
carrot
orange
Santa
Christmas
basket
candle
crayons
feather
after
early
every

WS

Many verbs (forget, pretend, etc.)
giraffe
balloon
around
canteen
maroon
TV
macaque
kaboom
baboon
raccoon
canoe
cassette
shampoo
Japan
motel
Vermont
above
before
behind
between

ŚWÒ/SWW

telephone
elephant
cowboy hat

music box
envelope
valentine
gasoline
hospital
ambulance
astronaut
pillowcase
tablecloth
magazine (dialectal)
photograph
ambulance
dinosaur
evergreen
library
medicine
calendar
cucumber
temperature
vegetable
alphabet
hamburger

ÒWŚ/WWS

violin
understand
chimpanzee
kangaroo
tangerine
engineer

WŚWÒ/WŚWW/ÒŚWW

thermometer
aquarium
speedometer
extinguisher
binoculars
librarian
material
harmonica
rhinoceros
asparagus
experiment
historian
biologist
comedian
custodian
peripheral
astronomy
cartographer
capitulate

WSẂ/WẂS̀

announcement
assignment
vacation
papaya
pajamas
potato
banana
tomato
spaghetti
umbrella
prescription
computer
eraser
tuxedo
mechanic
musician
detective
director
reporter
cartoonist
designer
bewildered
embarrassed
excited
endangered
terrific
burrito
fajitas
lasagna

ẂWS̀W

television
watercolors
secretary
radiator
elevator
caterpillar
supermarket
cauliflower
calculator
motorcycle
dictionary
peanut butter
alligator
watermelon

S̀WẂW/WWSW

macaroni
ravioli
perspiration
readjustment
disappointed
horizontal
satisfactory

S̀WẂWW

cafeteria
auditorium
hippopotamus
condominium

ẂS̀

Any "spondee" (e.g., hot dog, blackboard, baseball)

WẂWS̀W

refrigerator
contaminated
electrifying

APPENDIX C

International Phonetic Alphabet Symbols Used in This Book*

---

*For further information about International Phonetic Alphabet (IPA) symbols, see GK Pullum, WA Ladusaw. *Phonetic Symbol Guide.* Chicago: University of Chicago Press, 1986; and M Duckworth, G Allen, W Hardcastle, M Ball. Extensions to the International Phonetic Alphabet for the transcription of atypical speech. *Clinical Linguistics and Phonetics* 1990;4:273–280.

CONSONANTS

Orthographic Symbol	IPA Symbol	Key Word
ng	ŋ	ri**ng**
y	j	**y**es
th	θ	**th**in
th	ð	**th**en
sh	ʃ	ru**sh**
g	ʒ	rou**g**e
ch	tʃ	**ch**ur**ch**
j, g	dʒ	**j**u**dg**e
(Glottal stop)	ʔ	uh-oh
(Voiced velar fricative)	ɣ	a**g**ua (Spanish)
(Voiceless velar fricative)	x	A**ch**! (German)

VOWELS

Orthographic Symbol	IPA Symbol	Key Word
ee, ea, ie, y	i	b**ea**d
i	ɪ	b**i**d
a, ay, ai, a_e, ey	e	b**ay**
e	ɛ	b**e**d
a	æ	b**a**d
u, oo, u_e, ew	u	br**ew**
oo	ʊ	b**oo**k
o, oa, o_e, ough, ow	o	b**oa**t
aw, au, augh, ough	ɔ	b**ough**t
o	ɑ	b**o**p
u	ʌ	b**u**t
any vowel	ə	**a**bout
ir, ur, er	ɚ	b**ir**d, bett**er**
ow, ough, au	aʊ	b**ough**
i, i_e, y, uy	ɑɪ	b**uy**
oi, oy	ɔɪ	b**oy**

DIACRITICS

Acoustic Feature	IPA Diacritic Symbol	Example Word
Prolongation	ː	no: (no)
Aspiration	ʰ	tʰɪp (tip)
Flapped alveolar (d or t)	ɾ	bʌɾɚ (butter)
Nasalized	~	mæ̃n (man)
Voiceless	̥	bæd̥ (bad)
Unreleased	̚	tɪp̚ (tip)
Near-simultaneous articulation	‿	tʃ‿iz (cheese)
Dentalized	̪	s̪il (seal)

References

Akmajian A, Demers R, Harnish R. *Linguistics: An Introduction to Language and Communication.* Cambridge, MA: MIT Press, 1984.

Allen GD, Hawkins S. Phonological rhythm: Definition and development. In Yeni-Komshian GH, Kavanagh JF, Ferguson CA (eds). *Child Phonology.* New York: Academic Press, 1980, 227–256.

Archangeli D. Optimality theory: An introduction to linguistics in the 1990s. In Archangeli D, Langendoen DT (eds). *Optimality Theory: An Overview.* Malden, MA: Blackwell, 1997, 1–32.

Archangeli D, Langendoen DT. *Optimality Theory: An Overview.* Malden, MA: Blackwell, 1997.

Archibald J. The acquisition of stress. In Archibald J (ed). *Phonological Acquisition and Phonological Theory.* Hillsdale, NJ: Lawrence Erlbaum Associates, 1995, 81–109.

Baltaxe CAM. Use of contrastive stress in normal, aphasic, and autistic children. *Journal of Speech and Hearing Research* 1984;27:97–105.

Bankson NW, Bernthal JE. *Bankson-Bernthal Test of Phonology.* Chicago: Riverside Publishing, 1990.

Barlow JA. Variability and phonological knowledge. In Powell TW (ed). *Pathologies of Speech and Language: Contributions of Clinical Phonetics and Linguistics.* New Orleans: International Clinical Phonetics and Linguistics Association, 1996, 125–133.

Barton D. Phonemic perception in children. In Yeni-Komshian G, Kavanaugh J, Ferguson C (eds). *Child Phonology.* New York: Academic Press, 1980, 97–116.

Beckman J. Shona height harmony: Markedness and positional identity. In Beckman JN, Dickey LW, Urbanczyk S (eds). *University of Massachusetts Occasional Papers 18: Papers in Optimality Theory.* Amherst, MA: Graduate Linguistic Student Association, University of Massachusetts at Amherst, 1995, 53–75.

Beckman J. Syllable asymmetries in feature distribution: Evidence from Tamil. Presented to Rum J. Clam II, University of Massachusetts at Amherst, May 21, 1996.

Bedore LM, Leonard LB, Gandour J. The substitution of a click for sibilants: A case study. *Clinical Linguistics and Phonetics* 1994;8:283–293.

Beers M. Acquisition of Dutch phonological contrasts within the framework of Feature Geometry theory. In Bernhardt B, Gilbert J, Ingram D (eds). *Proceedings of the UBC International Conference on Phonological Acquisition.* Somerville, MA: Cascadilla Press, 1996, 28–41.

Bell A. Syllabic consonants. In Greenberg JH (ed). *Universals of Human Language.* Stanford, CA: Stanford University Press, 1978, 153–201.

Berman RA. Natural phonological processes at the one-word stage. *Lingua* 1977;43:1–21.

Bernhardt B. Application of nonlinear phonological theory to intervention with six phonologically disordered children. Ph.D. Thesis, University of British Columbia, 1990.

Bernhardt B. Developmental implications of nonlinear phonological theory. *Clinical Linguistics and Phonetics* 1992a;6:259–281.

Bernhardt B. The application of nonlinear phonological theory to intervention with one phonologically disordered child. *Clinical Linguistics and Phonetics* 1992b;6:283–316.

Bernhardt B, Stemberger JP. *Handbook of Phonological Development: From the Perspective of Constraint-Based Nonlinear Phonology.* San Diego: Academic Press, 1998.

Bernhardt BH, Stoel-Gammon C. Grounded phonology: Application to the analysis of disordered speech. In Ball MJ, Kent RD (eds). *The New Phonologies: Developments in Clinical Linguistics.* San Diego: Singular, 1997, 163–210.

Besnier N. An autosegmental approach to metathesis in Rotuman. *Lingua* 1987;73:201–223.

Bleile KM. *Child Phonology: A Book of Exercises for Students.* San Diego: Singular, 1991.

Bleile KM. *Manual of Articulation and Phonological Disorders.* San Diego: Singular, 1995.

Blevins J. The syllable in phonological theory. In Goldsmith JA (ed). *The Handbook of Phonological Theory.* Cambridge, MA: Blackwell, 1995, 206–244.

Borden G, Harris K. *Speech Science Primer: Physiology, Acoustics, and Perception of Speech.* Baltimore: Williams & Wilkins, 1994.

de Boysson-Bardies B, Vihman MM. Adaptation to language: Evidence from babbling and first words in four languages. *Language* 1991;67:297–319.

de Boysson-Bardies B, Bacri N, Sagart L, Poizat M. Timing in late babbling. *Journal of Child Language* 1981;8:525–539.

de Boysson-Bardies B, Sagart L, Halle P, Durand C. Acoustic investigations of cross-linguistic variability in babbling. In Lindblom B, Zetterstrom R (eds). *Precursors of Early Speech.* New York: Stockton Press, 1986, 113–126.

de Boysson-Bardies B, Vihman MM, Roug-Hellichius L, Durand C, Landberg I, Arao F. Material evidence of infant selection from target language: A cross-linguistic phonetic study. In Ferguson CA, Menn L, Stoel-Gammon C (eds). *Phonological Development: Models, Research, Implications.* Timonium, MD: York Press, 1992, 369–391.

Braine M. On what might constitute a learnable phonology. *Language* 1974;50:270–299.

Braine M. Review of 'The Acquisition of Phonology' by N. Smith. *Language* 1976;52:489–498.

Branigan G. Syllabic structure and the acquisition of consonants: The great conspiracy in word formation. *Journal of Psycholinguistic Research* 1976;5:117–133.

Browman CP, Goldstein LM. Towards an articulatory phonology. *Phonology Yearbook* 1986;3:219–252.

Browman CP, Goldstein L. Articulatory phonology: An overview. *Phonetica* 1992;49:155–180.

Bynon T. *Historical Linguistics.* Cambridge, MA: Cambridge University Press, 1977.

Chin SB, Dinnsen DA. Consonant clusters in disordered speech: Constraints and correspondence patterns. *Journal of Child Language* 1992;19:259–286.

Chomsky N, Halle M. *The Sound Pattern of English.* New York: Harper & Row, 1968.

Ciardi J. *A Browser's Dictionary and Native's Guide to the Unknown American Language.* New York: Harper & Row, 1980.

Clark J, Yallop C. *An Introduction to Phonetics and Phonology* (2nd ed). Cambridge, MA: Blackwell, 1995.

Cruttenden A. Assimilation in child language and elsewhere. *Journal of Child Language* 1978;5:376.

Crystal D. *The Cambridge Encyclopedia of Language.* New York: Cambridge University Press, 1987.

Crystal D. *A Dictionary of Linguistics and Phonetics* (3rd ed). Cambridge, MA: Basil Blackwell, 1991.

Davis BL, MacNeilage PF. Acquisition of correct vowel production: A quantitative case study. *Journal of Speech and Hearing Research* 1990;33:16–27.

Demuth K. The acquisition of tonal systems. In Archibald J (ed). *Phonological Acquisition and Phonological Theory.* Hillsdale, NJ: Lawrence Erlbaum Associates, 1995, 111–134.

Demuth K. The prosodic structure of early words. In Morgan JL, Demuth K (eds). *Signal to Syntax: Bootstrapping from Speech to Grammar in Early Acquisition.* Mahwah, NJ: Lawrence Erlbaum Associates, 1996, 171–186.

Demuth K, Fee JE. *Minimal Words in Early Phonological Development.* Ms., Brown University and Dalhousie University, 1995.

Dinnsen DA. Phonology: Implications and trends. In Naremore RC (ed). *Language Science: Recent Advances.* San Diego: College Hill, 1984, 181–209.

Dinnsen DA. Variation in developing and fully-developed phonologies. In Ferguson CA, Menn L, Stoel-Gammon C (eds). *Phonological Development: Models, Research, Implications.* Timonium, MD: York Press, 1992, 191–210.

Dinnsen DA. Context effects in the acquisition of fricatives. In Bernhardt B, Gilbert J, Ingram D (eds). *Proceedings of the UBC Interna-*

tional Conference on Phonological Acquisition. Somerville, MA: Cascadilla Press, 1996a, 136–148.

Dinnsen DA. Context-sensitive underspecification and the acquisition of phonemic contrasts. *Journal of Child Language* 1996b;23:57–80.

Dinnsen DA. Nonsegmental phonologies. In Ball MJ, Kent RD (eds). *The New Phonologies: Developments in Clinical Linguistics.* San Diego: Singular, 1997, 77–125.

Dinnsen DA, Elbert M. On the relationship between phonology and learning. In Elbert M, Dinnsen DA, Weismer G (eds). *Phonological Theory and the Misarticulating Child (ASHA Monograph No. 22).* Rockville, MD: American Speech-Language-Hearing Association, 1984, 59–68.

Donahue M. Phonological constraints on the emergence of two-word utterances. *Journal of Child Language* 1986;13:216.

Donegan PJ, Stampe D. The study of natural phonology. In Dinnsen DA (ed). *Current Approaches to Phonological Theory.* Bloomington, IN: Indiana University Press, 1979, 126–173.

Duckworth M, Allen G, Hardcastle W, Ball M. Extensions to the International Phonetic Alphabet for the transcription of atypical speech. *Clinical Linguistics and Phonetics* 1990;4:273–280.

Echols CH, Newport EL. The role of stress and position in determining first words. *Language Acquisition* 1992;2:189–220.

Edwards ML. Word position effects in the production of fricatives. In Bernhardt B, Gilbert J, Ingram D (eds). *Proceedings of the UBC International Conference on Phonological Acquisition.* Somerville, MA: Cascadilla Press, 1996, 149–158.

Eilers R, Oller DK. The role of speech discrimination in developmental sound substitutions. *Journal of Child Language* 1976;3:319–329.

Elbert M, Gierut J. *Handbook of Clinical Phonology: Approaches to Assessment and Treatment.* San Diego: College Hill, 1986.

Elbert M, Dinnsen DA, Powell TW. On the prediction of phonologic generalization learning patterns. *Journal of Speech and Hearing Disorders* 1984;49:309–317.

Farwell C. Some strategies in the early production of fricatives. *Papers and Reports in Child Language Development* 1976;12:97–104.

Fee EJ. Prosodic morphology in first language acquisition. Presented to Boston University Conference on Language Development, Boston, October 1991.

Fee EJ. Syllable structure and minimal words. In Bernhardt B, Gilbert J, Ingram D (eds). *Proceedings of the UBC International Conference on Phonological Acquisition.* Somerville, MA: Cascadilla Press, 1996, 85–98.

Ferguson CA. Learning to pronounce: The earliest stages of phonological development in the child. In Minifie F, Lloyd L (eds). *Communicative and Cognitive Abilities—Early Behavioral Assessment.* Baltimore: University Park Press, 1978, 273–297.

Ferguson CA, Farwell CB. Words and sounds in early language acquisition. *Language* 1975;51:419–439.

Fey M, Gandour J. Rule discovery in phonology acquisition. *Journal of Child Language* 1982;9:74–75.

Fikkert P. Well-formedness conditions in child phonology: A look at metathesis. Presented to Crossing Boundaries: Formal and Functional Determinants of Language Acquisition, Tübingen, Germany, October 1991.

Fikkert P. *On the Acquisition of Prosodic Structure.* The Hague: Holland Academic Graphics, 1994.

Fisichelli RM. An experimental study of the prelinguistic speech development of institutionalized infants. Ph.D. Thesis, Fordham University, 1950.

Freitas MJ. Onsets on early productions. In Bernhardt B, Gilbert J, Ingram D (eds). *Proceedings of the UBC International Conference on Phonological Acquisition.* Somerville, MA: Cascadilla Press, 1996, 76–84.

Fromkin V, Rodman R. *An Introduction to Language* (2nd ed). New York: Holt, Rinehart and Winston, 1978.

Fudala JB, Reynolds WM. *Arizona Articulation Proficiency Scale* (2nd ed). Los Angeles: Western Psychological Corporation, 1991.

Funk W. *Word Origins and Their Romantic Stories* (2nd ed). New York: Bell Publishing, 1978.

Gamkrelidze TV. On the correlation of stops and fricatives in a phonological system. *Lingua* 1975;35:231–261.

Gerken LA. The metrical basis for children's subjectless sentences. *Journal of Memory and Language* 1991;30:431–451.

Gerken LA. A metrical template account of children's weak syllable omissions from multisyllabic words. *Journal of Child Language* 1994a;21:565–584.

Gerken LA. Young children's representation of prosodic structure: Evidence from English-speakers' weak syllable omissions. *Journal of Memory and Language* 1994b;33:19–38.

Gerken LA, McIntosh BJ. The interplay of function morphemes and prosody in early language. *Developmental Psychology* 1993; 29:448–457.

Gierut JA. On the relationship between phonological knowledge and generalization learning in misarticulating children. Ph.D. Thesis, Indiana University, 1985.

Gierut JA. An experimental test of phonemic cyclicity. *Journal of Child Language* 1996a;23:81–102.

Gierut JA. Featural categories in English phonemic acquisition. In Bernhardt B, Gilbert J, Ingram D (eds). *Proceedings of the UBC International Conference on Phonological Acquisition.* Somerville, MA: Cascadilla Press, 1996b, 42–52.

Gierut JA, Simmerman CL, Neumann HJ. Phonemic structures of delayed phonological systems. *Journal of Child Language* 1994;21: 291–316.

Glucksman PH. *World-Wide German Dictionary.* Greenwich, CT: Fawcett, 1961.

Gnanadesikan AE. Markedness and faithfulness constraints in child phonology. Ms., University of Massachusetts at Amherst, 1995.

Goad H. Consonant harmony in child language: Evidence against coronal underspecification. In Bernhardt B, Gilbert J, Ingram D (eds). *Proceedings of the UBC International Conference on Phonological Acquisition.* Somerville, MA: Cascadilla Press, 1996, 187–200.

Goldman R, Fristoe M. *Goldman Fristoe Test of Articulation.* Circle Pines, MN: American Guidance Service, 1986.

Goldsmith J. *Autosegmental Phonology.* New York: Garland Press, 1979.

Goldsmith JA. *Autosegmental and Metrical Phonology.* Cambridge, MA: Basil Blackwell, 1990.

Goodell EW, Studdert-Kennedy M. Articulatory organization in early words: From syllable to phoneme. In de Boysson-Bardies B, de Schonen S, Jusczyk P, MacNeilage P, Morton J (eds). *XIIth International Congress of Phonetic Sciences, Vol. 4.* Aix-en-Provence, France: Université de Provence, 1991, 166–169.

Greenberg J. *Universals of Language. Volume 2: Phonology.* Stanford, CA: Stanford University Press, 1978.

Grunwell P. *The Nature of Phonological Disability in Children.* New York: Academic Press, 1981.

Grunwell P. *Clinical Phonology.* Rockville, MD: Aspen, 1982.

Grunwell P. *Phonological Assessment of Child Speech (PACS).* San Diego: College Hill, 1985.

Grunwell P. Developmental phonological disability: Order in disorder. In Hodson BW, Edwards ML (eds). *Perspectives in Applied Phonology.* Gaithersburg, MD: Aspen, 1997, 61–103.

Grunwell P. Natural phonology. In Ball MJ, Kent RD (eds). *The New Phonologies: Developments in Clinical Linguistics.* San Diego: Singular, 1997, 35–75.

Hammond M. Optimality theory and prosody. In Archangeli D, Langendoen DT (eds). *Optimality Theory: An Overview.* Malden, MA: Blackwell, 1997, 33–58.

Hargrove PM, Sheran CP. The use of stress by language-impaired children. *Journal of Communication Disorders* 1989;22:361–373.

Hayes B. *Metrical Stress Theory: Principles and Case Studies*. Chicago: University of Chicago Press, 1995.

Heselwood B. A case of nasal clicks for target sonorants: A feature geometry account. *Clinical Linguistics and Phonetics* 1997;11:43–61.

Hochberg J. First steps in the acquisition of Spanish stress. *Journal of Child Language* 1988;15:273–292.

Hockett C. *A Manual of Phonology*. Baltimore: Waverly Press, 1955.

Hodson B. *The Assessment of Phonological Processes, Revised*. Austin, TX: PRO-ED, 1986.

Hodson BW, Paden EP. Phonological processes which characterize unintelligible and intelligible speech in early childhood. *Journal of Speech and Hearing Disorders* 1981;46:369–373.

Hodson BW, Paden EP. *Targeting Intelligible Speech: A Phonological Approach to Remediation* (2nd ed). Austin, TX: PRO-ED, 1991.

Hoffman P, Stager S, Daniloff R. Perception and production of misarticulated /r/. *Journal of Speech and Hearing Disorders* 1983;48: 210–215.

Howard SJ. Articulatory constraints on a phonological system: A case study of cleft palate speech. *Clinical Linguistics and Phonetics* 1993;7:299–317.

Hyman LH. *Phonology: Theory and Analysis*. New York: Holt, Rinehart and Winston, 1975.

Ingram D. Fronting in child phonology. *Journal of Child Language* 1974;1:233–241.

Ingram D. Surface contrast in children's speech. *Journal of Child Language* 1975;2:287–292.

Ingram D. The role of the syllable in phonological development. In Bell A, Hooper J (eds). *Syllables and Segments*. Amsterdam: North-Holland Publishing, 1978, 143–155.

Ingram D. *Procedures for the Phonological Analysis of Children's Language*. Baltimore: University Park Press, 1981.

Ingram D. On children's homonyms. *Journal of Child Language* 1985;12:671–680.

Ingram D. *Phonological Disability in Children* (2nd ed). London: Cole and Whurr, 1989.

Ingram D. Some observations on feature assignment. In Bernhardt B, Gilbert J, Ingram D (eds). *Proceedings of the UBC International Conference on Phonological Acquisition*. Somerville, MA: Cascadilla Press, 1996, 53–61.

Ingram D. Generative phonology. In Ball MJ, Kent RD (eds). *The New Phonologies: Developments in Clinical Linguistics*. San Diego: Singular, 1997, 7–33.

Irwin OC. Infant speech: Consonantal sounds according to place of articulation. *Journal of Speech and Hearing Disorders* 1947;12:397–401.

Iverson G, Wheeler D. Hierarchical structures in child phonology. *Lingua* 1987;73:243–257.

Jaeger JJ. How to say 'Grandma': The problem of developing phonological representations. *First Language* 1997;17(Part 1):1–29.

Kehoe M. An investigation of rhythmic processes in English-speaking children's word productions. Ph.D. Thesis, University of Washington, 1995.

Kehoe M. Support for metrical stress theory in stress acquisition. Ms., Pennsylvania State University, 1996.

Kehoe M. Stress error patterns in English-speaking children's word productions. *Clinical Linguistics and Phonetics* 1997;11: 389–409.

Kehoe M, Stoel-Gammon C. The acquisition of prosodic structure: An investigation of current accounts of children's prosodic development. *Language* 1997a;73:113–144.

Kehoe M, Stoel-Gammon C. Truncation patterns in English-speaking children's word productions. *Journal of Speech Language and Hearing Research* 1997b;40:526–541.

Kenstowicz M. *Phonology in Generative Grammar*. Cambridge, MA: Blackwell, 1994.

Kenstowicz M, Kisseberth C. *Topics in Phonological Theory*. New York: Academic Press, 1977.

Kent RD. Gestural phonology: Basic concepts and applications in speech-language pathology. In Ball MJ, Kent RD (eds). *The New Phonologies: Developments in Clinical Linguistics*. San Diego: Singular, 1997, 247–265.

Khan L, Lewis N. *Khan-Lewis Phonological Analysis*. Circle Pines, MN: American Guidance Service, 1986.

Kingston J, Diehl RL. Phonetic knowledge. *Language* 1994;70:419–454.

Kisseberth CW. On the abstractness of phonology: The evidence from Yawelmani. *Papers in Linguistics* 1969;1:291–306. Cited by Hyman LH. *Phonology: Theory and Analysis*. New York: Holt, Rinehart, and Winston, 1975.

Konopczynski G. Acquisition de la proéminence dans le langage émergent. In de Boysson-Bardies B, de Schonen S, Jusczyk P, MacNeilage P, Morton J (eds). *Congrès International des Sciences Phonétiques XII, Vol. 1*. Aix-en-Provence, France: Université de Provence, 1991, 333–337.

Kornfeld J. Theoretical issues in child phonology. *Proceedings of the Chicago Linguistic Society* 1971;7:454–468.

Kresheck JD, Werner EO. *Structured Photographic Articulation Test Featuring Dudsberry*. Sandwich, IL: Janelle Publications, 1989.

Ladefoged P, Maddieson I. *The Sounds of the World's Languages*. Cambridge, MA: Blackwell, 1996.

Larson VL, McKinley N. *Language Disorders in Older Students: Preadolescents and Adolescents*. Eau Claire, WI: Thinking Publications.

Leonard LB. Models of phonological development and children with phonological disorders. In Ferguson CA, Menn L, Stoel-Gammon S (eds). *Phonological Development: Models, Research, and Implications*. Parkton, MD: York Press, 1992, 495–507.

Leonard LB, McGregor KK. Unusual phonological patterns and their underlying representations: A case study. *Journal of Child Language* 1991;18:261–272.

Leonard LB, Newhoff M, Mesalam L. Individual differences in early child phonology. *Applied Psycholinguistics* 1980;1:7–30.

Leonard LB, Schwartz RG, Allen GD, Swanson LA, Froem-Loeb D. Unusual phonological behavior and the avoidance of homonymy in children. *Journal of Speech and Hearing Research* 1989;32:583–590.

Leopold WF. *Speech Development of a Bilingual Child, 2: Sound-Learning in the First Two Years*. Evanston, IL: Northwestern University Press, 1947.

Lester L, Skousen R. The phonology of drunkenness. In Bruck A, Fox R, Lagaly M (eds). *Parasession on Natural Phonology*. Chicago: Chicago Linguistic Society, 1974, 233–239.

Levelt C. Consonant harmony: A reanalysis in terms of vowel-consonant interaction. Presented to Boston University Conference on Child Language Development, Boston, October 1992.

Levelt C. Consonant-vowel interactions in child language. In Bernhardt B, Gilbert J, Ingram D (eds). *Proceedings of the UBC International Conference on Phonological Acquisition*. Somerville, MA: Cascadilla Press, 1996, 229–239.

Levitt A. Babbling and child language acquisition: The transition from babbling to speech. Presented to New England Child Language Association, Northeastern University, Boston, April 1991.

Lindblom B. Phonological units as adaptive emergents of lexical development. In Ferguson CA, Menn L, Stoel-Gammon C (eds). *Phonological Development: Models, Research, Implications*. Timonium, MD: York Press, 1992, 131–163.

Lindblom B, Krull D, Stark J. Phonetic systems and phonological development. In de Boysson-Bardies B, de Schonen S, Jusczyk P, MacNeilage P, Morton J (eds). *Developmental Neurocognition: Speech and Face Processing in the First Year of Life*. Dordrecht, Holland: Kluwer, 1993, 399–409.

Lleó C. Homonymy and reduplication: On the extended availability of two strategies in phonological acquisition. *Journal of Child Language* 1990;17:267–278.

Lleó C. A parametrical view of harmony and reduplication processes in child phonology. Ms., Universität Hamburg, 1992.

Lleó C. To spread or not to spread: Different styles in the acquisition of Spanish phonology. In Bernhardt B, Gilbert J, Ingram D (eds).

Proceedings of the UBC International Conference on Phonological Acquisition. Somerville, MA: Cascadilla Press, 1996, 215–228.

Lleó C, Prinz M. Consonant clusters in child phonology and the directionality of syllable structure assignment. *Journal of Child Language* 1996;23:31–56.

Locke J. The inference of speech perception in the phonologically disordered child. *Journal of Speech and Hearing Disorders* 1980;45: 431–468.

Locke J. *Phonological Acquisition and Change.* New York: Academic Press, 1983.

Lowe RJ. *Assessment Link Between Phonology and Articulation–Revised (ALPHA-R).* Mifflinville, PA: Alpha Speech and Language Resources, 1995.

Macken MA. Individual differences in phonological acquisition: Strategies versus cognitive styles. Stanford Child Language Seminar Series. Stanford, CA: Stanford University, April 1976. Cited by Ingram D. The role of the syllable in phonological development. In Bell A, Hooper J (eds). *Syllables and Segments.* Amsterdam: North-Holland, 1978, 143–155.

Macken MA. Permitted complexity in phonological development: One child's acquisition of Spanish consonants. *Papers and Reports on Child Language Development* 1978;11:1–27.

Macken MA. The child's lexical representation: The 'puzzle-puddle-pickle' evidence. *Papers and Reports in Child Language Development* 1979;16:26–41.

Macken M. Developmental changes in the acquisition of phonology. In de Boysson-Bardies B, de Schonen S, Jusczyk P, MacNeilage P, Morton J (eds). *Developmental Neurocognition: Speech and Face Processing in the First Year of Life.* Dordrecht, Holland: Kluwer, 1993, 435–449.

Macken MA. Prosodic constraints on features. In Bernhardt B, Gilbert J, Ingram D (eds). *Proceedings of the UBC International Conference on Phonological Acquisition.* Somerville, MA: Cascadilla Press, 1996, 159–172.

Macken MA, Barton D. The acquisition of the voicing contrast in English: A study of voice onset time in word-initial stop consonants. *Journal of Child Language* 1979;7:41–74.

MacNeilage PF, Davis BL. Acquisition of speech production: Frames, then content. In Geannerod M (ed). *Motor Representation and Control.* Hillsdale NJ: Lawrence Erlbaum Associates, 1990, 453–475.

Maddieson I. *Patterns of Sounds.* Cambridge, MA: Cambridge University Press, 1984.

Maddieson I, Precoda K. Updating UPSID. *Journal of the Acoustic Society of America* 1989;86:S19.

Marantz A. Re: Reduplication. *Linguistic Inquiry* 1982;13:435–482.

Matthei EH. Crossing boundaries: More evidence for phonological constraints on early multi-word utterances. *Journal of Child Language* 1989;16:41–54.

Maxwell E, Weismer G. The contribution of phonological, acoustic, and perceptual techniques to the characterization of a misarticulating child's voice contrast for stops. *Applied Psycholinguistics* 1982;3:29–43.

McCarthy JJ. Feature geometry and dependency: A review. *Phonetica* 1988;43:84–108.

McCarthy JJ. Linear order in phonological representation. *Linguistic Inquiry* 1989;20:71–99.

McCarthy JJ. L'infixation réduplicative dans les langages secrets. *Langages* 1991;101:11–29.

McCarthy JJ, Prince AS. Prosodic morphology. Ms., University of Massachusetts and Brandeis University, 1986 (in progress).

McCarthy JJ, Prince AS. Foot and word in prosodic morphology: The Arabic broken plural. *Natural Language and Linguistic Theory* 1990;8:209–283.

McCarthy JJ, Prince AS. Generalized alignment. In Booji G, van Marle J (eds). *Yearbook of Morphology 1993.* Dordrecht, Holland: Kluwer, 1993, 79–153.

McCarthy JJ, Prince AS. The emergence of the unmarked: Optimality in prosodic morphology. In Gonzàlez M (ed). *Proceedings of the North East Linguistic Society 24.* Amherst, MA: Graduate Linguistic Student Association, University of Massachusetts at Amherst, 1994, 333–379.

McCarthy JJ, Prince AS. Faithfulness and reduplicative identity. In Beckman JN, Dickey LW, Urbanczyk S (ed). *Papers in Optimality Theory.* Amherst, MA: Graduate Linguistic Student Association, University of Massachusetts at Amherst, 1995, 249–384.

McCarthy J, Prince AS. *Prosodic Morphology I: Constraint Interaction and Satisfaction.* Cambridge, MA: MIT Press (in press).

McCune L, Vihman MM. Vocal motor schemes. *Papers and Reports on Child Language Development* 1987;26:72–79.

McDonough J, Myers S. Consonant harmony and planar segregation in child language. Ms., University of California, Los Angeles and University of Texas at Austin, 1991.

McLeod S, van Doorn J, Reed VA. Realizations of consonant clusters by children with phonological impairments. *Clinical Linguistics and Phonetics* 1997;11:85–113.

Menn L. *Pattern, Control, and Contrast in Beginning Speech: A Case Study in the Development of Word Form and Word Function.* Bloomington, IN: Indiana University Linguistics Club, 1978a.

Menn L. Phonological units in beginning speech. In Bell A, Hooper JB (eds). *Syllables and Segments.* Amsterdam: North-Holland Publishing, 1978b, 157–171.

Menn L. Development of articulatory, phonetic, and phonological capabilities. In Butterworth B (ed). *Language Production.* London: Academic Press, 1983, 3–50.

Menn L, Matthei E. The 'two-lexicon' account of child phonology: Looking back, looking ahead. In Ferguson CA, Menn L, Stoel-Gammon C (eds). *Phonological Development: Models, Research, Implications.* Parkton, MD: York Press, 1992, 211–247.

Mester RA, Itô J. Feature predictability and underspecification: Palatal prosody in Japanese mimetics. *Language* 1989;65:258–293.

Monty Python and the Holy Grail. 1974. Directed by Terry Gilliam and Terry Jones. 89 minutes. Columbia Pictures USA. Videocassette.

Moskowitz B. The acquisition of fricatives: A study in phonetics and phonology. *Journal of Phonetics* 1975;3:141–150.

Naiman A. *Every Goy's Guide to Common Jewish Expressions.* New York: Ballantine Books, 1981.

Ohala D. A unified theory of final consonant deletion in early child speech. Ms., University of Arizona, 1991.

Otomo K, Stoel-Gammon C. The acquisition of unrounded vowels in English. *Journal of Speech and Hearing Research* 1992;35:604–616.

Pater J, Paradis J. Truncation in early child phonology: Alignment and correspondence. Presented to BU Conference on Language Development, Boston, November 1995.

Pendergast K, Dickey S, Selmar J, Soder A. *Photo Articulation Test (PAT)* (2nd ed). Danville, IL: Interstate Printers and Publishers, 1984.

Pierce JE, Hanna IV. *The Development of a Phonological System in English Speaking American Children.* Portland, OR: HaPi Press, 1974.

Pollock KE. Individual preferences: Case study of a phonologically delayed child. *Topics in Language Disorders* 1983;3:10–23.

Pollock KE, Hall P. An analysis of the vowel misarticulations of five children with developmental apraxia of speech. *Clinical Linguistics and Phonetics* 1991;5:207–224.

Pollock KE, Keiser NJ. An examination of vowel errors in phonologically disordered children. *Clinical Linguistics and Phonetics* 1990;4: 161–178.

Poser WJ. Phonological representation and action-at-a-distance. In van der Hulst H, Smith N (eds). *The Structure of Phonological Representations: Part II.* Dordrecht, Holland: Foris, 1982, 121–158.

Prather EM, Hedrick DL, Kern CA. Articulation development in children aged two to four years. *Journal of Speech and Hearing Disorders* 1975;40:179–191.

Priestly TMS. One idiosyncratic strategy in the acquisition of phonology. *Journal of Child Language* 1977;4:45–65.

Prince A, Smolensky P. *Optimality Theory: Constraint Interaction in Generative Grammar.* Cambridge, MA: MIT Press (in press).

Pullum GK, Ladusaw WA. *Phonetic Symbol Guide.* Chicago: University of Chicago Press, 1986.

Queller K. Excrescence and modification: Intrasystemic sources for innovative word and syllable structures in early speech. Presented to 15th Annual Child Phonology Conference, Sun Valley, Idaho, May 1994.

Queller K. Templates and melodies: A typology of ordering constraints in early child phonology. In Palek B (ed). *Item Order in Natural Languages; Proceedings of LP'94.* Prague: Charles University Press, 1995, 94–124.

Reid TR. Karaoke popular in Japanese and U.S. Clubs. National Public Radio, October 12, 1992.

Return of the Jedi. 1983. Directed by Richard Marquand. 134 minutes. 20th Century Fox. Videocassette. Cited by Crystal D. *The Cambridge Encyclopedia of Language.* New York: Cambridge University Press, 1987.

Rice K. Aspects of variability in child language acquisition. In Bernhardt B, Gilbert J, Ingram D (eds). *Proceedings of the UBC International Conference on Phonological Acquisition.* Somerville, MA: Cascadilla Press, 1996, 1–14.

Rice K, Avery P. Variability in a deterministic model of language acquisition: A theory of segmental elaboration. In Archibald J (ed). *Phonological Acquisition and Phonological Theory.* Hillsdale, NJ: Lawrence Erlbaum Associates, 1995, 23–42.

Robb MP, Bleile KM. Consonant inventories of young children from 8 to 25 months. *Clinical Linguistics and Phonetics* 1994;8:295–320.

Robb MP, Saxman JH. Syllable durations of preword and early word vocalizations. *Journal of Speech and Hearing Research* 1990;33: 583–593.

Rosenhouse J. Intonation problems of hearing-impaired Hebrew-speaking children. *Language and Speech* 1986;29(Part 1):69–92.

Ruhlen M. *A Guide to the Languages of the World.* Stanford, CA: Stanford University Press, 1976.

Schwartz RG, Goffman L. Metrical patterns of words and production accuracy. *Journal of Speech and Hearing Research* 1995;38:876–888.

Schwartz RG, Leonard LB. Do children pick and choose? An examination of phonological selection and avoidance in early lexical acquisition. *Journal of Child Language* 1982;9:319–336.

Schwartz RG, Leonard LB, Froem-Loeb D, Swanson LA. Attempted sounds are sometimes not: An expanded view of phonological selection and avoidance. *Journal of Child Language* 1987;14:411–418.

Schwartz RG, Leonard LB, Wilcox MJ, Folger MK. Again and again: Reduplication in child phonology. *Journal of Child Language* 1980;7:75–87.

Secord W. *Test of Minimal Articulation Competence (T-MAC).* USA: Psychological Corporation, 1981.

Shattuck-Hufnagel S, Klatt D. The limited use of distinctive features and markedness in speech production: Evidence from speech error data. *Journal of Verbal Learning and Verbal Behavior* 1979;18:41–55.

Shriberg LD, Kent RD. *Clinical Phonetics* (2nd ed). Boston: Allyn & Bacon, 1995.

Shriberg LD, Kwiatkowski J. *Natural Process Analysis (NPA).* New York: John Wiley & Sons, 1980.

Shriberg LD, Aram DM, Kwiatkowski J. Developmental Apraxia of Speech: I. Descriptive and theoretical approaches. *Journal of Speech Language and Hearing Research* 1997a;40:273–285.

Shriberg LD, Aram DM, Kwiatkowski J. Developmental Apraxia of Speech: II. Toward a diagnostic marker. *Journal of Speech Language and Hearing Research* 1997b;40:286–312.

Shriberg LD, Aram DM, Kwiatkowski J. Developmental Apraxia of Speech: III. A subtype marked by inappropriate stress. *Journal of Speech Language and Hearing Research* 1997c;40:313–337.

Shriberg LD, Kwiatkowski J, Rasmussen C, Lof GL, Miller JF. *The Prosody-Voice Screening Profile (PVSP): Psychometric Data and Reference Information for Children.* Tucson, AZ: Communication Skill Builders, 1992.

Simpson JA, Weiner ESC. *Oxford English Dictionary* (2nd ed). Oxford: Clarendon Press, 1989.

Smit AB, Hand L, Freilinger JJ, Bernthal JE, Bird A. The Iowa articulation norms project and its Nebraska replication. *Journal of Hearing and Speech Disorders* 1990;55:779–798.

Smith K. *Delayed Sensory Feedback and Behavior.* Philadelphia: Saunders, 1962.

Smith NV. *The Acquisition of Phonology: A Case Study.* Cambridge, MA: Cambridge University Press, 1973.

Snow D, Stoel-Gammon C. Intonation and final lengthening in early child language. In Yavas M (ed). *First and Second Language Phonology.* San Diego: Singular, 1994, 81–105.

Sproat R, Fujimura O. Allophonic variation in English /l/ and its implications for phonetic implementation. *Journal of Phonetics* 1993;21:291–311.

Stampe D. The acquisition of phonetic representation. In Bruck A, Fox R, Lagaly M (eds). *Papers from the Fifth Regional Meeting of the Chicago Linguistic Society: Parasession on Natural Phonology.* Chicago: Chicago Linguistic Society, 1969, 443–454.

Stampe D. *A Dissertation on Natural Phonology.* New York: Garland, 1979.

Stemberger JP. Between-word processes in child phonology. *Journal of Child Language* 1988;15:39–61.

Stemberger JP. Default onsets and constraints in language acquisition. Ms., University of Minnesota, 1993.

Stemberger JP. Syllable structure in English, with emphasis on codas. In Bernhardt B, Gilbert J, Ingram D (eds). *Proceedings of the UBC International Conference on Phonological Acquisition.* Somerville, MA: Cascadilla Press, 1996, 62–75.

Stemberger JP, Bernhardt BH. Optimality theory. In Ball MJ, Kent RD (eds). *The New Phonologies: Developments in Clinical Linguistics.* San Diego: Singular, 1997, 211–245.

Stemberger JP, Stoel-Gammon C. The underspecification of coronal: Evidence from language acquisition and performance errors. In Paradis C, Prunet J-F (eds). *The Special Status of Coronals.* Dordrecht, Holland: Foris, 1991, 181–199.

Steriade D. Underspecification and markedness. In Goldsmith JA (ed). *The Handbook of Phonological Theory.* Cambridge, MA: Blackwell, 1995, 114–174.

Stevens KN. Quantal nature of speech. In David EE, Denes PB (eds). *Human Communication: A Unified View.* New York: McGraw-Hill, 1972, 51–66.

Stevens KN. On the quantal nature of speech. *Journal of Phonetics* 1989;17:3–45.

Stoel-Gammon C. Constraints on consonant-vowel sequences in early words. *Journal of Child Language* 1983;10:455–457.

Stoel-Gammon C. Phonetic inventories, 15–24 months: A longitudinal study. *Journal of Speech and Hearing Research* 1985;28:505–512.

Stoel-Gammon C. Phonological skills of 2-year-olds. *Language Speech and Hearing Services in the Schools* 1987;18:323–329.

Stoel-Gammon C. On the acquisition of velars in English. In Bernhardt B, Gilbert J, Ingram D (eds). *Proceedings of the UBC International Conference of Phonological Acquisition.* Somerville, MA: Cascadilla Press, 1996, 201–214.

Stoel-Gammon C, Herrington P. Vowel systems of normally developing and phonologically disordered children. *Clinical Linguistics and Phonetics* 1990;4:145–160.

Stoel-Gammon C, Stemberger JP. Consonant harmony and phonological underspecification in child speech. In Yavas M (ed). *First and Second Language Phonology.* San Diego: Singular, 1994, 63–80.

Stoel-Gammon C, Stone JR. Assessing phonology in young children. *Clinics in Communication Disorders* 1991;1:25–39.

Stonham J. Current issues in morphological theory. Ph.D. Thesis, Stanford University, 1990. Cited by Bernhardt B. Developmental implications of nonlinear phonological theory. *Clinical Linguistics and Phonetics* 1992a;6:259–281.

Studdert-Kennedy M, Goodell EW. Gestures, features, and segments in early child speech. *Haskins Laboratories Status Report on Speech Research* 1992;SR-111/112:1–14.

Tyler AA, Langsdale TE. Consonant-vowel interaction in early phonological development. *First Language* 1996;16(Part 2):159–191.

Velleman DJ. *How To Prove It: A Structured Approach*. Cambridge, UK: Cambridge University Press, 1994.

Velleman SL. The role of linguistic perception in later phonological development. *Applied Psycholinguistics* 1988;9:221–236.

Velleman SL. A nonlinear model of harmony and metathesis. Presented to Linguistic Society of America, Philadelphia, January 1992.

Velleman SL. The interaction of phonetics and phonology in developmental verbal dyspraxia: Two case studies. *Clinics in Communication Disorders* 1994;4:67–78.

Velleman SL. The development of phonology and mental representations in a child with pervasive developmental disorder. In Powell TP (ed). *Pathologies of Speech and Language: Contributions of Clinical Phonetics and Linguistics*. New Orleans: International Clinical Phonetics and Linguistics Association, 1996a, 27–36.

Velleman SL. Metathesis highlights feature-by-position constraints. In Bernhardt B, Gilbert J, Ingram D (eds). *Proceedings of the UBC International Conference on Phonological Acquisition*. Somerville, MA: Cascadilla Press, 1996b, 173–186.

Velleman SL, Shriberg LD. Syllabic stress constraints in a subtype of developmental apraxia of speech. Ms., Elms College and University of Wisconsin—Madison (in preparation).

Velleman SL, Strand K. Developmental verbal dyspraxia. In Bernthal JE, Bankson NW (eds). *Child Phonology: Characteristics, Assessment, and Intervention with Special Populations*. New York: Thieme, 1994, 110–139.

Velleman SL, Huntley R, Lasker J. Is it developmental verbal dyspraxia or is it phonology? Presented to American Speech-Hearing-Language Association, Atlanta, November 1991.

Velten J. The growth of phonemic and lexical patterns in infant language. *Language* 1943;19:281–292. Cited in Ingram D. *Procedures for the Phonological Analysis of Children's Language*. Baltimore, University Park Press, 1981.

Vihman MM. From prespeech to speech: On early phonology. *Papers and Reports on Child Language Development* 1976;12:230–244.

Vihman MM. Consonant harmony: Its scope and function in child language. In Greenberg JH (ed). *Universals of Human Language*. Stanford, CA: Stanford University Press, 1978, 281–334.

Vihman MM. Phonology and the development of the lexicon: Evidence from children's errors. *Journal of Child Language* 1981;8:239–264.

Vihman MM. Early syllables and the construction of phonology. In Ferguson CA, Menn L, Stoel-Gammon C (eds). *Phonological Development: Models, Research, Implications*. Parkton, MD: York Press, 1992, 393–422.

Vihman MM. *Phonological Development: The Origins of Language in the Child*. Cambridge, MA: Blackwell, 1996.

Vihman MM, McCune L. When is a word a word? *Journal of Child Language* 1994;21:517–542.

Vihman MM, Velleman SL. Phonological reorganization: A case study. *Language and Speech* 1989;32:149–170.

Vihman MM, DePaolis RA, Davis BL. Is there a "trochaic bias" in early word learning? Evidence from infant production in English and French. Ms., University of Wales at Bangor and University of Texas at Austin, 1997.

Vihman MM, Ferguson C, Elbert M. Phonological development from babbling to speech: Common tendencies and individual differences. *Applied Psycholinguistics* 1986;7:3–40.

Vihman MM, Velleman SL, McCune L. How abstract is child phonology? Towards an integration of linguistic and psychological approaches. In Yavas M (ed). *First and Second Language Phonology*. San Diego: Singular, 1994, 9–44.

Waterson N. Child phonology: A prosodic view. *Journal of Linguistics* 1971;7:179–221.

Weiner FF. *Phonological Process Analysis*. Austin, TX: PRO-ED, 1979.

Weismer G, Dinnsen D, Elbert M. A study of the voicing distinction associated with omitted, word-final stops. *Journal of Speech and Hearing Disorders* 1981;46:320–328.

Wiig E, Secord W, Semel E. *Clinical Evaluation of Language Fundamentals—Preschool (CELF-P)*. San Antonio: Psychological Corporation, 1992.

Williams AL, Dinnsen DA. A problem of allophonic variation in a speech disordered child. *Innovations in Linguistic Education* 1987;5:85–90.

Yavas M. Feature enhancement and phonological acquisition. *Clinical Linguistics and Phonetics* 1997;11:153–172.

Yule G. *The Study of Language* (2nd ed). New York: Cambridge University Press, 1996.

Index